SAM W. BANKS, M.D.

Associate Professor of Orthopaedic Surgery, Northwestern University Medical School; Attending Orthopaedic Surgeon, Chicago Wesley Memorial Hospital and the VA Research Hospital

HAROLD LAUFMAN, M.D., Ph.D.

Director, The Institute for Surgical Studies, Montefiore Hospital and Medical Center; Professor of Clinical Surgery, Albert Einstein College of Medicine, New York City; formerly Professor of Surgery and Director of Experimental Surgery, Northwestern University Medical School.

An Atlas of

Surgical Exposures of the Extremities

552 Illustrations on 179 Plates

W. B. SAUNDERS COMPANY · *PHILADELPHIA, LONDON*

W. B. Saunders Company: West Washington Square
Philadelphia, Pa. 19105

1 St. Anne's Road
Eastbourne, East Sussex BN21 3UN England

833 Oxford Street
Toronto, Ontario M8Z 5T9, Canada

Listed here is the latest translated edition of this book together with the language of the translation and the publisher.

Spanish (*1st Edition*)—Editorial Beta,
Buenos Aires, Argentina

An Atlas of Surgical Exposure of the Extremities ISBN 0-7216-1530-9

Press of W. B. Saunders Company. Library of Congress catalog card number 52-12872.

Print No.: 15 14 13

DEDICATED TO
THE PIONEERS OF SCIENCE
MANY KNOWN–MANY OBSCURE–SOME FORGOTTEN
WHO JOINED UNDERSTANDING OF ANATOMIC FUNCTION
WITH NEW SURGICAL SKILL AND DARING
TO BUILD EFFECTIVE KNOWLEDGE
OF INCISIONAL TECHNICS

Preface

The need for a comprehensive atlas of surgical incisions of the extremities has existed for many years. The available textbooks on the various surgical specialties, including those on orthopedics, devote much space to pathology, treatment and other aspects of lesions of the extremities, but give little attention to the details of surgical exposure, which is, in many instances, the major task of the operation. This pictorial atlas is designed to serve the student and resident in surgery as an introduction to the most frequently used exposures of the extremities, and to be a timely "refresher" to the experienced surgeon who operates on the extremities only occasionally. In order to attain the widest range of usefulness, many of the simplest as well as the more complicated incisions have been included in this volume and the descriptive text has been kept to a minimum.

The authors consider the surgical approaches illustrated in this atlas to be both practicable and anatomically correct, with emphasis on the preservation of function. The illustrations are the result of a process which began in the laboratory. Dissections were made on cadavers, and each step of an exposure was photographed while a description of the procedure was dictated. The photographs depicting each surgical approach were then collated and the important structures were labeled. The sets of photographs served as the basis for the rough drawings, and in no instance were individual structures or their relationships altered from the original photographs. Each final drawing is therefore a faithful representation of the anatomical findings encountered at surgery.

No illustration has been borrowed or adapted from other textbooks, but no claim is made by the authors of having originated any incision described in this atlas. Proper names have been avoided in designating the various incisions, because it was felt that an anatomical description would be preferable from the standpoint of clarity, and because the priority for the original description is in most instances unknown or controversial.

We have enjoyed the cooperation of many people in the creation of this work.We are especially grateful to Dr. Edward A. Evans, of Salt Lake City, and to Dr. John Caserta, of Chicago, for invaluable assistance with the dissections. Mr. Clark Moore, Jr., photographed each step of the exposures and deserves much credit for his fine work and great patience. The major portion of the art work was done by Miss Jean McConnell, medical artist of Northwestern University Medical School. Her excellent draftsmanship and incredible capacity for work have been largely instrumental in bringing this volume to completion. Mr. Melford Diedrick, medical artist of the University of Buffalo Medical School, in addition to preparing a number of drawings, did much to create the pattern of the layout for the atlas. Mrs. Mary Dixon Elder, of Northwestern University Medical School, prepared a number of the illustrations.

Major credit for the hand-lettering in the illustrations goes to Miss Rosamonde Howland, of Northwestern University Medical School, and to Miss Harriette E. Story and Miss Lillian Hunter, who assisted her.

Publication of this atlas would have been impossible except for the encouragement and splendid cooperation of the publisher, W. B. Saunders Company. Dr. Loyal Davis, Chairman of the Department of Surgery, and Dr. Philip Lewin, Chairman of the Department of Bone and Joint Surgery, of Northwestern University Medical School, gave us every encouragement in the development of this work. The typing of the manuscript and its various revisions was ably done by Mrs. Orell F. Jenkins, and editorial help in preparing the text matter was expertly rendered by Mr. Walter Thiele. Mr. C. T. E. Schultze photographed the finished plates in the preparation of the layouts.

It is with gratitude that we acknowledge the importance of the contributions of those who have worked with us so faithfully and patiently the past five years during which this work has been in progress. Our highest hope is that the usefulness of the atlas will have deserved their collaboration.

SAM W. BANKS

HAROLD LAUFMAN

Contents

Region of the Shoulder Girdle

Region of the Shoulder Joint

Region of the Shaft of the Humerus

Region of the Elbow Joint

Region of the Radius and Ulna

Region of the Wrist Joint and Hand

Region of the Hip Joint

Region of the Femur

Region of the Knee Joint

Region of the Tibia and Fibula

Region of the Ankle Joint and Foot

An Atlas of Surgical Exposures of the Extremities

Section I

Region of the Shoulder Girdle

EXPOSURE OF THE SPINE OF THE SCAPULA THROUGH A POSTERIOR HORIZONTAL INCISION

Indications: 1. Excision of Benign Tumors

2. Local Resection of Malignant Tumors

3. Partial Ostectomy for Osteomyelitis

Plate 1: Description of Procedure

A The incision begins over the acromion process and extends posteriorly for the desired distance, centering on the spine of the scapula.

B The skin flaps are mobilized, the deep fascia is opened and the anterior margin of the trapezius muscle is identified in the posterior portion of the wound. This muscle may be transected in line with the skin incision, or its margin may be mobilized and retracted toward the midline. The posterior portion of the deltoid muscle lies distal to the spine of the scapula in the lateral portion of the wound. Medial to it is the infraspinatus muscle.

C An incision is made through the fascia and periosteum to the spine of the scapula. The bone is exposed subperiosteally by elevating the trapezius and supraspinatus muscles from the proximal surface and the deltoid and infraspinatus muscles from the inferior surface of the scapular spine.

NOTE: The suprascapular nerve passes around the base of the spine of the scapula into the infraspinatus fossa to enter the deep surface of the infraspinatus muscle, which it innervates. The nerve is accompanied by the transverse scapular artery.

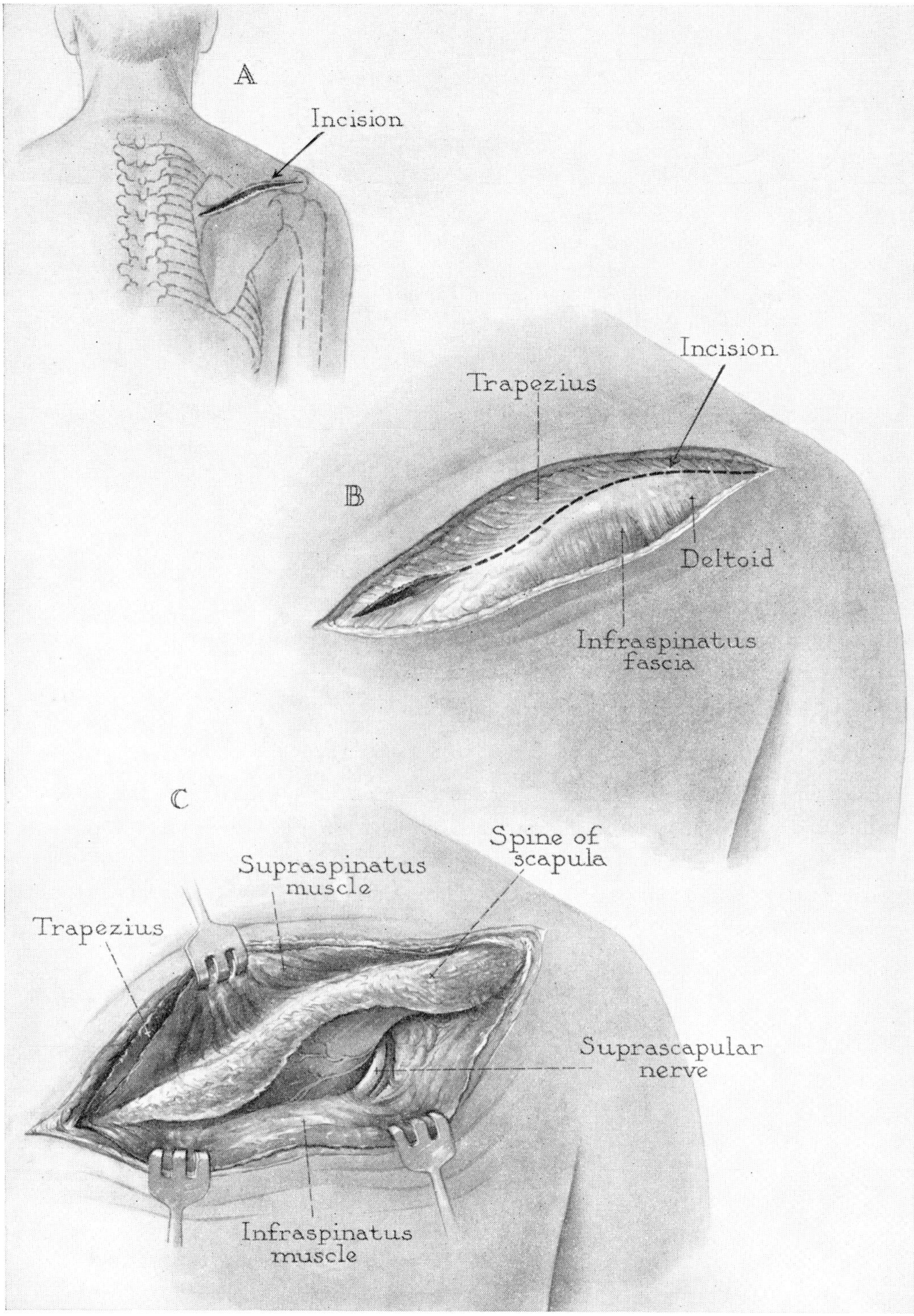

Exposure of the spine of the scapula through a posterior horizontal incision

EXPOSURE OF THE SUPRASPINATUS FOSSA THROUGH A LINEAR INCISION OVER THE SPINE OF THE SCAPULA

Indications: 1. Removal of Benign Tumors

2. Partial Ostectomy for Chronic Osteomyelitis

Plate 2: Description of Procedure

A The incision is made over the spine of the scapula. It starts just posterior to the acromion and ends at the vertebral margin of the scapula. The skin margins are undermined and retracted.

B The incision is deepened through the fascia and periosteum to the spine of the scapula. The margin of the trapezius muscle is raised to permit exposure of the supraspinatus muscle, which lies deep to it. An incision made across the trapezius muscle, as outlined in the illustration, will facilitate the exposure of the base of the scapular spine. Detachment of the deltoid and infraspinatus muscles from the inferior margin of the spine of the scapula is not necessary, unless indicated otherwise.

C The superior surface of the spine of the scapula and the supraspinatus fossa are exposed by elevating the supraspinatus muscle subperiosteally from the bone. The suprascapular nerve and the transverse scapular artery which supply the supraspinatus muscle are located in the lateral portion of the wound and must not be sectioned.

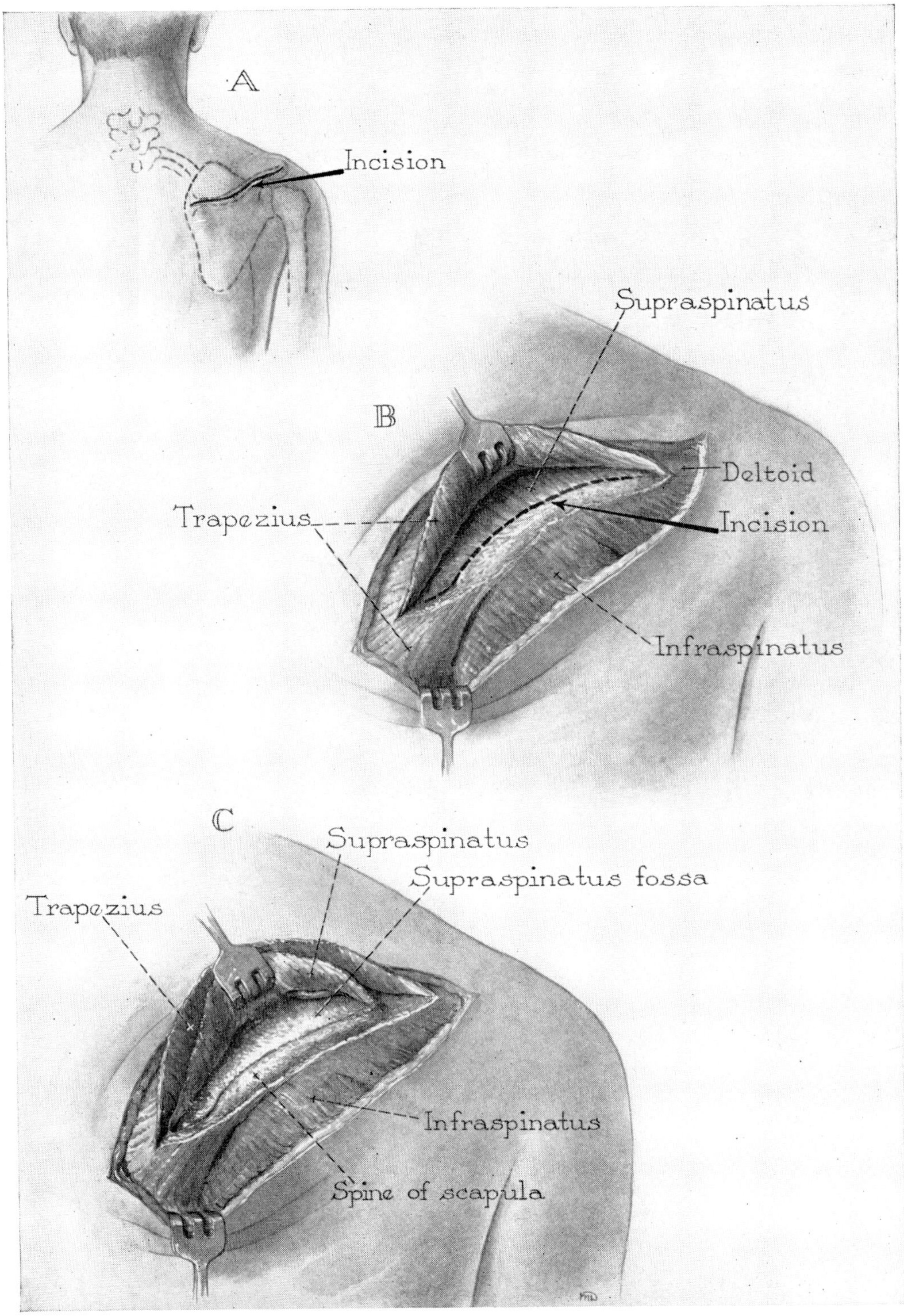

Exposure of the supraspinatus fossa through a linear incision over the spine at the scapula

EXPOSURE OF THE INFRASPINATUS FOSSA THROUGH A CURVED INCISION OVER THE SPINE AND VERTEBRAL MARGIN OF THE SCAPULA

Indications: 1. Removal of Benign Tumors

2. Treatment of Recent Fractures

3. Partial Ostectomy for Osteomyelitis

Plate 3: Description of Procedure

A After palpation of the spine and lower two-thirds of the vertebral margin of the scapula, a skin incision is made centrally over these structures, as illustrated. The skin margins then are retracted, and identification is made of the posterior third of the deltoid and infraspinatus muscles distal to the spine and lateral to the vertebral margin of the scapula. The rhomboid major muscle is located along the medial margin of the vertebral border.

B The fascia and periosteum are incised down to the spine of the scapula, after which the dissection is continued along the vertebral margin between the rhomboid major and infraspinatus muscles.

C Next, the infraspinatus fossa is exposed by elevating the infraspinatus muscle subperiosteally from the posterior surface of the scapula. The origin of the deltoid muscle is detached from the scapular spine, and then this muscle, together with the infraspinatus muscle, is retracted downward and outwardly. The suprascapular nerve and transverse scapular artery must be identified and protected as they enter the infraspinatus fossa from the greater scapular notch.

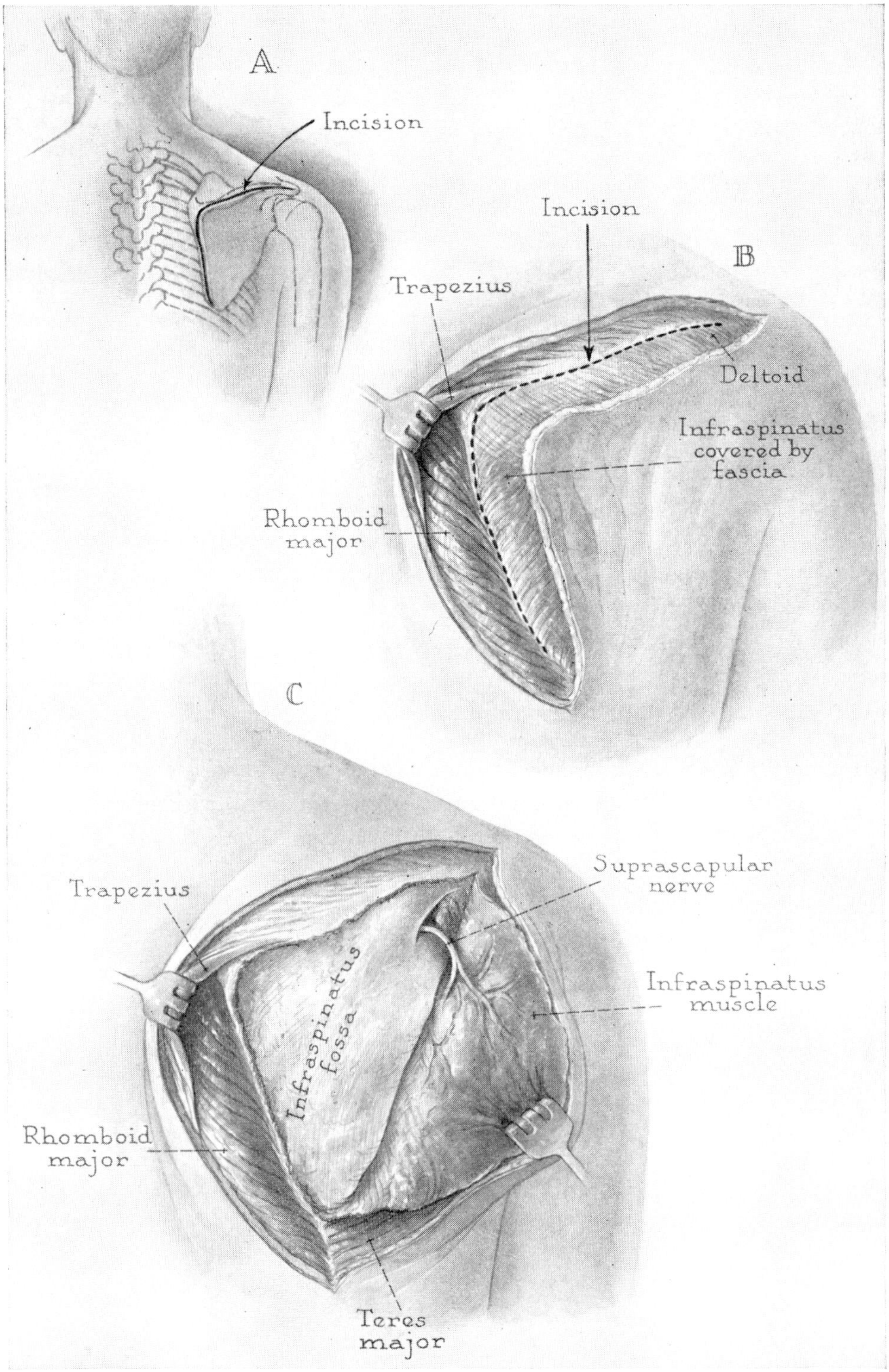

Exposure of the infraspinatus fossa through a curved incision over the spine and vertebral margin of the scapula

EXPOSURE OF THE SUPRASPINATUS AND THE INFRASPINATUS FOSSAE THROUGH A CURVED INCISION REFLECTING THE SUPRA-SPINATUS AND INFRASPINATUS MUSCLES

Indications: 1. Excision of Benign Tumors

2. Excision of Malignant Tumors

3. Partial Ostectomy for Osteomyelitis

4. Open Reduction of Fractures

Plate 4: Description of Procedure

A The incision begins at the anterior end of the spine of the scapula and extends posteriorly over it to the vertebral margin where it curves downward in the interval between the rhomboid major and infraspinatus muscles, terminating at the inferior angle of the scapula.

B The skin margins are mobilized and the deep fascia is opened. The fibers of the trapezius muscle, which run obliquely upward and outward to terminate at the medial end of the spine of the scapula, are isolated at their free margin. The trapezius muscle is retracted upward and toward the midline. Its free margin may be transected if exposure will be facilitated thereby. The rhomboid major muscle must be identified at its attachment along the vertebral margin of the scapula. (Procedure continued on Plate 5.)

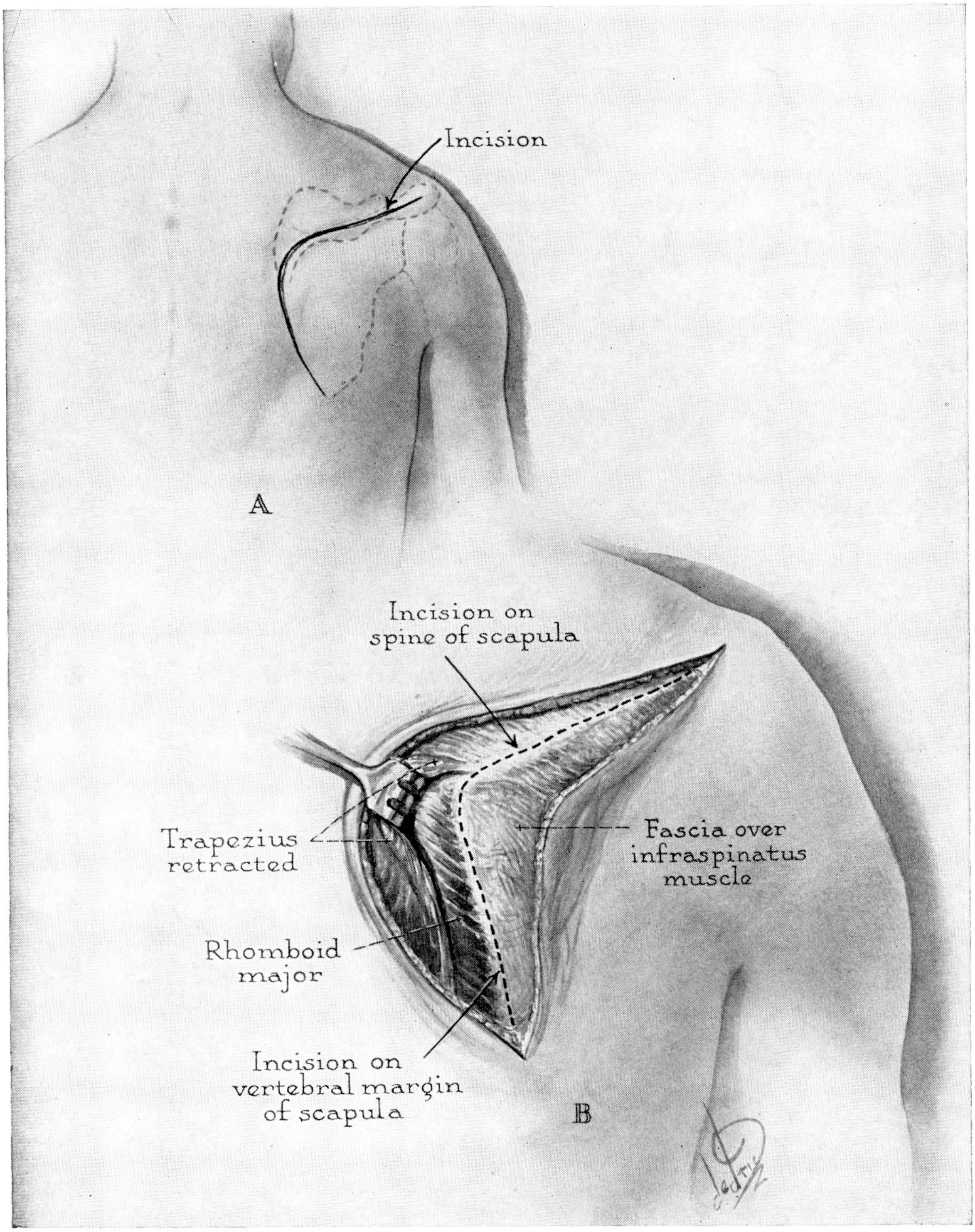

Exposure of the supraspinatus and infraspinatus fossae through a curved incision, reflecting the supraspinatus and infraspinatus muscles

EXPOSURE OF THE SUPRASPINATUS AND THE INFRASPINATUS FOSSAE THROUGH A CURVED INCISION REFLECTING THE SUPRASPINATUS AND INFRASPINATUS MUSCLES *(Continued)*

Plate 5: Description of Procedure

C An incision is made through the soft tissues and the periosteum, down to the spine and vertebral margin of the scapula. The infraspinatus muscle is reflected subperiosteally away from the scapula, and then is retracted downward and forward to expose the entire posterior aspect of the scapula distal to its spine (infraspinatus fossa).

The suprascapular nerve and its accompanying vessels emerge from the supraspinatus fossa at the posterior surface of the neck and beneath the spine of the scapula and then enter the infraspinatus muscle; they must not be injured.

D The supraspinatus fossa is exposed by the subperiosteal and upward reflection of the trapezius and supraspinatus muscles from the spine and dorsal surface of the scapula above it.

The suprascapular nerve and the accompanying transverse scapular artery must be protected

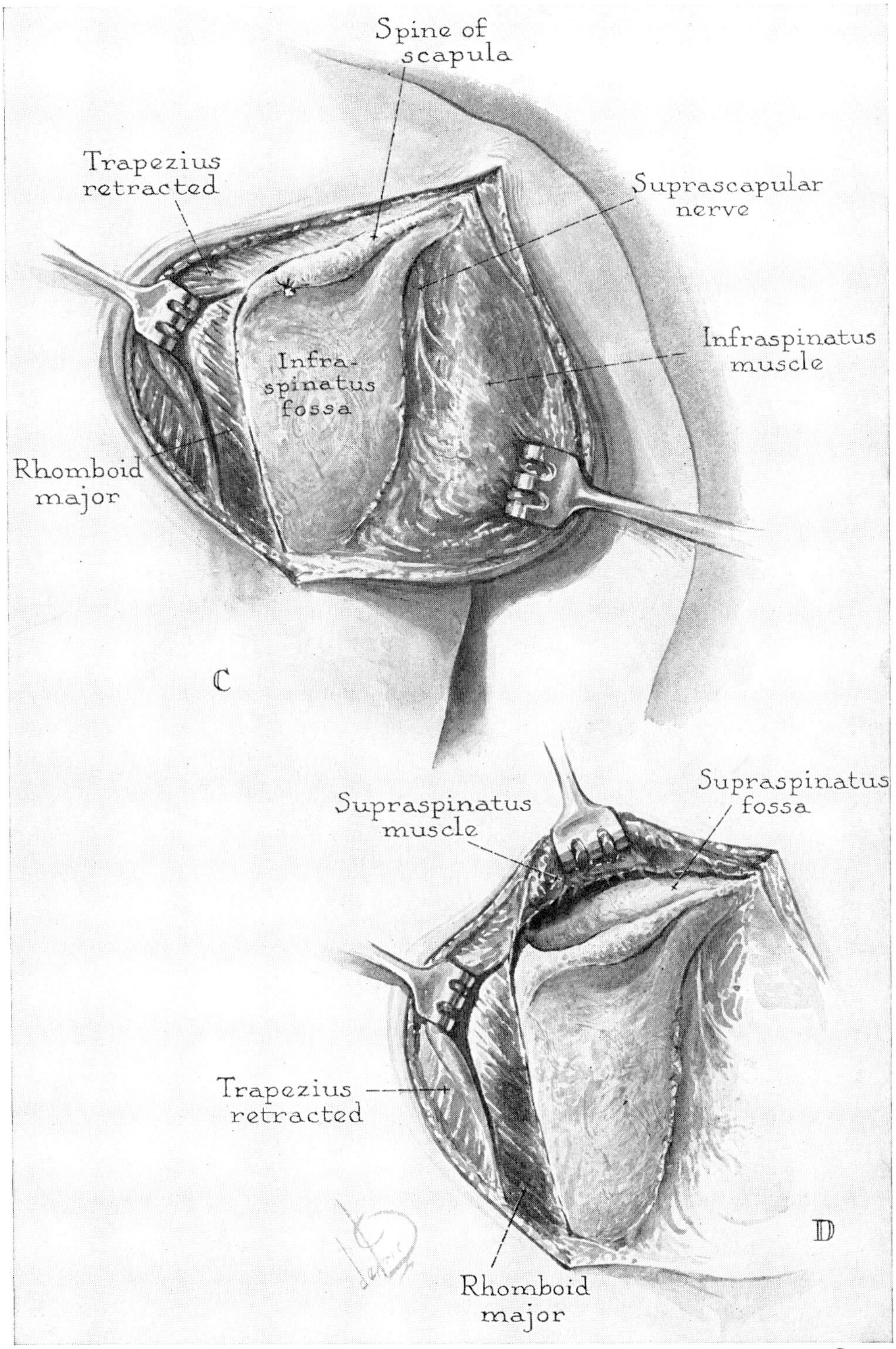

Exposure of the supraspinatus and infraspinatus fossae through a curved incision reflecting the supraspinatus and infraspinatus muscles

EXPOSURE OF THE SUBSCAPULAR FOSSA THROUGH AN INCISION OVER THE VERTEBRAL MARGIN OF THE SCAPULA

Indications: 1. Removal of Benign Tumors

2. Resection of Small Malignant Tumors

Plate 6: Description of Procedure

A A straight incision is made, starting at the superior angle of the scapula and extending downward along the vertebral margin to the inferior angle. The skin margins are mobilized and retracted.

B The free margin and the adjacent portion of the trapezius muscle are separated from the underlying structures, so that the muscle can be retracted upward and toward the midline. If necessary, its outer fibers may be cut along the line indicated in the illustration, which permits retraction of the muscle and affords wider exposure. The vertebral margin of the scapula is then palpated, and note is made of the rhomboid muscles attached to its medial edge, and of the infraspinatus and supraspinatus muscles at its lateral edge.

C The incision then is developed down to the vertebral margin of the scapula by a cut through the fibers of attachment of the adjacent muscles and the periosteum.

D The costal surface of the scapula is exposed by detaching the rhomboid muscles and by raising the subscapularis subperiosteally. Access to the subscapular fossa is facilitated by placing a sharp retractor on the vertebral margin of the scapula and pulling the bone to the side, laterally.

NOTE: The incision is free from danger. The dorsal scapular nerve and the descending branch of the transverse scapular artery are located in the rhomboid muscles just medial to their attachment to the vertebral margin of the scapula. Subperiosteal mobilization of the rhomboid muscles away from the scapula will preserve this nerve and artery from injury. Exposure of the supraspinatus and infraspinatus fossae may be obtained by elevation of the corresponding muscles.

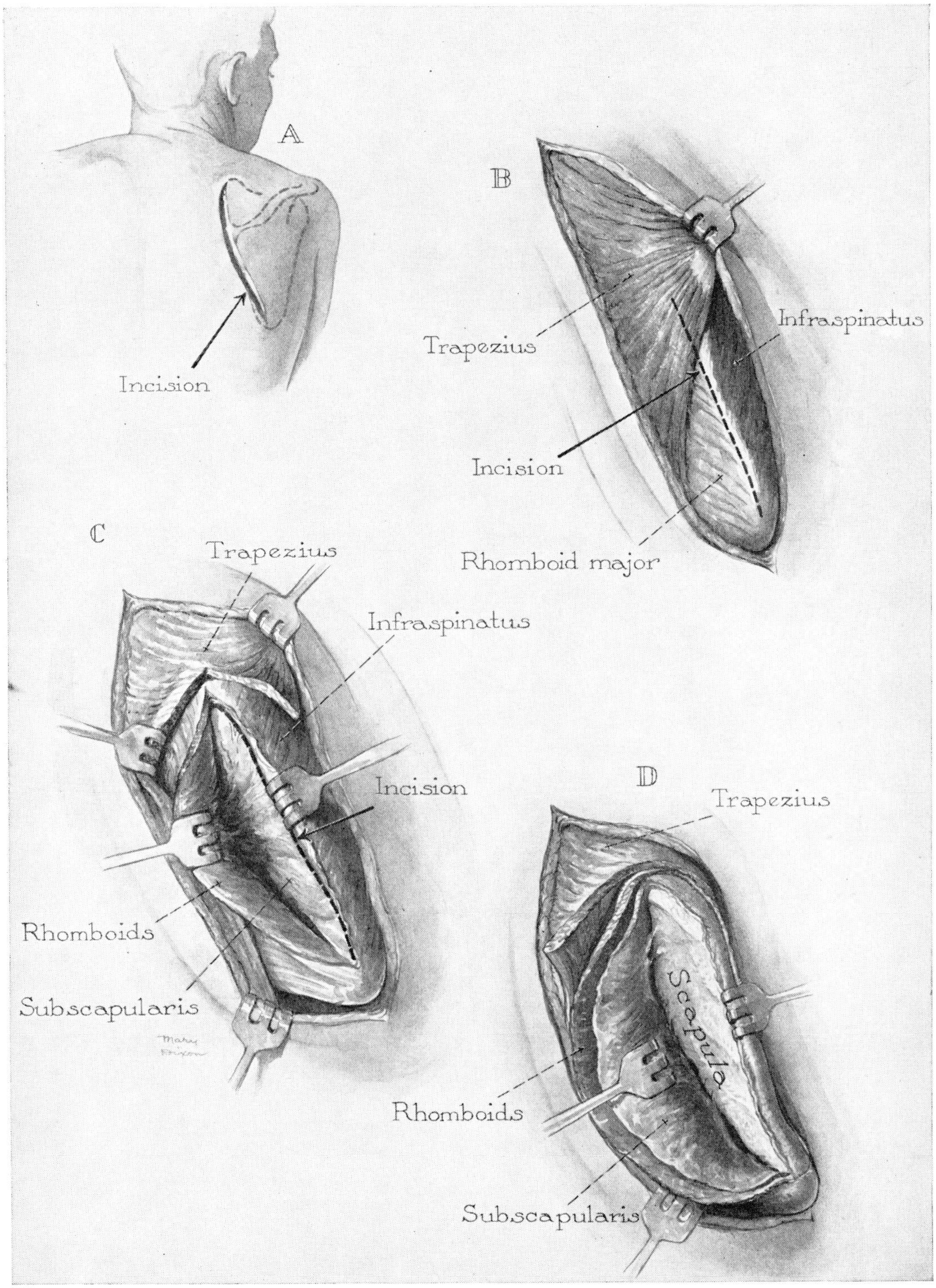

Exposure of the subscapular fossa through an incision over the vertebral margin of the scapula

EXPOSURE OF THE SUPRASPINATUS, INFRASPINATUS AND SUBSCAPULAR FOSSAE THROUGH A POSTERIOR LONGITUDINAL INCISION

Indications 1. Resection of Tumors

2. Open Reduction of Fractures

3. Correction of Congenital Elevation of the Scapula

Plate 7: Description of Procedure

A The incision extends from the superior angle to the inferior angle of the scapula, skirting its vertebral margin. The skin flaps are widely mobilized and retracted.

B The lower fibers of the trapezius muscle are cut to gain access to the proximal portion of the vertebral margin of the scapula. The supraspinatus, infraspinatus and rhomboid muscles are then identified.

C The rhomboid major and minor muscles are detached from the scapula to expose the subscapularis muscle.

D Subperiosteal elevation of the supraspinatus, infraspinatus and subscapularis muscles will lay bare corresponding portions of the scapula.

NOTE: Retraction of the lateral skin flap will permit exposure of the greater portion of the spine and also of the dorsal surface of the scapula. The suprascapular nerve lies on the undersurface of the supraspinatus and infraspinatus muscles and must be protected.

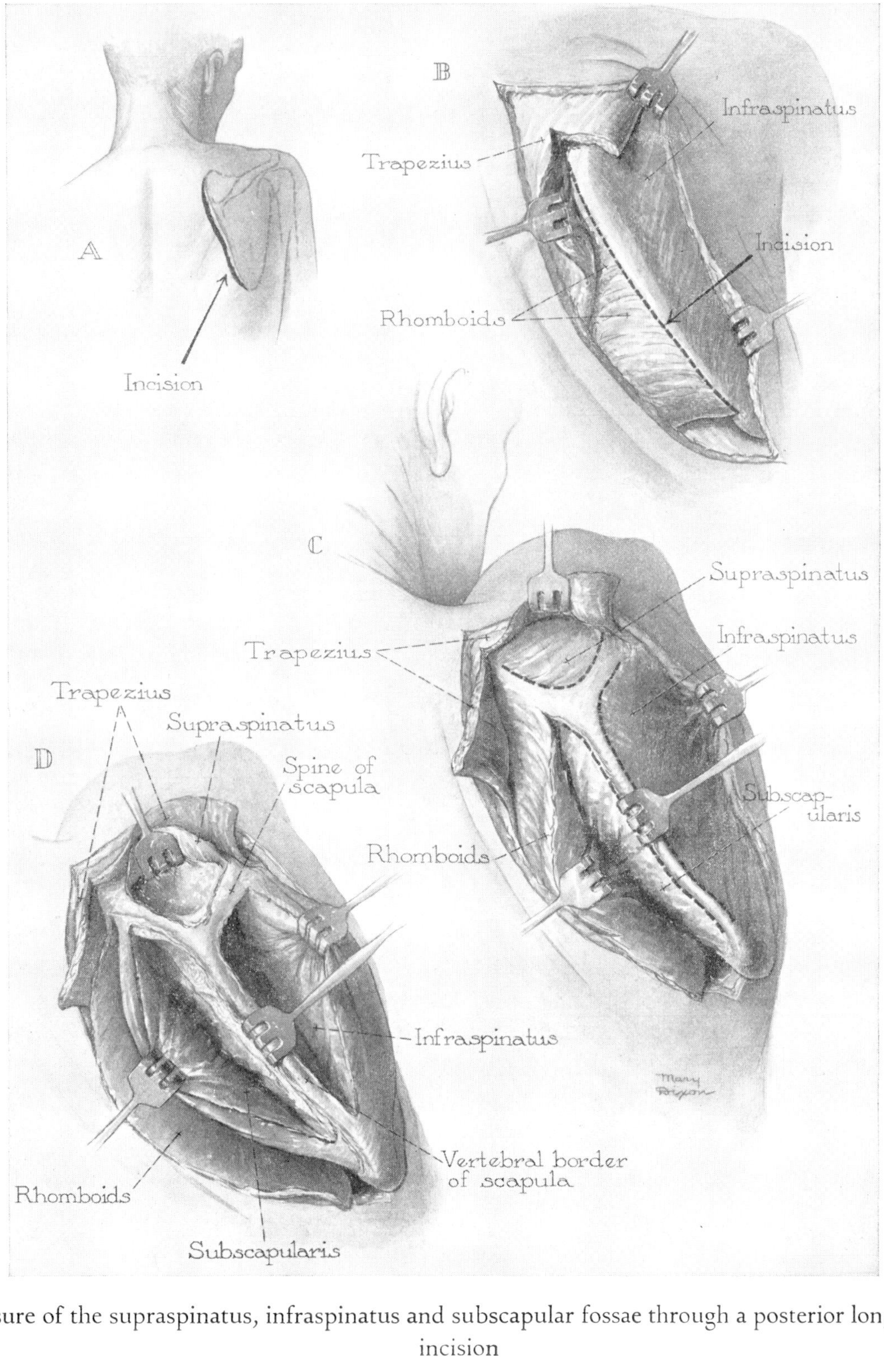

Exposure of the supraspinatus, infraspinatus and subscapular fossae through a posterior longitudinal incision

EXPOSURE OF THE DISTAL HALF OF THE AXILLARY MARGIN OF THE SCAPULA

Indications: 1. Removal of Benign and Malignant Tumors

2. Treatment of Acute and Chronic Infections

Plate 8: Description of Procedure

A The inferior angle and the distal half of the axillary margin of the scapula are identified by palpation. The incision begins at the inferior angle and extends upward for the desired distance, by skirting the axillary margin of the scapula in the interval between the infraspinatus and teres major muscles.

B The fascia is opened and the lower margin of the infraspinatus muscle is separated from the teres major. The dissection then is developed down to the bone and the periosteum of the scapula is incised.

C The infraspinatus muscle is reflected subperiosteally from the dorsal surface of the scapula and retracted proximally and medially. The teres major muscle is retracted downward and forward as the axillary margin of the scapula is exposed subperiosteally. Exposure of the adjacent deep surface of the scapula is obtained by mobilization of the nearby portion of the subscapular muscle.

NOTE: The nerve supply to the infraspinatus muscle (suprascapular nerve) enters its deep surface posteriorly to the neck of the scapula, but is not shown in the illustration. The teres major muscle is innervated from its axillary surface by the lower subscapular nerve; damage to this nerve can be avoided by careful subperiosteal mobilization of this muscle.

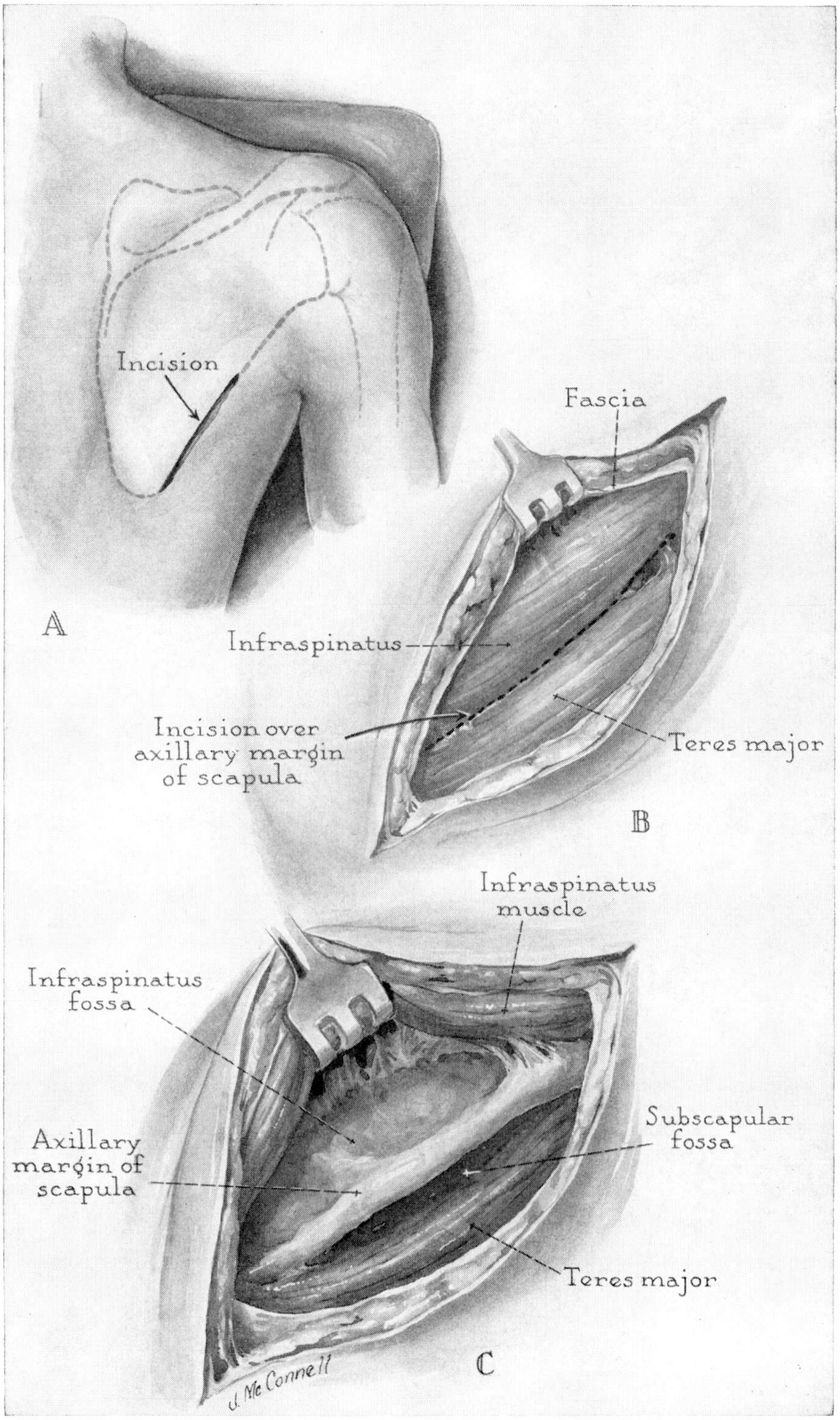

Exposure of the distal half of the axillary margin of the scapula

EXPOSURE OF THE PROXIMAL HALF OF THE AXILLARY MARGIN OF THE SCAPULA, INCLUDING THE SHOULDER JOINT

Indications: 1. Resection of New Growths, Benign and Malignant

2. Partial Ostectomy of the Scapula for Osteomyelitis

3. Arthrodesis of the Shoulder Joint in Some Instances

Plate 9: Description of Procedure

A The incision extends from the posterior margin of the deltoid muscle downward over the axillary margin of the scapula as far as necessary.

B The deep fascia is opened and the posterior margin of the deltoid muscle (it occupies the proximal triangle of the wound) is identified. The interval between the infraspinatus and teres minor muscles is determined by palpation, and an incision is made through it and the periosteum down to the axillary border of the scapula.

C The infraspinatus muscle is raised from the scapula and retracted upward, thereby exposing the infraspinatus fossa and the posterior capsule of the shoulder joint. The teres minor muscle is mobilized downward. Exposure of the tendinous origin of the long head of the triceps muscle from the infraglenoid tuberosity of the scapula may be effected as illustrated.

D The head of the humerus can be exposed through a linear incision which opens the shoulder joint, the deltoid muscle being retracted laterally.

NOTE: No important vessels or nerves are encountered in this dissection. The axillary nerve lies distal to the lateral margin of the teres minor, and deep to the long head of the triceps muscles. The circumflex scapular artery can be ligated at the scapular margin without producing ill effects.

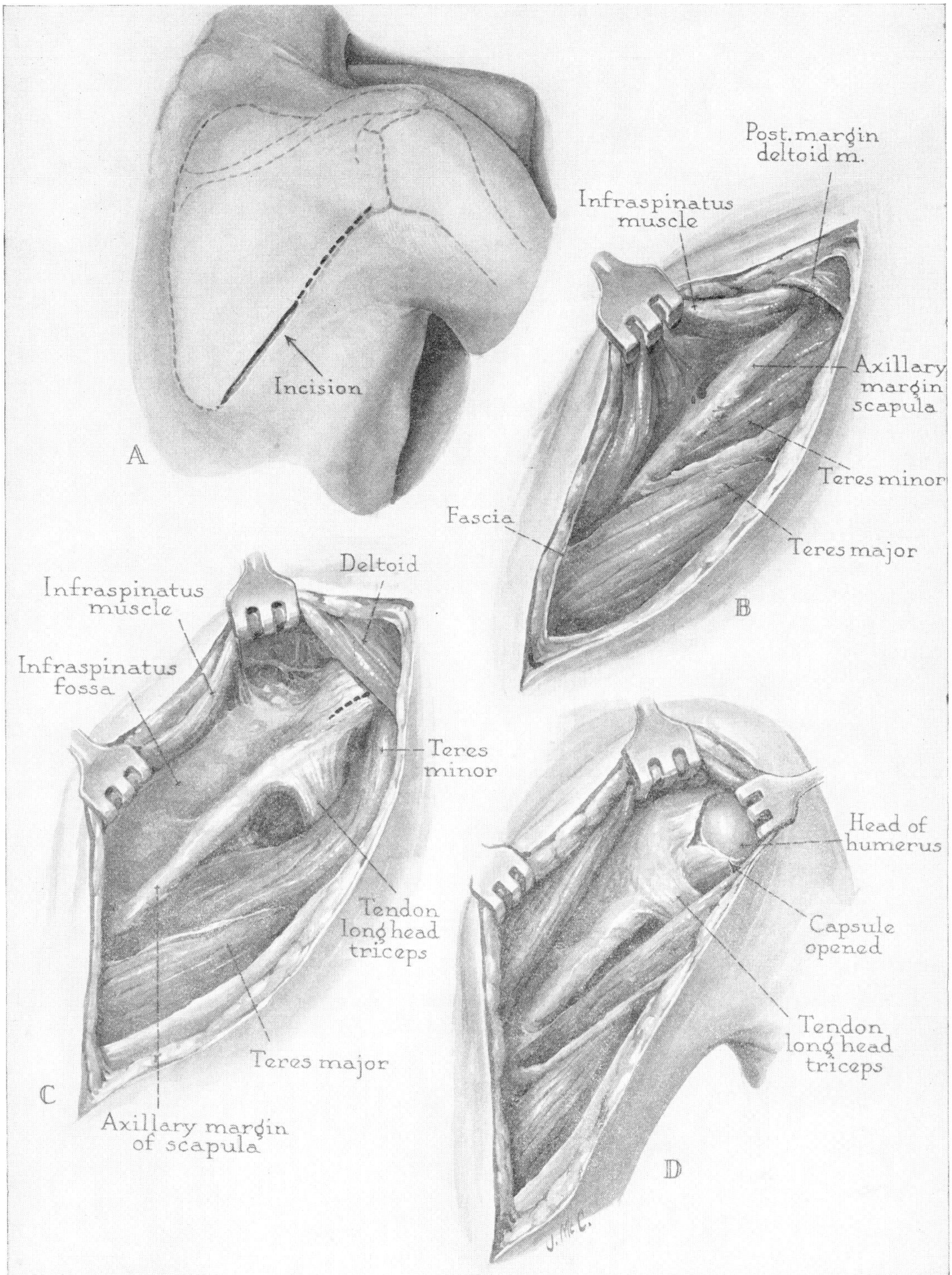

Exposure of the proximal half of the axillary margin of the scapula, including the shoulder joint

EXPOSURE OF THE ACROMIOCLAVICULAR JOINT THROUGH A CORONAL INCISION

Indications: 1. Open Reduction of Acute Dislocations of the Acromioclavicular Joint

2. Treatment of Chronic Dislocations of the Acromioclavicular Joint

3. Excision of Benign Tumors

4. Treatment of Chronic Infections

Plate 10: Description of Procedure

A The curved incision begins approximately 1 1/2 inches short of the lateral end of the clavicle and extends posteriorly around the free margin of the acromion, ending posteriorly one inch over the spine of the scapula.

B The skin flaps are undermined widely and retracted, bringing into view the clavicle with the attached deltoid muscle covered by fascia distally, and the attached fibers of the trapezius muscle proximally. The acromioclavicular joint is identified, and a linear incision is made which centers on the joint and extends laterally over the acromion process and medially onto the clavicle, for the necessary distance.

C The acromion and the end of the clavicle are exposed subperiosteally, and the capsule of the joint, which is reinforced by the anterior acromioclavicular ligament, is opened and its margins are retracted proximally and distally. The acromioclavicular joint is exposed together with the interposed cartilaginous disk (*Note* that the latter has been removed in the illustration).

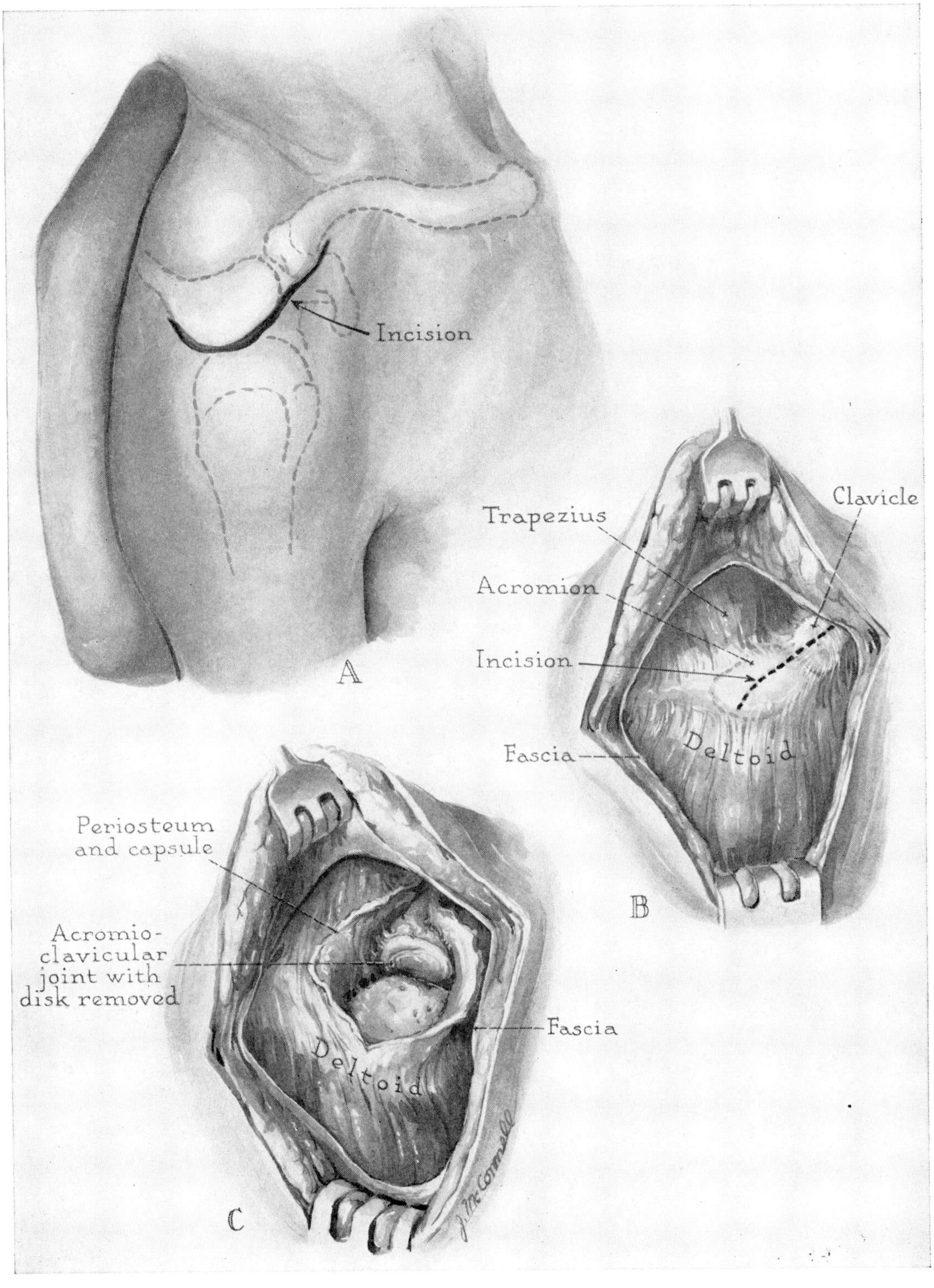

Exposure of the acromioclavicular joint through a coronal incision

EXPOSURE OF THE ACROMIOCLAVICULAR JOINT AND THE CORACO-CLAVICULAR LIGAMENTS THROUGH A CORONAL INCISION REFLECTING THE DELTOID MUSCLE DOWNWARD

Indications: 1. Open Reduction of Acute Dislocations of the Acromioclavicular Joint with Rupture of the Ligaments

2. Open Reduction of Chronic Dislocations of the Acromioclavicular Joint with High Displacement of the Clavicle

3. Repair of the Coracoclavicular Ligaments

Plate 11: Description of Procedure

A The curved incision runs along the lower margin of the clavicle, beginning approximately 3-inches from the lateral end, and then skirts posteriorly around the acromioclavicular joint and the acromion, to terminate over the adjacent portion of the spine of the scapula.

B The skin flaps are undermined widely to expose the clavicle, the acromion and the trapezius and deltoid muscles.

C A linear incision is made centrally over the outer end of the clavicle, the capsule of the acromioclavicular joint and the acromion. Adequate exposure is obtained by opening the joint and by dissecting the adjacent bone subperiosteally. The deltoid muscle is reflected downward from the outer end of the clavicle and the acromion. The coracoid process is found by palpation, and the coracoclavicular ligaments are identified as they pass in a fan-like manner from the superior surface of the coracoid process to the deep surface of the outer end of the clavicle and the acromium. The coraco-acromial ligament, it may be noted, greatly adds to the stability of the acromioclavicular joint.

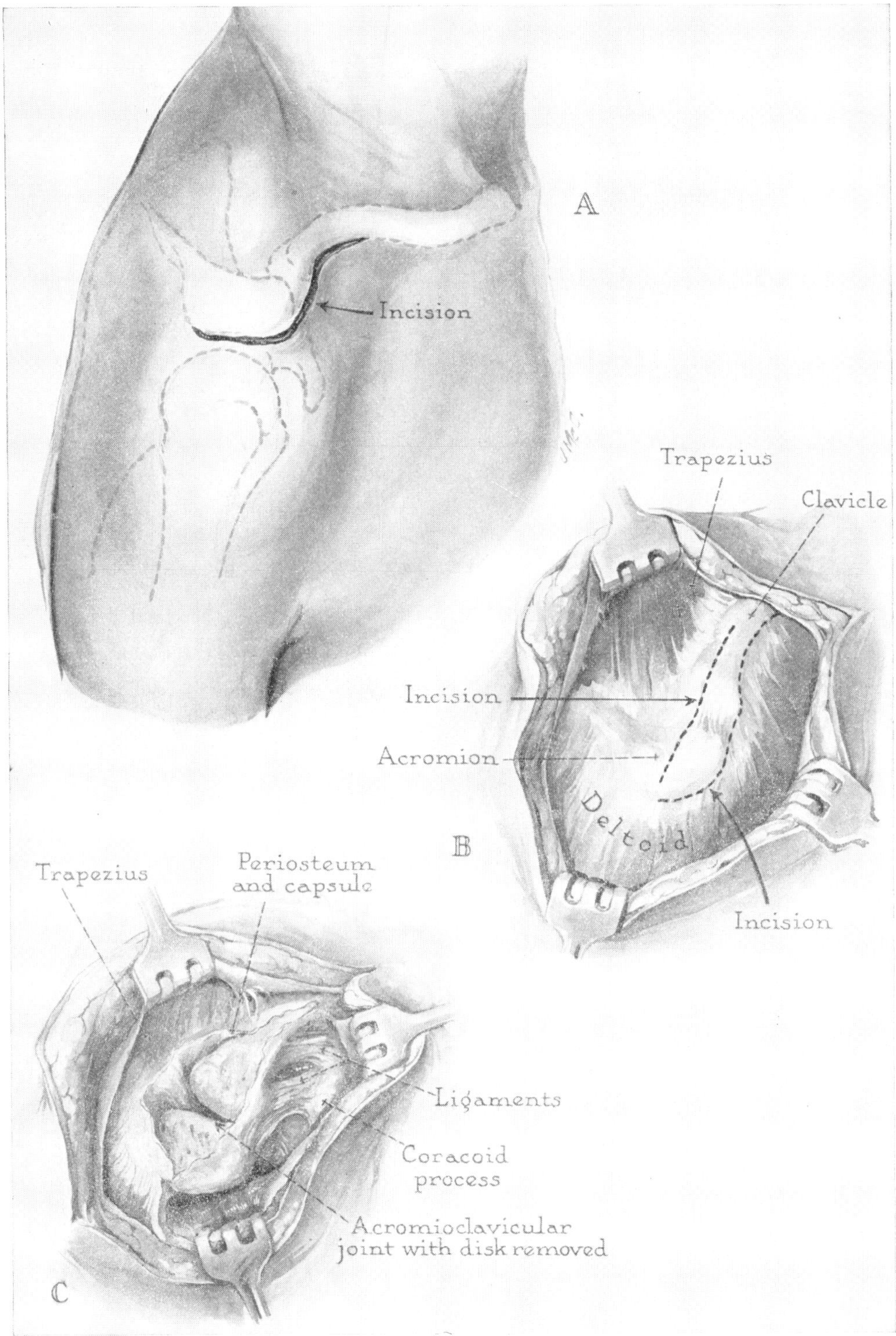

Exposure of the acromioclavicular joint and the coracoclavicular ligaments through a coronal incision reflecting the deltoid muscle downward

EXPOSURE OF THE MIDDLE PORTION OF THE CLAVICLE THROUGH AN ANTERIOR INCISION

Indications: 1. Open Reduction of Recent and Old Fractures

2. Treatment of Benign and Malignant Tumors

Plate 12: Description of Procedure

A An incision is made for the desired distance along the anterior inferior aspect of the clavicle, which can be palpated subcutaneously.

B The deep fascia is opened and the fibers of the platysma are transected in line with the incision.

C The periosteum is opened and reflected from the clavicle. Care must be exercised in the dissection posteriorly, so as to preclude an injury to the subclavian artery and the pleura. The fibers of the pectoralis and subclavius muscles will be encountered in the wound along the anterior aspect of the clavicle. The trapezius will be seen superiorly if the dissection continues to the outer third of the clavicle and the sternocleidomastoid tendon is uncovered when the wound extends to the sternum.

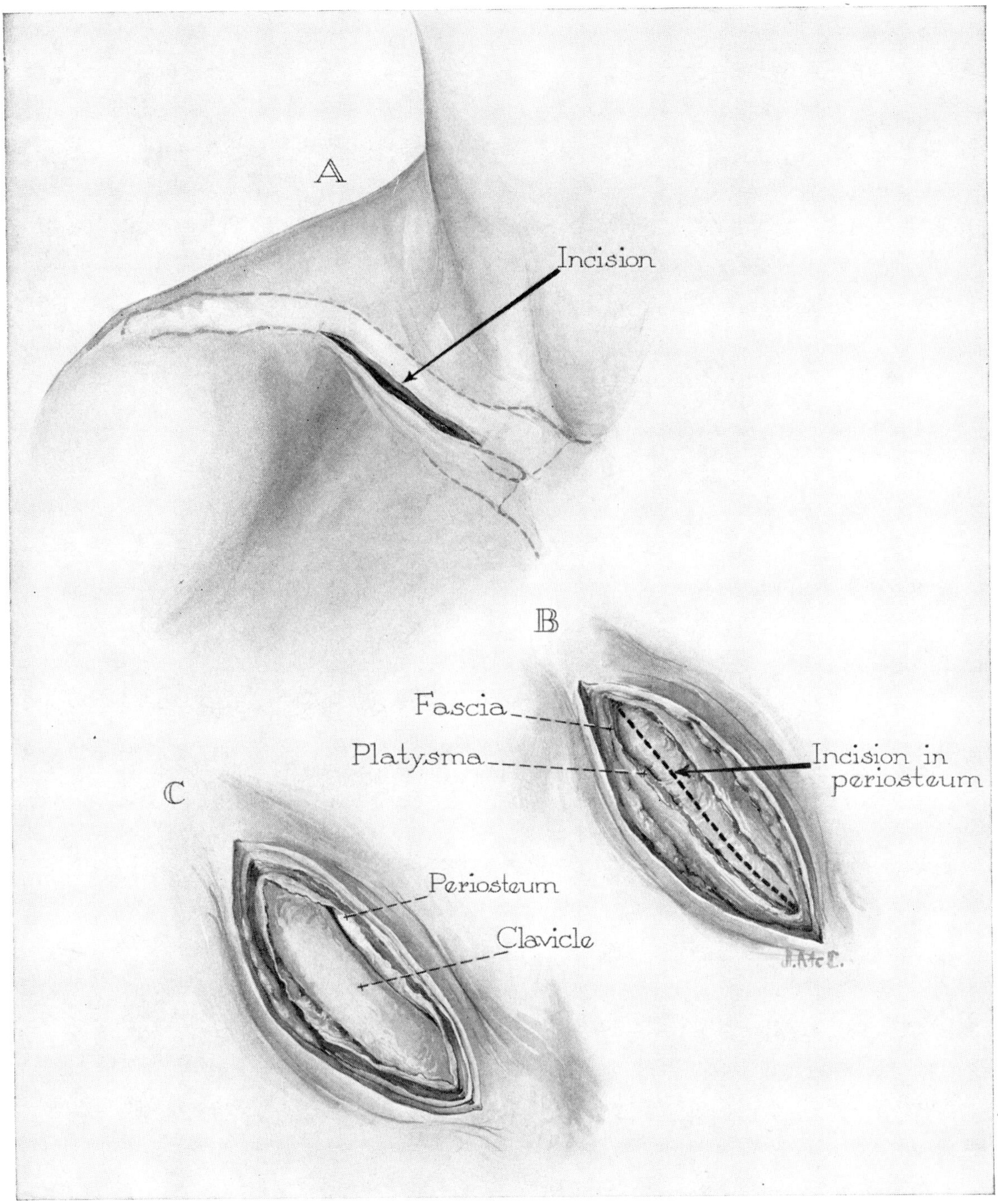

Exposure of the middle portion of the clavicle through an anterior incision

EXPOSURE OF STERNOCLAVICULAR JOINT THROUGH ANTERIOR CLAVICLE-STERNAL INCISION

Indications: 1. Open Reduction of Acute Dislocations of the Sternoclavicular Joint

2. Open Reduction of Chronic Dislocations of the Sternoclavicular Joint

3. Resection of Benign Tumors of the Sternal End of the Clavicle

4. Treatment of Chronic Infections

Plate 13: Description of Procedure

A A curved incision is made over the anterior aspect of the inner fourth of the clavicle and then extends downward across the sternoclavicular joint, terminating over the manubrium.

B The fascia is incised, and the fibers of the platysma muscle in the clavicular portion of the wound are severed.

C The dissection is carried down to the clavicle, which is exposed subperiosteally. It should be recalled that the subclavian artery lies posteriorly to it. Medially, the interval between the tendon of the sternocleidomastoid and pectoralis major muscles is developed by sharp dissection. The incision is carried down to the sternoclavicular joint, which is opened to expose the cartilaginous disk between the end of the clavicle and the articular surface of the sternum. The adjacent portion of the manubrium is exposed subperiosteally.

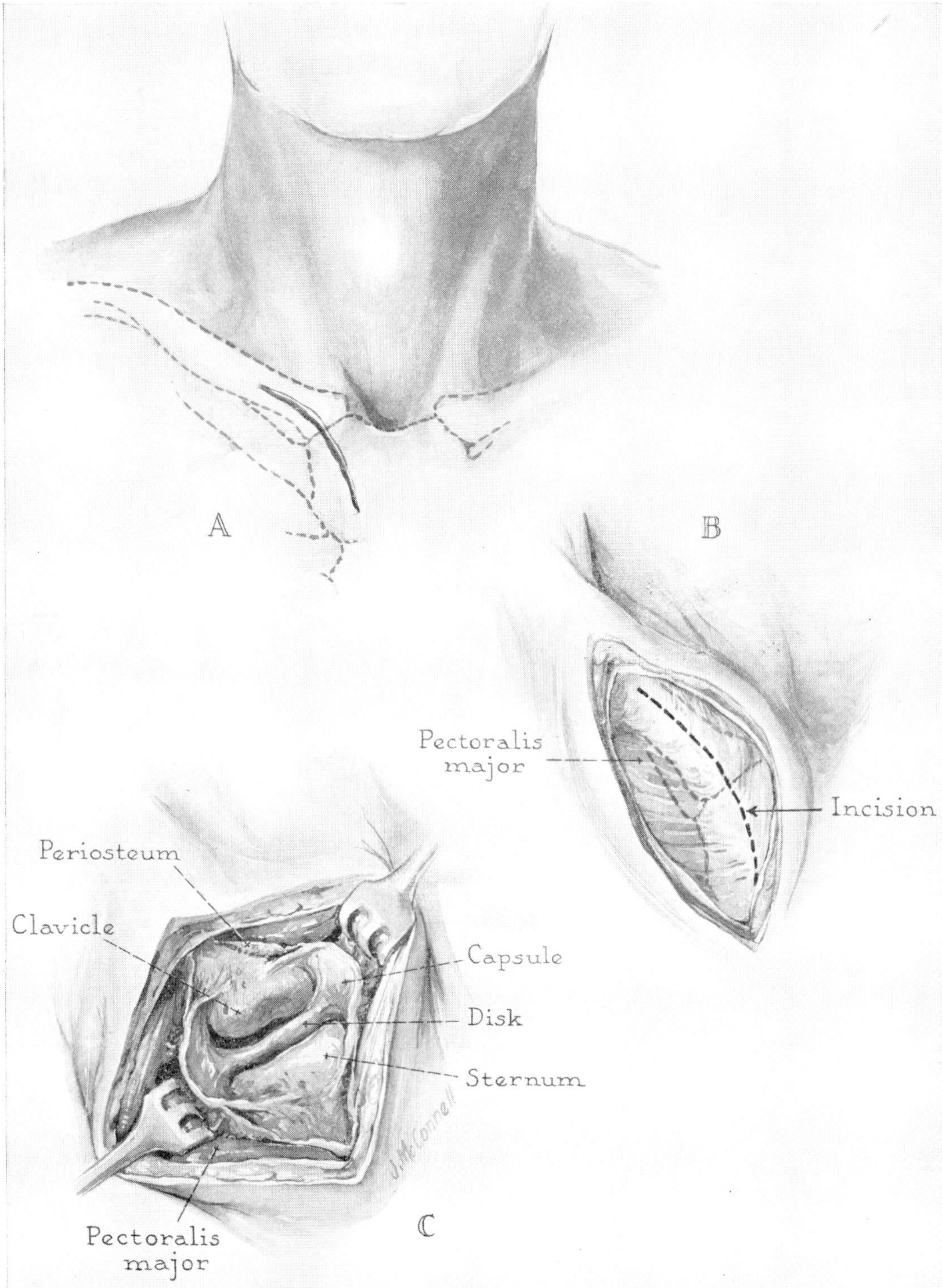

Exposure of the sternoclavicular joint through an anterior clavicle-sternal incision

Section II

Region of the Shoulder Joint

EXPOSURE OF THE SHOULDER JOINT THROUGH AN ANTERIOR DELTOID INCISION

Indications: 1. Release of Adhesions

2. Removal of Loose Bodies

3. Arthrodesis of the Shoulder Joint

4. Biopsy of the Synovia

Plate 14: Description of Procedure

A The incision begins over the coracoid process at the lower margin of the clavicle, and extends downward along the anterior margin of the deltoid muscle for a distance of approximately 5 inches.

B The cephalic vein is identified in the interval between the deltoid and pectoralis major muscles and must be protected as the fascia is opened in line with the skin incision. The vein may be retracted to either side of the wound, but is preferably brought inward if the tributaries from the deltoid are neither large nor numerous. Both development of the wound and protection of this vein can be facilitated, however, by leaving a thin band of deltoid muscle attached to the vein and retracting them with the pectoralis major muscle, medially. The separated band of deltoid muscle must be kept down to minimal size because it is isolated from its nerve supply and will undergo atrophy and fibrosis. (Procedure continued on Plate 15.)

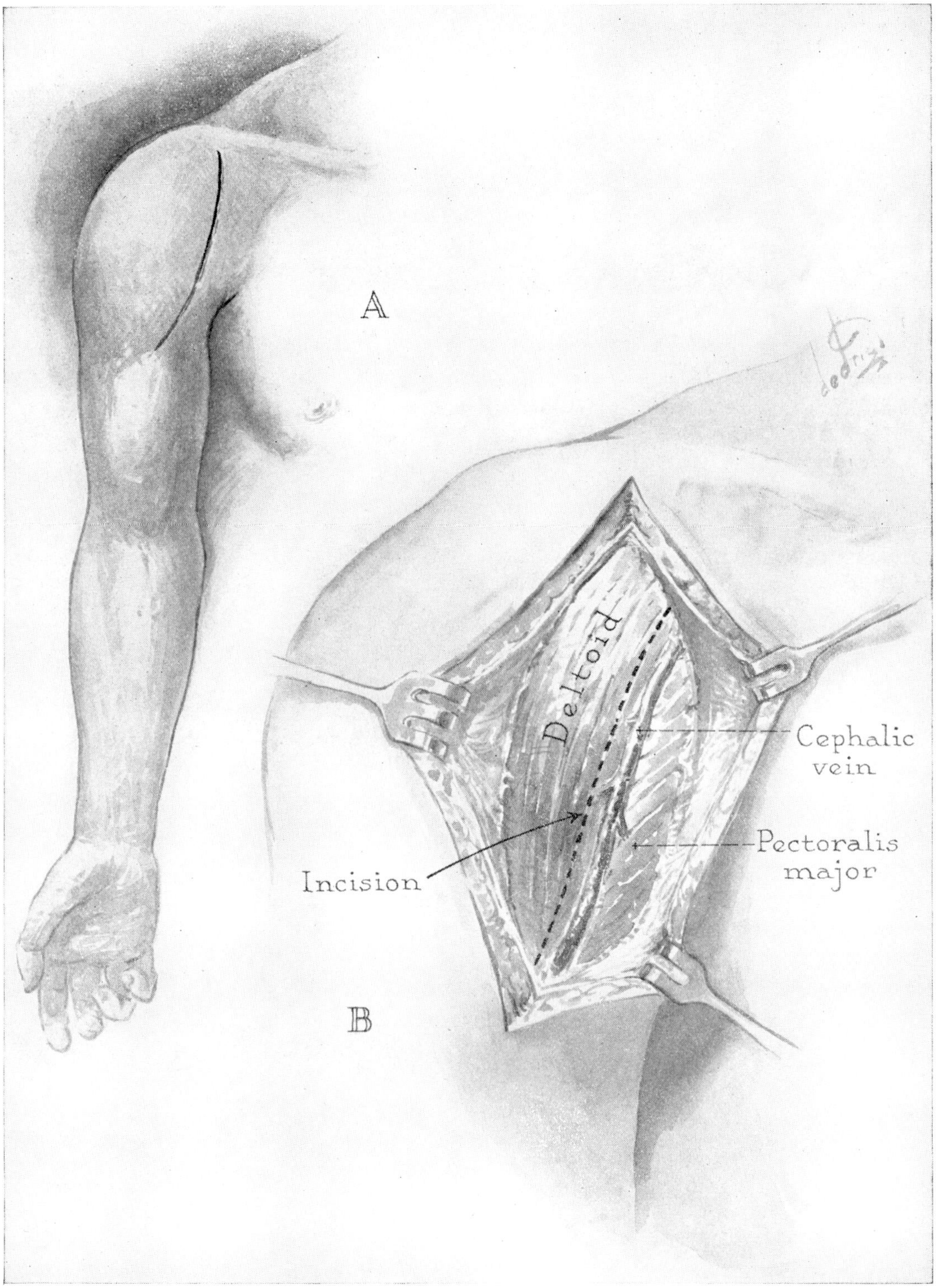

Exposure of the shoulder joint through an anterior deltoid incision

EXPOSURE OF THE SHOULDER JOINT THROUGH AN ANTERIOR DELTOID INCISION *(Continued)*

Plate 15: Description of Procedure

C A portion of the anterior fibers of the deltoid muscle are separated from the clavicle, and the muscle is retracted laterally to bring into view the short head of the biceps and the coracobrachialis muscles. It must be kept in mind that the axillary nerve is situated on the deep surface of the deltoid muscle and must be protected. Distally, the pectoralis major muscle and tendon pass laterally to gain their insertion onto the humerus. The fascia over the short head of the biceps muscle is incised along its lateral edge and the muscle together with the coracobrachialis is retracted toward the midline.

D An incision is made in the superior medial portion of the shoulder joint capsule. The intracapsular portion of the tendon of the long head of the biceps muscle is located directly lateral to the opening and must be protected.

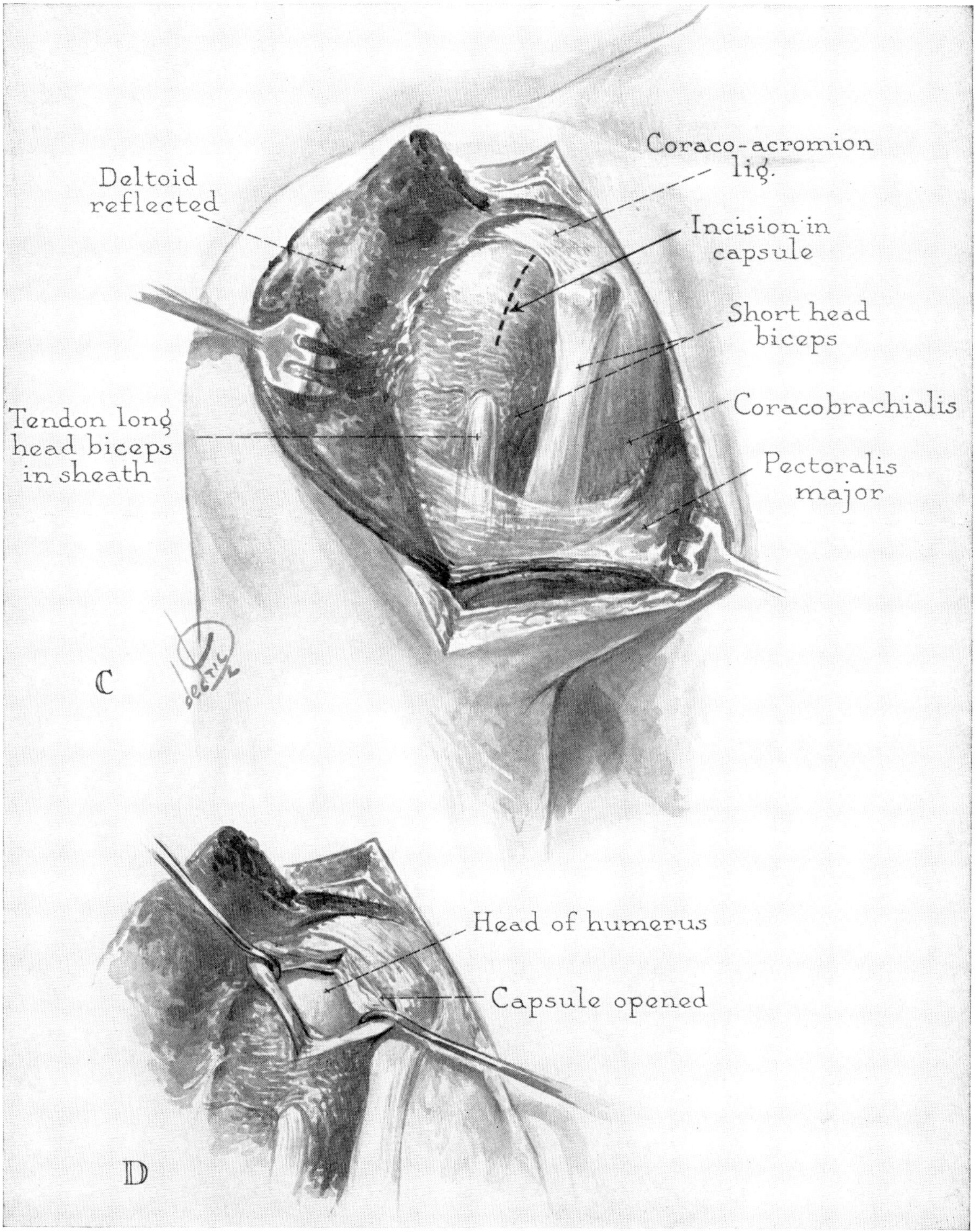

Exposure of the shoulder joint through an anterior deltoid incision

EXPOSURE OF THE LONG AND SHORT HEADS OF THE BICEPS MUSCLE THROUGH AN ANTERIOR DELTOID INCISION

Indications: 1. Transplantation of the Long Head of the Biceps Tendon in the Treatment of Recurrent Dislocation of the Shoulder

2. Repair of Ruptures of the Long Head of the Biceps Tendon

3. Treatment of Chronic Tenosynovitis of the Tendon of the Long Head of the Biceps Muscle

Plate 16: Description of Procedure

A The lower margin of the clavicle, the coracoid process and the anterior margin of the deltoid muscle are the landmarks for the skin incision. The incision begins at the clavicle and extends downward over the interval between the pectoralis major and deltoid muscles for a distance of approximately 5 inches.

B The fascia is opened in line with the skin incision, and the cephalic vein is isolated and retracted to the medial side of the wound, together with the inner fibers of the deltoid muscle. If the tributaries from the latter muscle are large and numerous, it may be better to retract the cephalic vein laterally. (Procedure continued on Plate 17.)

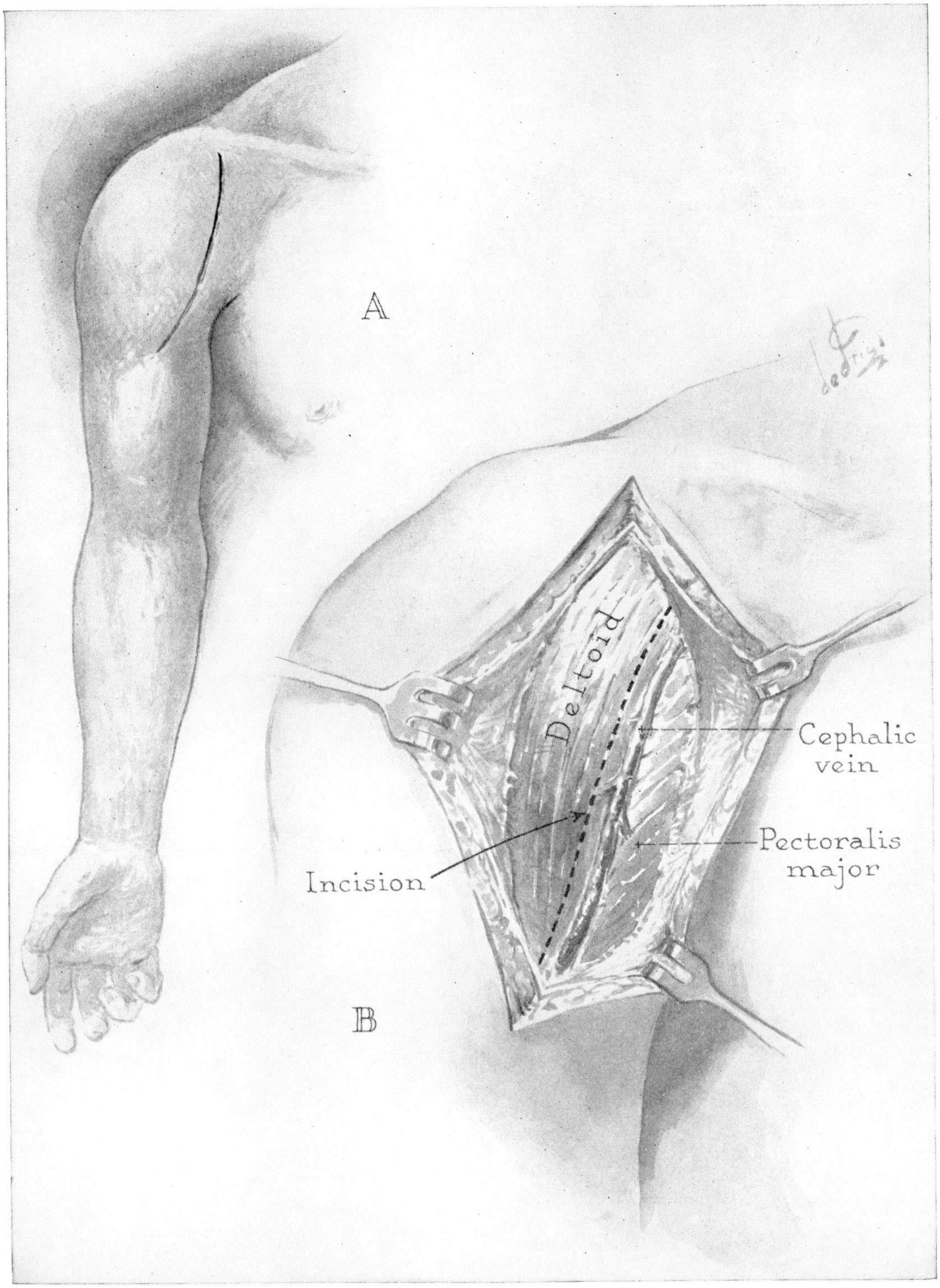

Exposure of the long and short heads of the biceps muscle through an anterior deltoid incision

EXPOSURE OF THE LONG AND SHORT HEADS OF THE BICEPS MUSCLE THROUGH AN ANTERIOR DELTOID INCISION *(Continued)*

Plate 17: Description of Procedure

C The shiny aponeurotic surface of the short head of the biceps is brought into view by retracting the edges of the wound. Distally, this muscle passes beneath the pectoralis major tendon as the latter gains its insertion at the medial side of the shaft of the humerus. The long head of the biceps muscle is exposed by rotating the arm internally and by firmly retracting the deltoid muscle.

D It is located along the anterior surface of the proximal portion of the humerus. It disappears distally beneath the pectoralis major tendon, and passes proximally into the capsule of the shoulder joint from beneath the transverse humeral ligament. The long head of the biceps tendon is exposed by a longitudinal incision into its tendon sheath. The transverse humeral ligament must be cut to mobilize the tendon when it is transplanted.

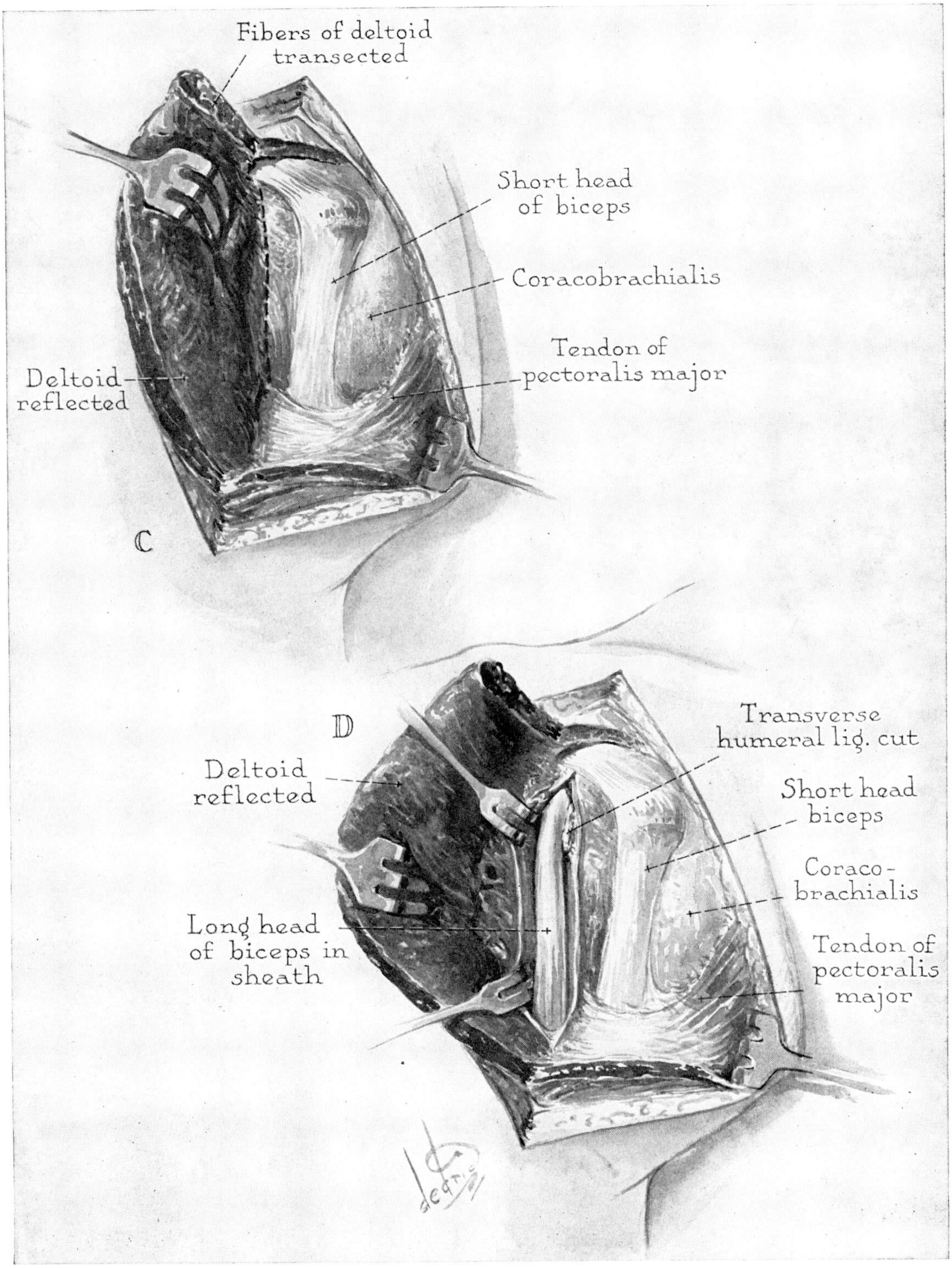

Exposure of the long and short heads of the biceps muscle through an anterior deltoid incision

EXPOSURE OF THE SUBSCAPULAR MUSCLE AND TENDON THROUGH AN ANTERIOR DELTOID INCISION

Indication: 1. Tenotomy of the Subscapular Tendon in the Treatment of Internal Rotation Contracture Following Birth Palsy

Plate 18: Description of Procedure

A An incision, which is made between the deltoid and pectoralis major muscles, begins at the anterior margin of the clavicle over the coracoid process, and extends downward for a distance of approximately 4 inches.

B The fascia is opened in line with the skin incision, and the cephalic vein is isolated and retracted medially with the pectoralis major muscle. A narrow strip of deltoid is retracted medially together with the vein and pectoralis muscle in some instances. The size of the strip must be kept at a minimum because it is deprived of its nerve supply and will undergo atrophy. (Procedure continued on Plate 19.)

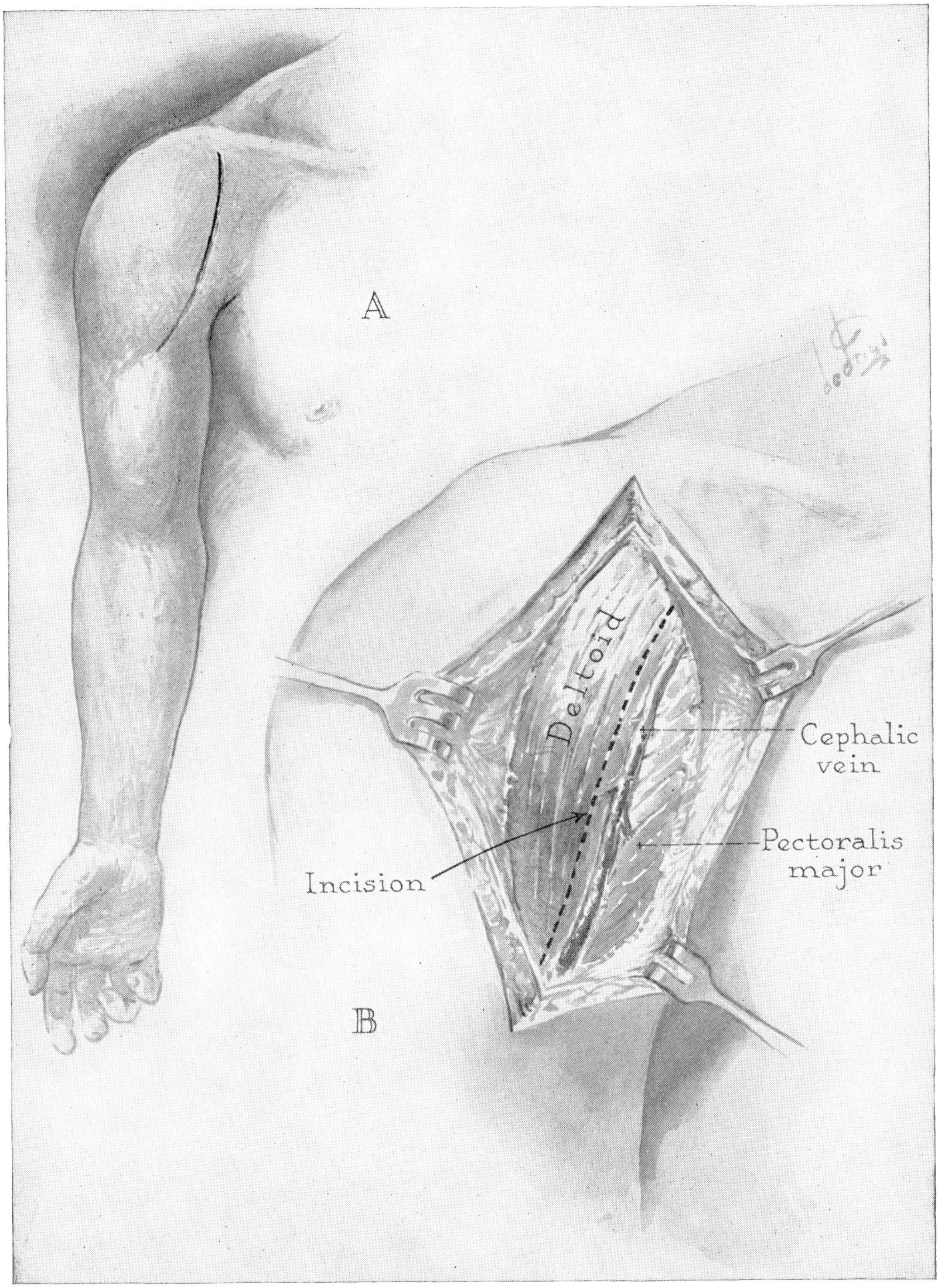

Exposure of the subscapular muscle and tendon through an anterior deltoid incision

EXPOSURE OF THE SUBSCAPULAR MUSCLE AND TENDON THROUGH AN ANTERIOR DELTOID INCISION *(Continued)*

Plate 19: Description of Procedure

C The outer margin of the short head of the biceps is isolated and firmly retracted medially to expose the subscapularis muscle which lies under it.

D A director is carefully placed beneath the subscapular tendon in order to separate this muscle from the anterior aspect of the capsule of the shoulder joint to which it may be intimately connected. The tendon is transected over the director.

NOTE: Care must be taken when retracting the short head of the biceps and the coracobrachialis muscles that no injury is done to the musculocutaneous nerve which enters the coracobrachialis along its axillary margin.

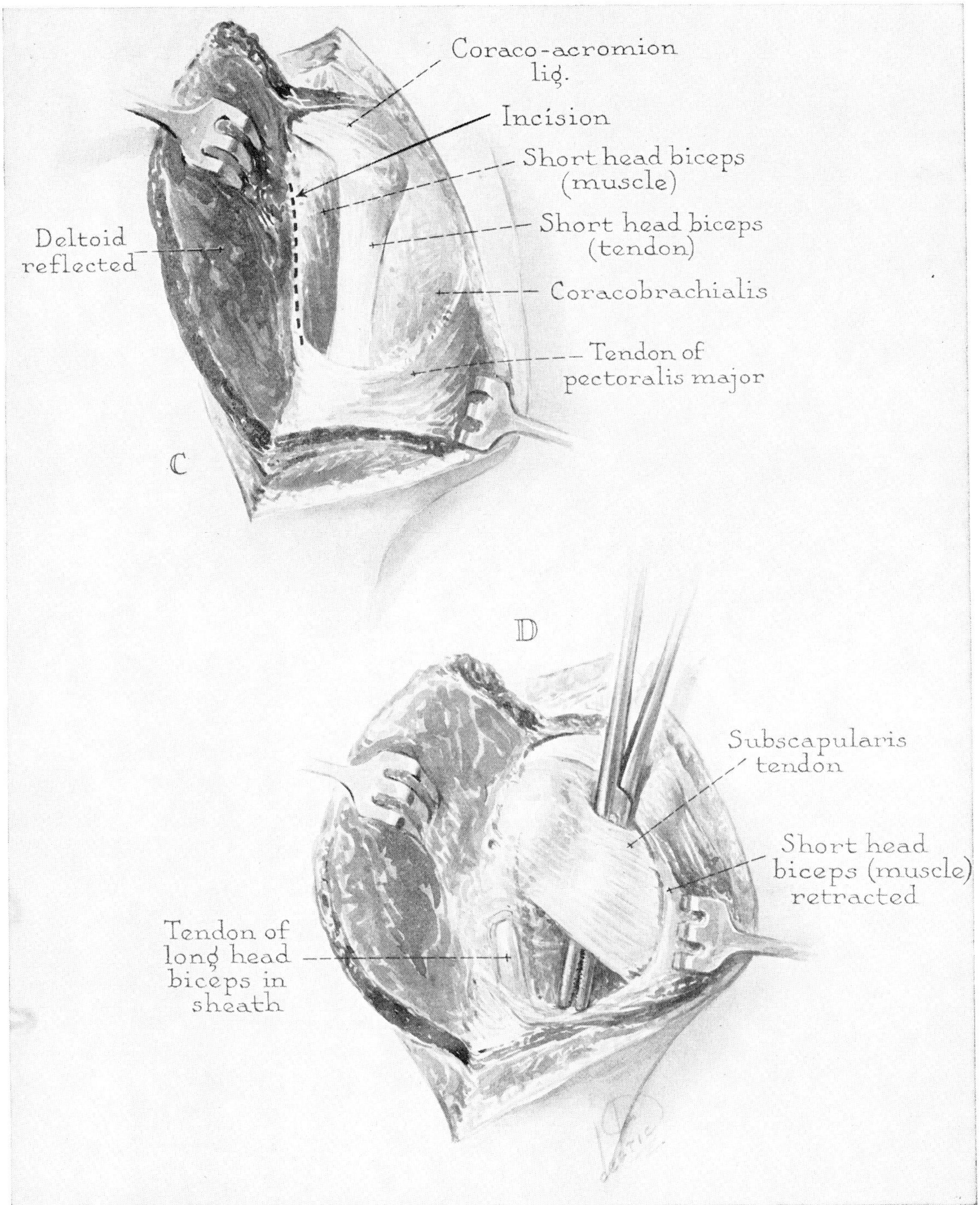

Exposure of the subscapular muscle and tendon through an anterior deltoid incision

EXPOSURE OF THE ANTERIOR ASPECT OF THE SHOULDER JOINT AND THE GLENOID FOSSA THROUGH AN ANTERIOR DELTOID INCISION WITH OSTEOTOMY OF THE CORACOID PROCESS

Indications: 1. Capsular Repair for Recurrent Anterior Dislocations of the Shoulder Joint

2. Reduction of Old Unreduced Dislocations of the Shoulder Joint

3. Reduction of a Dislocation of the Head of the Humerus Associated with a Fracture of the Proximal End of the Shaft

Plate 20: Description of Procedure

A The incision starts at the level of the lower border of the clavicle, and follows the anterior margin of the deltoid muscle down to its insertion onto the tuberosity of the humerus.

B The cephalic vein is identified. This vein courses over and along the interval between the deltoid and the pectoralis major muscles and serves therefore to identify this interval. The vein and pectoralis major muscle are retracted medially. If large and numerous tributaries from the deltoid muscle are encountered, it is preferable to separate by blunt dissection a thin marginal slice of this muscle and to retract it together with the cephalic vein and pectoralis major muscle. The deltoid muscle proper is retracted laterally.

C Ample room is desirable for this exposure and can be obtained by cutting across the anterior portion of the deltoid muscle near the clavicle. Bleeding from the deltoid branches of the thoraco-acromial artery is controlled by ligation. The short head of the biceps is recognized in the floor of the wound by its white glistening surface. It should be noted that some of its muscle fibers project from the lateral margin of the tendon. The coracobrachialis muscle is located medial to the short head of the biceps. The fascia over these muscles is opened laterally, and the coracoid process is osteotomized in an oblique manner approximately 3/8 inch from its end, but leaving the pectoralis minor tendon attached to the base. (Procedure continued on Plate 21.)

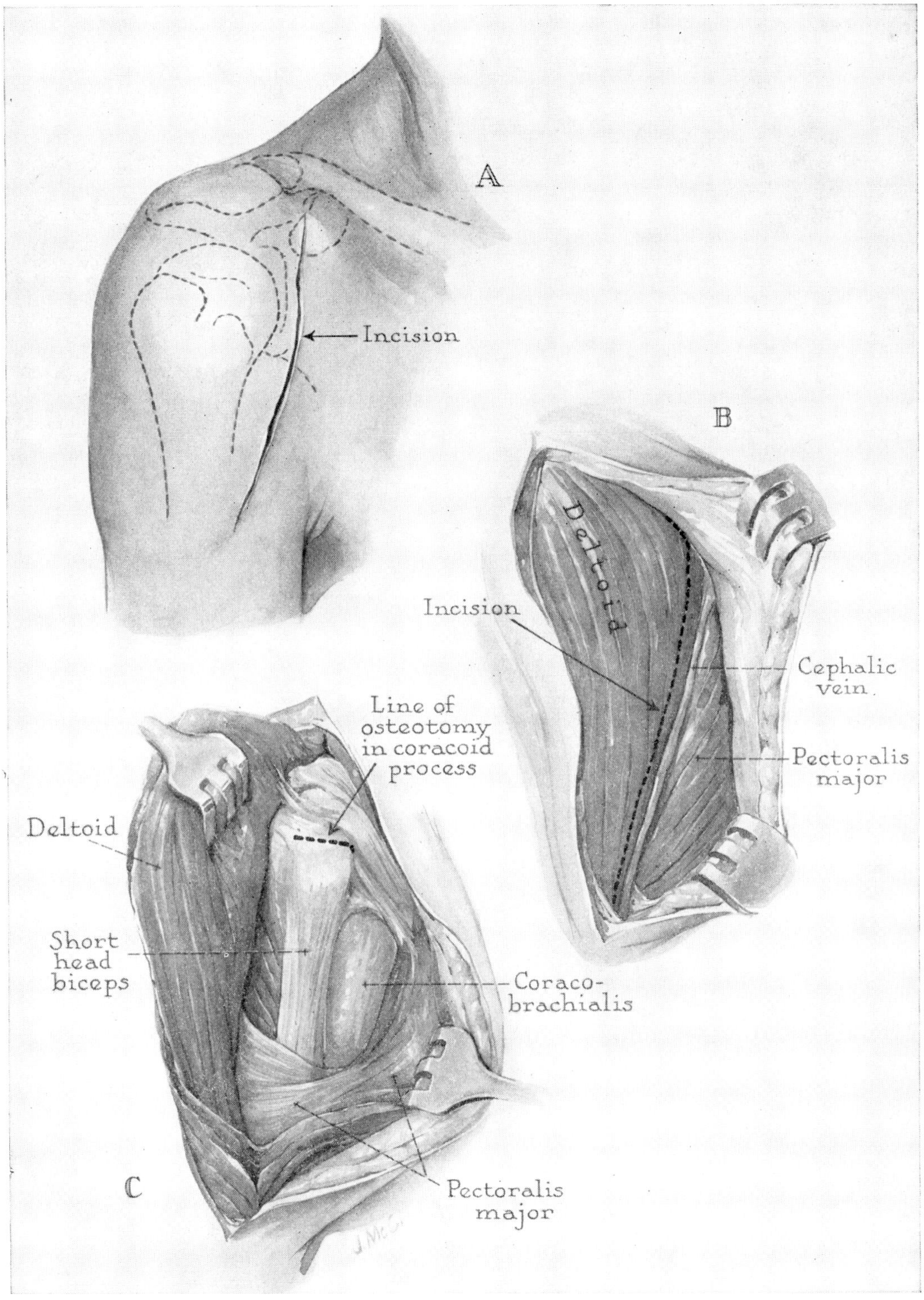

Exposure of the anterior aspect of the shoulder joint and the glenoid fossa through an anterior deltoid incision with osteotomy of the coracoid process

EXPOSURE OF THE ANTERIOR ASPECT OF THE SHOULDER JOINT AND THE GLENOID FOSSA THROUGH AN ANTERIOR DELTOID INCISION WITH OSTEOTOMY OF THE CORACOID PROCESS (*Continued*)

Plate 21: Description of Procedure

D The tip of the coracoid process and the attached short head of the biceps and coracobrachialis muscles are dissected from the surrounding loose areolar tissue and reflected downward and medially. These muscles must not be subjected to undue tension, because it may result in tearing the musculocutaneous nerve which enters the coracobrachialis muscle along its axillary margin.

E The subscapularis muscle is seen as it passes forward and outward to gain its insertion onto the lesser tubercle of the humerus. External rotation of the arm will facilitate the next step. The tendon is separated from the underlying anterior capsule of the shoulder joint with the aid of a director, and two sutures are placed at the musculotendinous junction. The scapularis muscle is transected near the lesser tubercle, over the director, and the muscle is reflected medially and forward to expose the anterior aspect of the shoulder joint. The anterior humeral circumflex artery is located directly distal to the tendon and must not be sectioned.

F The capsule of the shoulder joint is opened by a curved incision running parallel with the anterior margin of the glenoid, but at a distance approximately 3/4 inch forward to the latter. The head of the humerus is brought into view by rotating the arm externally.

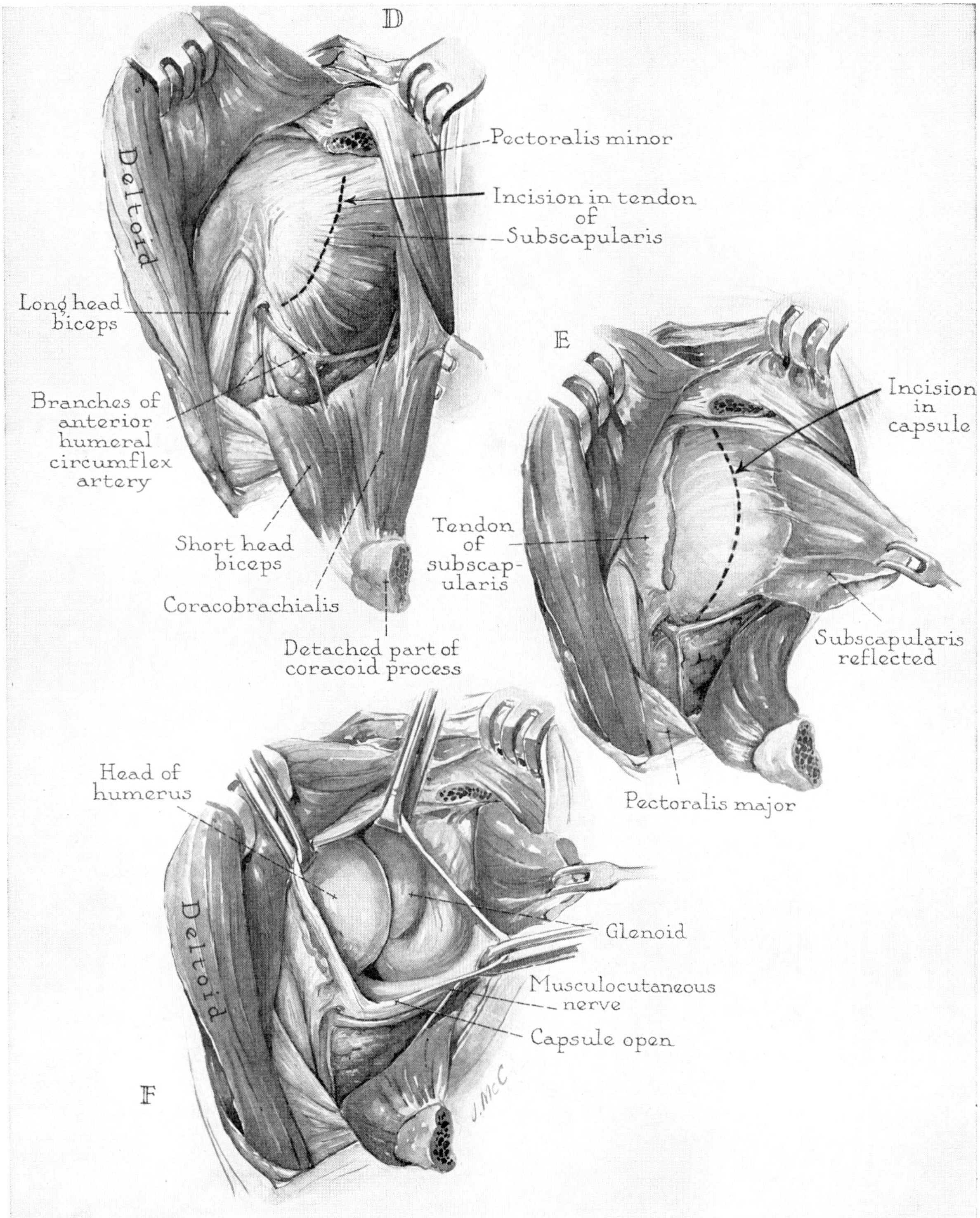

Exposure of the anterior aspect of the shoulder joint and the glenoid fossa through an anterior deltoid incision with osteotomy of the coracoid process

EXPOSURE OF THE AXILLARY SURFACE OF THE SCAPULA THROUGH AN ANTERIOR DELTOID INCISION WITH OSTEOTOMY OF THE CORACOID PROCESS

Indication: 1. Excision of Benign Tumors Which Cannot Be Exposed through an Incision over the Vertebral Margin of the Scapula

Plate 22: Description of Procedure

EXPLANATORY NOTE: Only the final illustration of this exposure is shown here; the preceding steps are shown in "Exposure of the Anterior Aspect of the Shoulder Joint and the Glenoid Fossa through an Anterior Deltoid Incision with Osteotomy of the Coracoid Process" (Illustrations A, B, C, D and E of Plates 20 and 21).

The incision begins over the coracoid process and extends in a curved manner along the anterior margin of the deltoid down to the attachment of this muscle to the humerus. The deep fascia is incised in line with the skin incision. The cephalic vein is identified in the interval between the deltoid and the pectoralis major muscles.

A linear strip of muscle approximately 1/4 inch wide is separated from the main portion of the deltoid and is retracted medially with the vein and the pectoralis major muscle as the wound is deepened. The deltoid is retracted laterally.

The short head of the biceps muscle is now identified by its white aponeurotic surface and is traced up to its attachment to the coracoid process. The coracobrachialis and the pectoralis minor muscles are medial to the short head of the biceps. The coracoid process is osteotomized, and its tip with the attached short head of the biceps and the coracobrachialis muscle are reflected downward, as illustrated.

The subscapularis muscle is now tenotomized near its insertion into the lesser tubercle of the humerus, and retracted medially. The capsule of the shoulder joint may be adherent to the subscapularis muscle and tendon, and must not be opened during the operation. The medial surface of the scapula is palpated in the floor of the wound. The subscapular fossa is exposed subperiosteally.

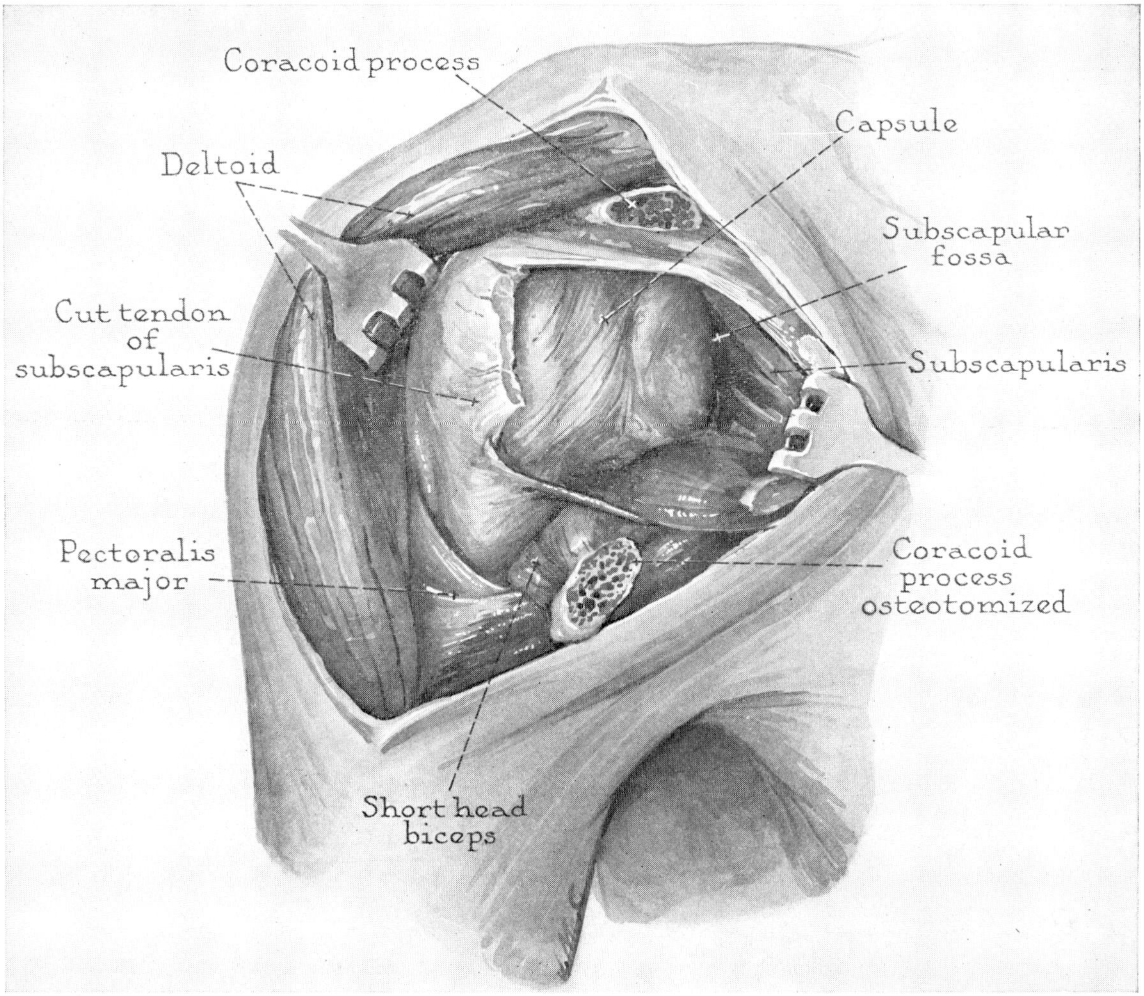

Exposure of the axillary surface of the scapula through an anterior deltoid incision with osteotomy of the coracoid process

EXPOSURE OF THE SHOULDER JOINT THROUGH A POSTERIOR DELTOID INCISION

Indications: 1. Removal of Loose Bodies in the Posterior Aspect of the Shoulder Joint

2. Repair of Recurrent Posterior Dislocations of the Shoulder

3. Resection of Pathological Lesions of the Posterior Glenoid Region of the Scapula

Plate 23: Description of Procedure

A The patient is placed on the operating table in the prone position with a sandbag beneath the shoulder. The U shaped skin incision begins at the tip of the acromion process and extends 3 inches posteriorly along the inferior margin of the spine of the scapula, and then continues distally for another 3 inches along the posterior margin of the deltoid muscle.

B The fascia is incised, and the posterior margin of the deltoid muscle is isolated. The muscle is then detached from the spine of the scapula and reflected downward and forward. The axillary nerve is not encountered, but full awareness of its location is necessary.

C The thick fascial covering of the infraspinatus and teres minor muscles can now be seen. The fascia is incised longitudinally over the interval between these muscles. (Procedure continued on Plate 24.)

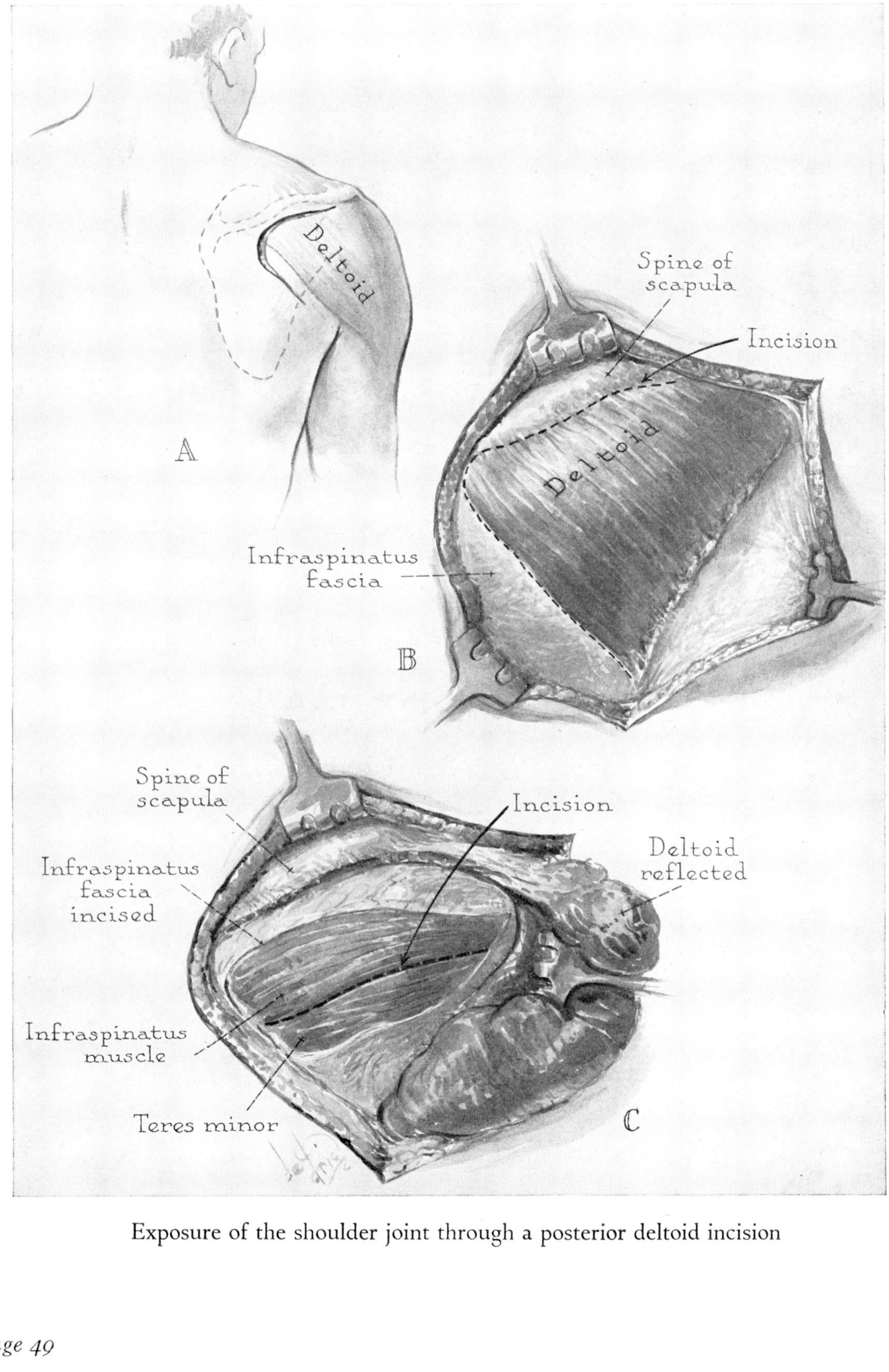

Exposure of the shoulder joint through a posterior deltoid incision

EXPOSURE OF THE SHOULDER JOINT THROUGH A POSTERIOR DELTOID INCISION *(Continued)*

Plate 24: Description of Procedure

D The infraspinatus muscle is mobilized from the scapula and capsule of the shoulder joint and retracted upward. The suprascapular nerve is located on the under surface of this muscle. It emerges from beneath the spine of the scapula and must not be injured. The teres minor muscle is pulled downward. The nerve supply of this muscle is not endangered, since it is located along the opposite or inferior margin of the muscle.

E The capsule of the shoulder joint is incised to expose the humeral head. The incision may be made parallel with the glenoid margin, as shown in the illustration, or may be T shaped.

F The posterior surface of the neck and adjacent portion of the scapula can be exposed by additional mobilization of the infraspinatus and teres minor muscles, as shown in the illustration.

NOTE: Care must be taken not to injure the suprascapular nerve as it passes around the base of the spine of the scapula to gain entrance to the infraspinatus fossa and to supply the infraspinatus muscle. The axillary nerve is protected by the teres minor muscle. A branch of this nerve enters the inferior aspect of the latter muscle before the nerve passes forward under the deltoid muscle to innervate it. The axillary nerve lies at a level distal to the dissection described in this exposure, and this nerve will not be exposed to danger if the deep exposure is kept superior to the proximal margin of the teres minor muscle.

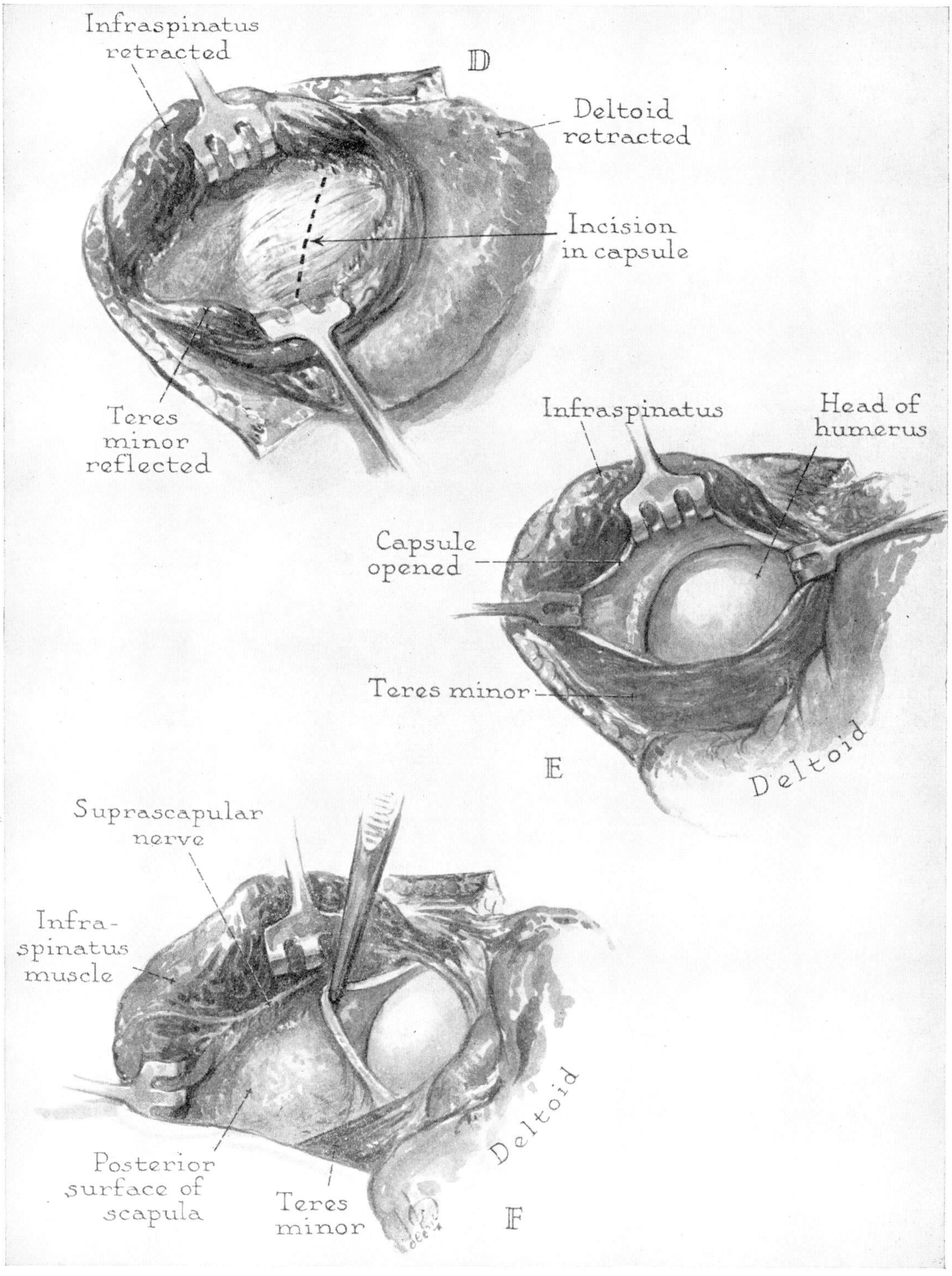

Exposure of the shoulder joint through a posterior deltoid incision

EXPOSURE OF THE SUBDELTOID BURSA AND GREATER TUBERCLE OF THE HUMERUS THROUGH A LATERAL INCISION SPLITTING THE DELTOID MUSCLE IN ITS PROXIMAL PORTION

Indications: 1. Evacuation of the Subdeltoid Bursa

2. Removal of Deposits of Calcium from the Supraspinatus Tendon and Subdeltoid Bursa

3. Open Reduction of Avulsion Fracture of the Greater Tubercle of the Humerus

4. Biopsy of Pathological Lesions of the Greater Tubercle Area of the Humerus

Plate 25: Description of Procedure

A An incision approximately 1 3/4 inches in length is made which begins at the tip of the acromion process and extends distally in a linear fashion over the deltoid muscle.

B The margins of the wound are retracted. The fascia over the deltoid muscle is incised the length of the incision, and the deltoid fibers are separated in a linear manner by careful blunt dissection to expose the underlying structures.

C The subdeltoid bursa is encountered in the depth of the wound, directly below the deltoid muscle. The distinct roof of this bursa must be incised before it can be entered. The supraspinatus tendon is brought into view by cutting through the floor of the bursa which overlies it

NOTE: This incision cannot be extended distally to any significant degree without the risk of cutting the axillary nerve which runs forward beneath the middle third of the deltoid muscle which it supplies.

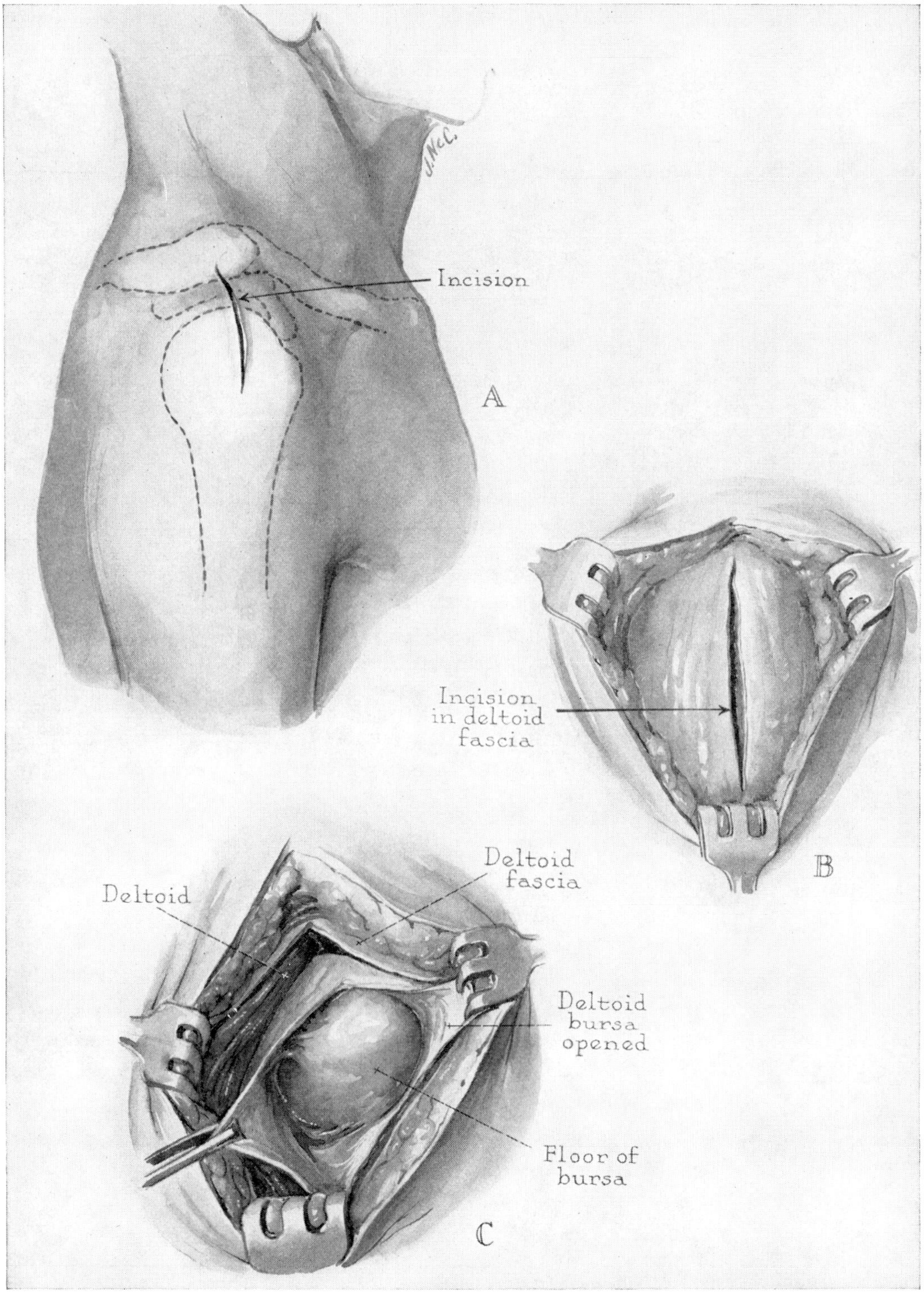

Exposure of the subdeltoid bursa and the greater tubercle of the humerus through a lateral incision splitting the deltoid muscle in its proximal portion

EXPOSURE OF THE SUBDELTOID BURSA AND SUPRASPINATUS TENDON THROUGH A TRANSVERSE SHOULDER ANTERIOR DELTOID INCISION, DETACHING THE ORIGIN OF THE DELTOID MUSCLE

Indications: 1. Repair of Ruptures of the Supraspinatus Tendon (or Musculotendinous Cuff)

2. Open Reduction of Fractures of the Greater Tubercle of the Humerus

Plate 26: Description of Procedure

A An inverted U shaped incision begins at the lateral extremity of the spine of the scapula and extends forward and around the lateral margin of the acromion and the anterior edge of the clavicle, to the deltopectoral triangle, and thence continues distally over the deltoid muscle for approximately 1 1/2 inches. The incision is crosshatched to permit accurate approximation of the skin flaps when the wound is closed.

B The deltoid fascia is cut in line with the incision and the cephalic vein is exposed in the deltopectoral groove. The vein is mobilized together with the most mesial fibers of the deltoid muscle, and both are retracted toward the midline with the pectoralis major muscle. The origin of the deltoid muscle is separated from the clavicle and the acromion and also from the exposed portion of the spine of the scapula, and then is retracted downward and outward.

C The subdeltoid bursa, the coraco-acromial ligament and the coracoid process, with the attachments of the short head of the biceps and the coracobrachialis and pectoralis minor muscles, can be seen in the wound. An incision is made in the roof and the floor of the subdeltoid bursa to expose the greater tubercle and the common tendinous attachment of the supraspinatus, the infraspinatus and the teres minor muscles. The hemostat which is shown in the illustration beneath the supraspinatus tendon is lifting the tendon forward after having made an opening in the musculotendinous cuff with its pointed end. Although this particular step in the procedure would be unnecessary for the repair of a rupture of the cuff or the removal of calcium deposits, it has been included in the illustration to emphasize the course and location of the supraspinatus tendon beneath the acromion process. Ample additional space for the suture of ruptures can be obtained by removal of the acromion process and the sectioning of the coraco-acromial ligament, the latter being left unsutured.

NOTE: Adequate exposure is afforded for performing the above procedures without extending the wound distally in the deltopectoral interval, at least for the experienced surgeon. Only very little additional operating time will be required to make the incision which is illustrated. The less experienced operator would find the extra working space particularly advantageous, especially in muscular patients with tendon ruptures.

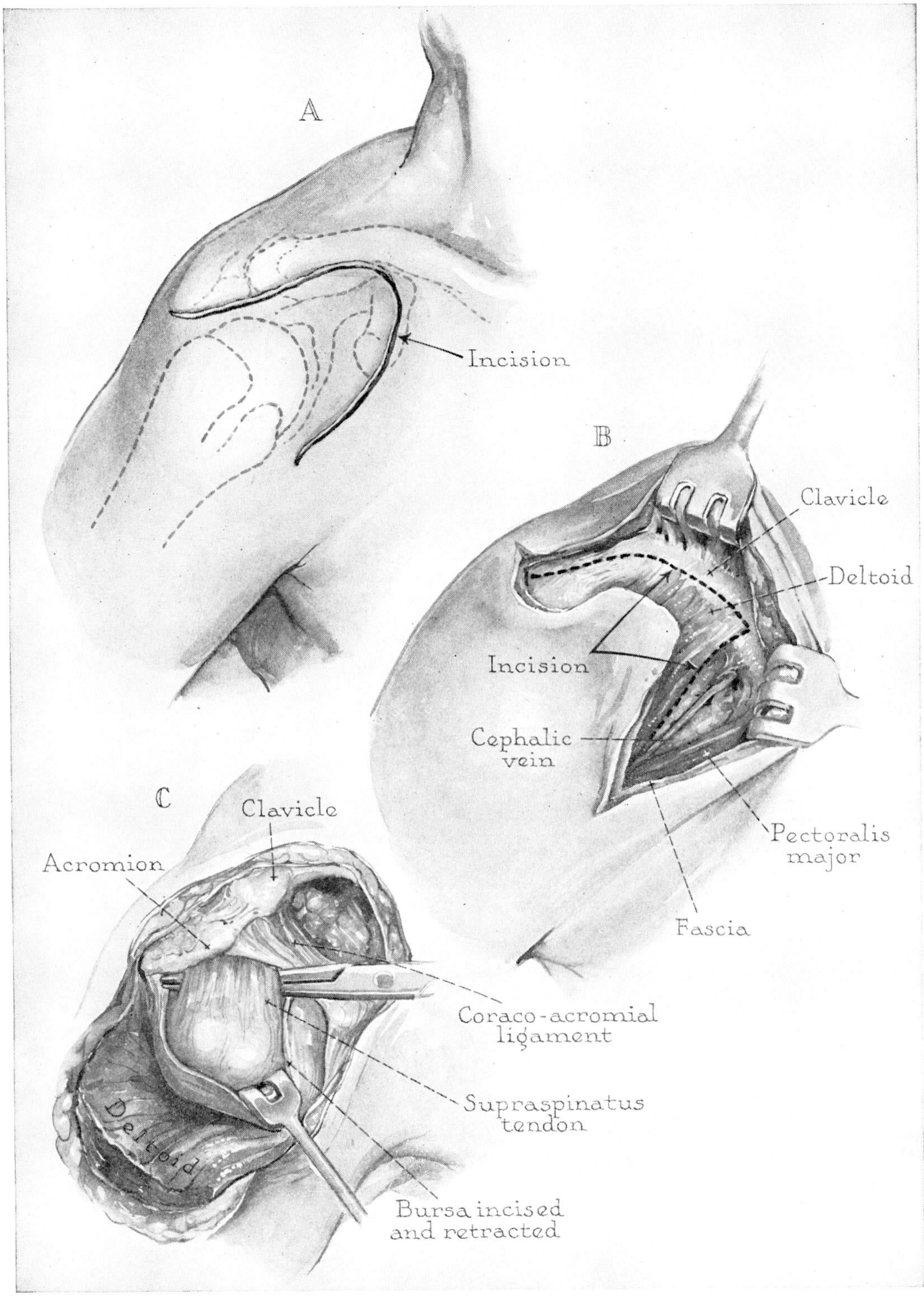

Exposure of the subdeltoid bursa and the supraspinatus tendon through a transverse shoulder anterior deltoid incision, detaching the origin of the deltoid muscle

EXPOSURE OF THE FIRST PORTION OF THE AXILLARY ARTERY

Indications: 1. Sling Control for Surgery of the Axillary Artery

2. Access to Arteriovenous Aneurysms Following Trauma

Plate 27: Description of Procedure

A The skin incision is made one inch below the clavicle from the coracoid process to about an inch lateral to the sternoclavicular joint. The length of the incision may be shorter in thin individuals.

B The anterior thoracic nerves span the operative field in a more or less vertical direction as the superficial fascia is cut and retracted and the fibers of the pectoralis major muscle are separated. Laterally, a portion of the deltoid muscle will be seen in well developed individuals. The brachial plexus runs diagonally downward in the upper lateral portion of the wound and can be seen through a thin fascia over it. In some instances the upper border of the pectoralis minor may be retracted downward with the lower lateral portion of the pectoralis major for additional exposure.

C The thoraco-acromial is isolated in the lateral third of the wound and is clamped and ligated if the vessel cannot be retracted laterally out of the way.

D Gentle dissection will reveal the axillary vein. The cephalic vein joins it at about the middle ot the wound from a lateral direction. At this point the axillary vein dips inferiorly. If the axillary vein cannot be retracted downward with ease, it can be cut and doubly ligated. The axillary artery lies superior to and slightly deeper than the axillary vein. A sling can now be placed on the artery at this point. If the pectoralis minor muscle has a high attachment, better vision can be obtained by cutting through its tendinous attachment. The brachial plexus lies in close approximation to the axillary artery in the lateral portions of the wound. Therefore, it is preferable to isolate the artery as far medially as possible.

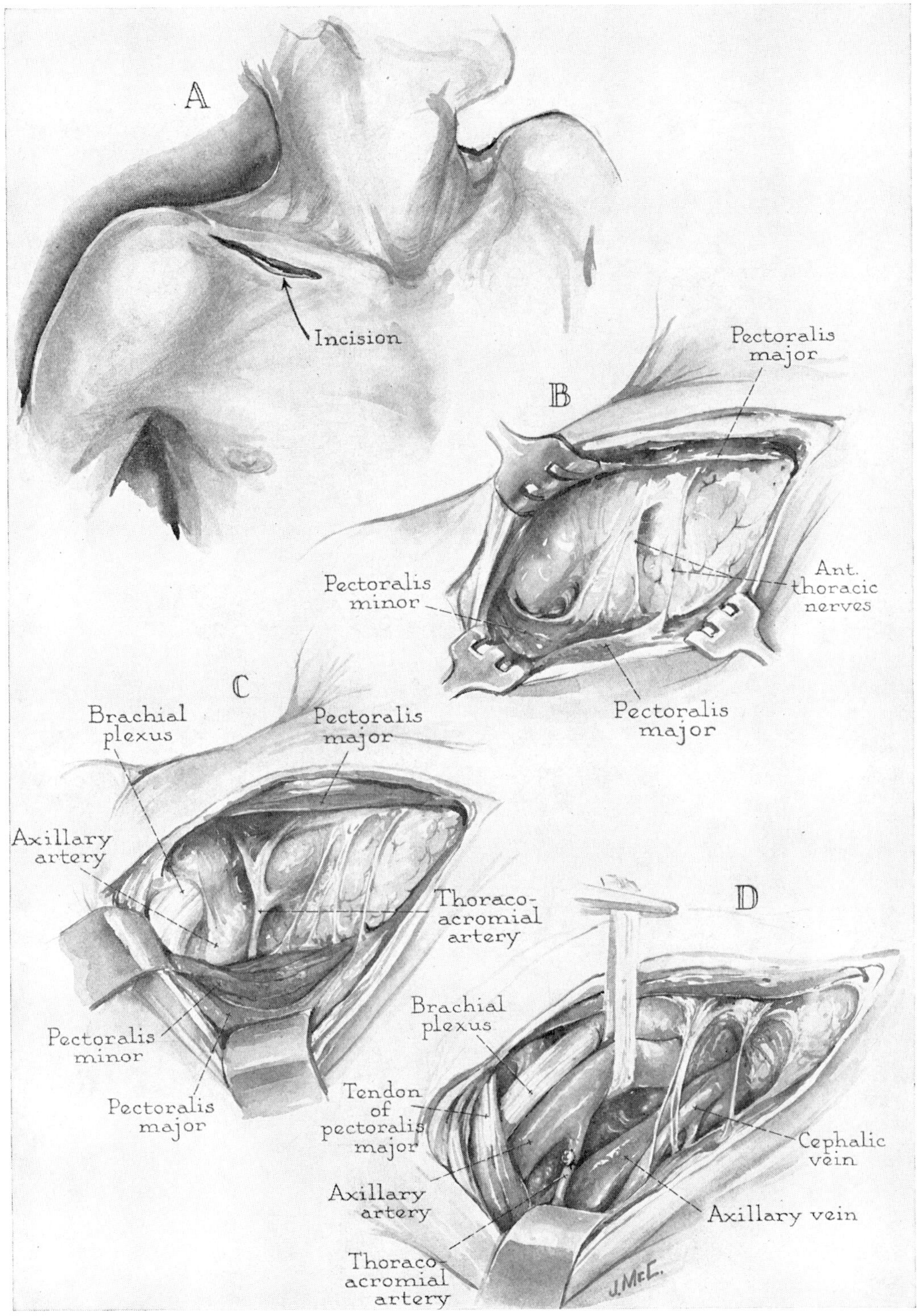

Exposure of the first portion of the axillary artery

EXPOSURE OF THE BRACHIAL ARTERY IN THE PROXIMAL PORTION OF THE ARM THROUGH A MEDIAL INCISION

Indication: 1. Sling Control for Surgery of the Brachial Artery in the Arm

Plate 28: Description of Procedure

A The arm is extended at right angles to the trunk of the body; the palm of the hand is turned upward. The skin incision begins at the lower margin of the pectoralis major muscle, and extends along the inner border of the coracobrachialis muscle on the line which joins the midpoint of the clavicle with the tendon of the biceps muscle at the elbow. It may be extended in either direction if desired.

B The deep fascia is incised and opened along the line of the incision to uncover the coracobrachialis muscle. This muscle then is retracted sufficiently to expose the musculocutaneous nerve which enters it medially. The axillary artery is hugged closely by the median nerve above, and by the ulnar nerve below. The axillary vein courses in the lower portion of the wound; it is considerably more superficial than is the artery with its accompanying nerves.

C Gentle dissection of the nerves away from the axillary artery will permit a sling to be placed upon it. On the other hand, the sling on the brachial vein shown in the illustration need not be used unless it will facilitate access to the artery.

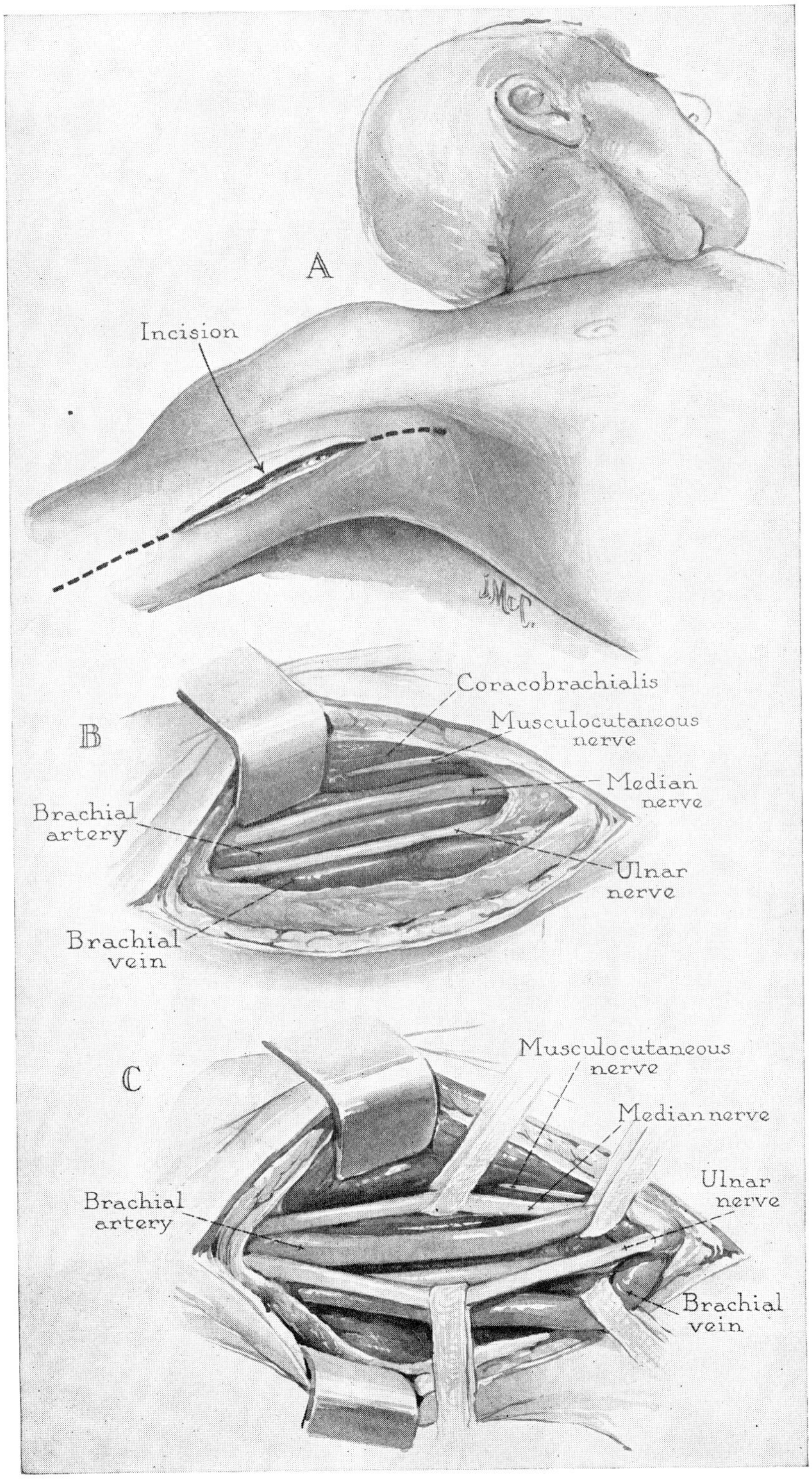

Exposure of the brachial artery in the proximal portion of the arm through a medial incision

Section III

Region of the Shaft of the Humerus

EXPOSURE OF THE PROXIMAL FOURTH OF THE SHAFT OF THE HUMERUS, INCLUDING THE SHOULDER JOINT, THROUGH AN ANTERIOR INCISION, REFLECTING THE DELTOID MUSCLE FROM THE CLAVICLE

Indications: 1. Open Reduction of Recent Fractures

2. Treatment of Non-union of Fractures

3. Resection of Benign and Malignant Tumors

Plate 29: Description of Procedure

A An incision is made directly posterior to the acromion process and extended forward along the free margin of this process and of the clavicle up to the deltopectoral triangle from where it is directed distally in the groove between the pectoralis major and deltoid muscles, for the desired distance.

B The deep fascia is then opened in the line of the incision and the cephalic vein is isolated in the depression between the deltoid and pectoralis major muscles. In order to protect this vein, a 1/4 inch longitudinal strip of deltoid muscle is left attached to the pectoralis major when these two muscles are separated. The deltoid muscle is next detached from the clavicle and the acromion process to permit its reflection laterally and posteriorly. The axillary nerve can then be seen on the undersurface of the midportion of the deltoid muscle as it emerges from behind the proximal end of the humerus. The long and short heads of the biceps as well as the coracoid process should be identified.

C The humerus is rotated inward to bring the anterior and lateral surfaces of the shaft and greater tubercle into the wound. There are no deep structures covering this portion of the shaft. A periosteal incision is made to expose the bone beneath. The shoulder joint may be opened through an incision either anterior or posterior to the intracapsular portion of the tendon of the long head of the biceps. The anterior incision offers greater exposure.

The greater portion of the articular surface of the head of the humerus can be exposed by an incision in the anterior capsule, after the sectioning of the coracoid process and of the subscapularis tendon. The anterior circumflex humeral artery is contacted at the junction of the shaft and the head of the humerus, and may be ligated to obtain a subperiosteal exposure of the bone.

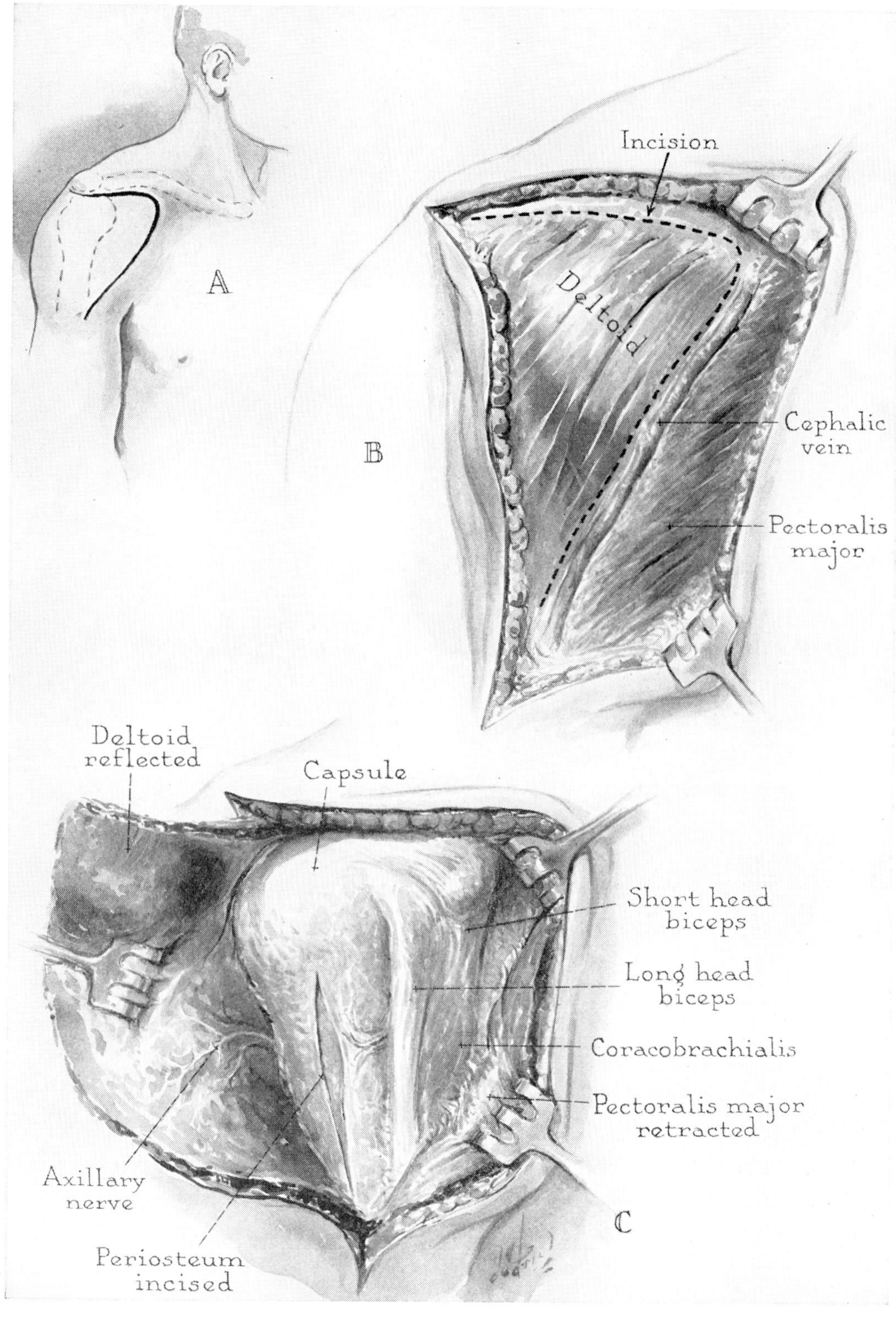

Exposure of the proximal fourth of the shaft of the humerus, including the shoulder joint, through an anterior incision, reflecting the deltoid muscle from the clavicle

EXPOSURE OF THE PROXIMAL THIRD OF THE ANTERIOR AND LATERAL SURFACES OF THE HUMERUS THROUGH AN ANTERIOR DELTOID INCISION

Indications: 1. Open Reduction of Recent Fractures

2. Treatment of Non-union of Fractures of the Humerus

3. Partial Ostectomy for Osteomyelitis

4. Resection of Benign and Malignant Tumors

Plate 30: Description of Procedure

A The skin incision begins at the lower margin of the clavicle near the coracoid process, and extends downward over the anterior margin of the deltoid muscle for a distance of 5 inches.

B The fascia is opened along the line of the incision, and the cephalic vein is isolated and retracted to one side of the wound, preferably toward the inside. If the tributaries from the deltoid muscle are large and numerous, it is better to separate a strip of this muscle approximately 1/4 inch wide and to retract it medially with the vein and the pectoralis major muscle. This strip must be kept narrow because it is deprived of its nerve supply and subject to atrophy.

C The deltoid muscle is firmly retracted to the lateral side to bring into view the distal portion of the broad tendon of the pectoralis major muscle near its insertion into the humerus. The deltoid branches of the thoraco-acromial artery cross the field just above the superior margin of the pectoralis major tendon and must be ligated. The short head of the biceps may be identified proximally by its shiny surface. It should be noted that its muscle fibers extend laterally between the tendon and the humerus.

D The arm is rotated inward, and the location of the tendon of the long head of the biceps is determined by palpating it along the proximal anterior surface of the humerus. At the lower end of the wound this tendon is no longer visible because it is beneath the pectoralis major tendon.

The humerus then is exposed by incising the periosteum on its anterior surface along the dotted line shown in the illustration. This incision is lateral to the long head of the biceps muscle above, and the insertion of the pectoralis major muscle below. The anterior circumflex artery is encountered in its course around the humerus just distal to the neck, and may be ligated if necessary.

NOTE: The axillary nerve is located on the undersurface of the deltoid muscle and must not be injured by retractors.

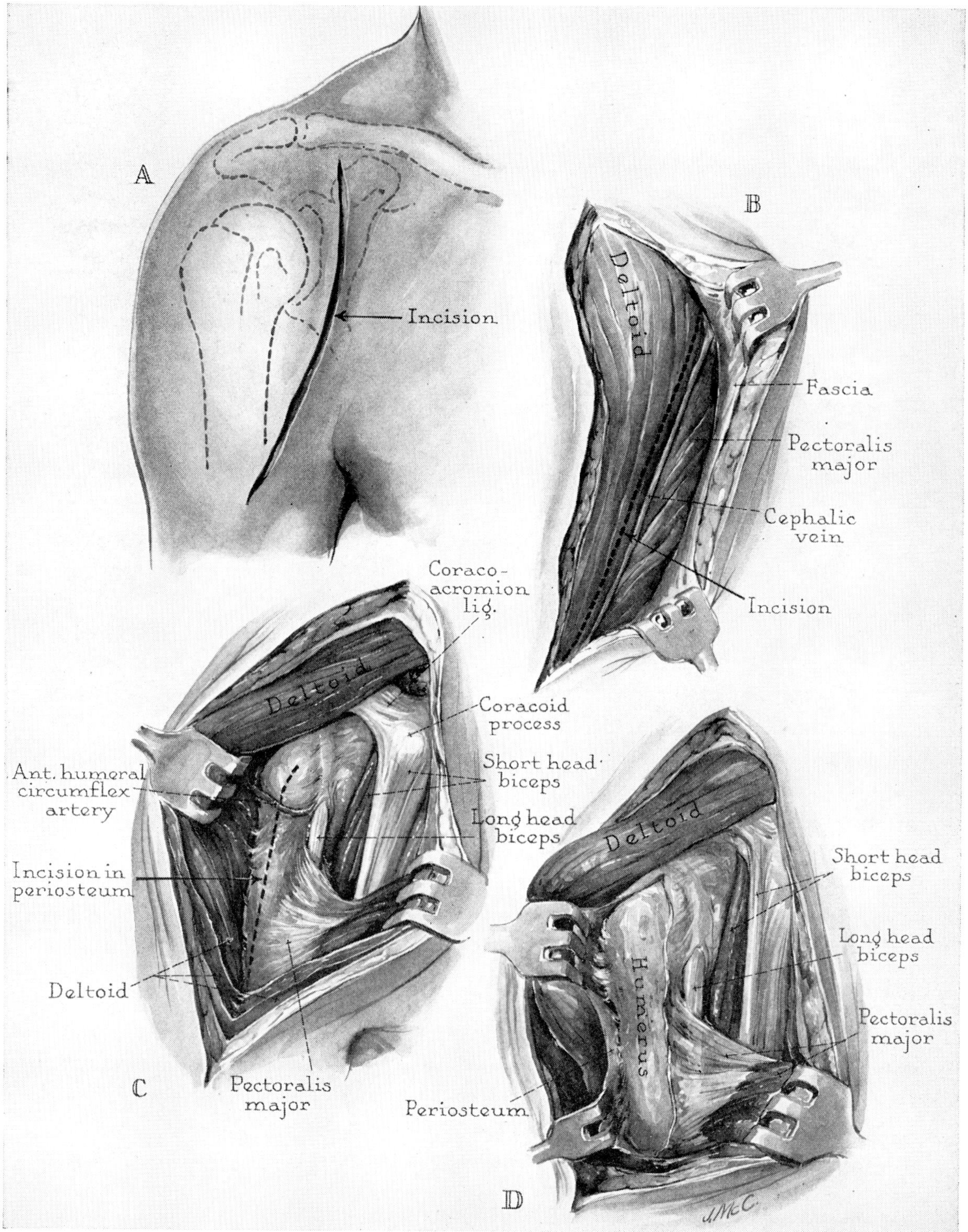

Exposure of the proximal third of the anterior and lateral surfaces of the humerus through an anterior deltoid incision

EXPOSURE OF MIDDLE AND PROXIMAL THIRDS OF THE HUMERUS THROUGH AN ANTERIOR DELTOID-LATERAL BICEPS INCISION

Indications: 1. Open Reduction of Acute Fractures of the Humerus

2. Treatment of Un-united Fractures of the Humerus

3. Excision of Benign Tumors

4. Local Resection of Malignant Tumors

5. Treatment of Osteomyelitis

Plate 31: Description of Procedure

A The incision begins about 2 inches below the clavicle and extends distally and laterally along the medial margin of the deltoid muscle as far as its insertion on the humerus, from whence it curves distally along the lateral aspect of the arm in the interval between the triceps and brachialis muscles.

B The deep fascia is incised throughout the length of the incision. The cephalic vein is isolated in the proximal third of the wound and retracted toward the midline together with the pectoralis major muscle and tendon. The wound is enlarged by sharp dissection between the pectoralis major and deltoid muscle, which is retracted outward. Distally to the insertion of the deltoid muscle the interval is developed between the brachialis muscle and the lateral head of the triceps, where the dissection is carried down to the humerus. The periosteum then is incised throughout the length of the incision, including the few fibers of the brachialis muscle which are located proximally and laterally to the deltoid insertion. Biceps and brachialis muscles are located medially in the lower half of the wound.

C The humerus is exposed subperiosteally. The insertions of the deltoid and pectoralis major tendons may be separated from the humerus if exposure of the whole circumference of the latter is desired. Care must be taken not to injure the radial nerve, which here extends downward in a lateral curve behind the bone. This danger can be forestalled by wholly subperiosteal dissection. When the wound is next extended to the junction of the middle and distal thirds of the humerus, identification of the radial nerve must be made as it emerges in the interval between the brachialis and brachioradialis muscles. A linear and lateral strip of the brachialis muscle can be left in place to protect the radial nerve while the main portion of the latter muscle is retracted medially.

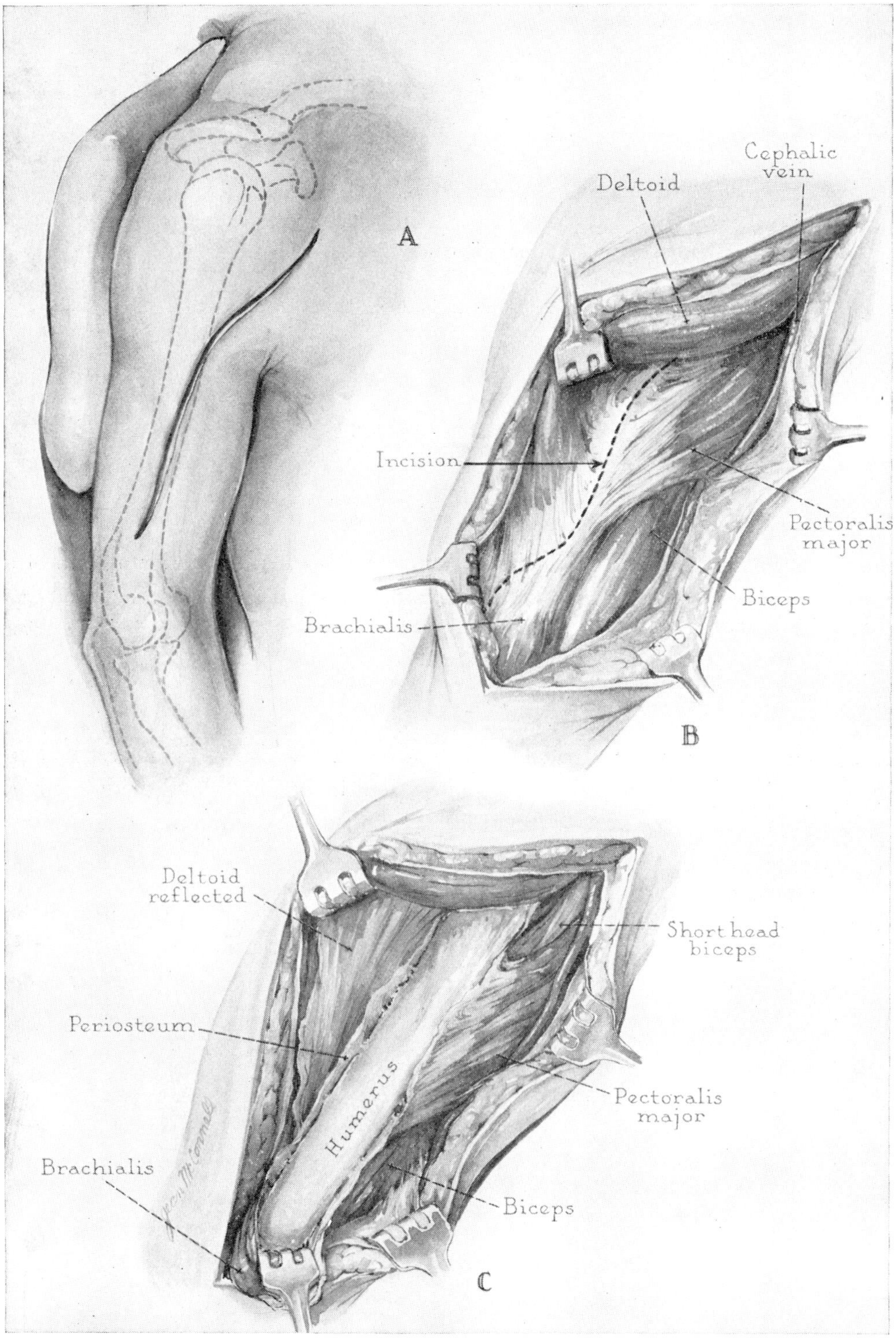

Exposure of the middle and proximal thirds of the humerus through an anterior deltoid-lateral biceps incision

EXPOSURE OF THE MIDDLE THIRD OF THE HUMERUS THROUGH A LATERAL INCISION

Indications: 1. Open Reduction of Recent Fractures

2. Application of Bone Grafts for Non-union of Fractures

3. Partial Ostectomy for Chronic Osteomyelitis

4. Resection of Benign and Malignant Tumors

Plate 32: Description of Procedure

A An incision approximately 6 1/2 inches in length begins at the anterior margin of the distal 2 inches of the deltoid muscle and curves downward and parallel with the lateral margin of the brachialis muscle, terminating over the interval between the brachialis and brachioradialis muscles.

B The deep fascia is incised and the flaps are undermined. The radial nerve then is isolated at the lower end of the wound in the groove between the brachialis and the brachioradialis muscles. A hernia tape placed around the nerve will permit its positioning so as to prevent injury.

C The lateral margin of the brachialis muscle is th n mobilized so that it and the overlying biceps muscle can be retracted medially, as a preliminary step to the subperiosteal exposure of the humerus. The back of the humerus is exposed by raising the triceps muscles subperiosteally.

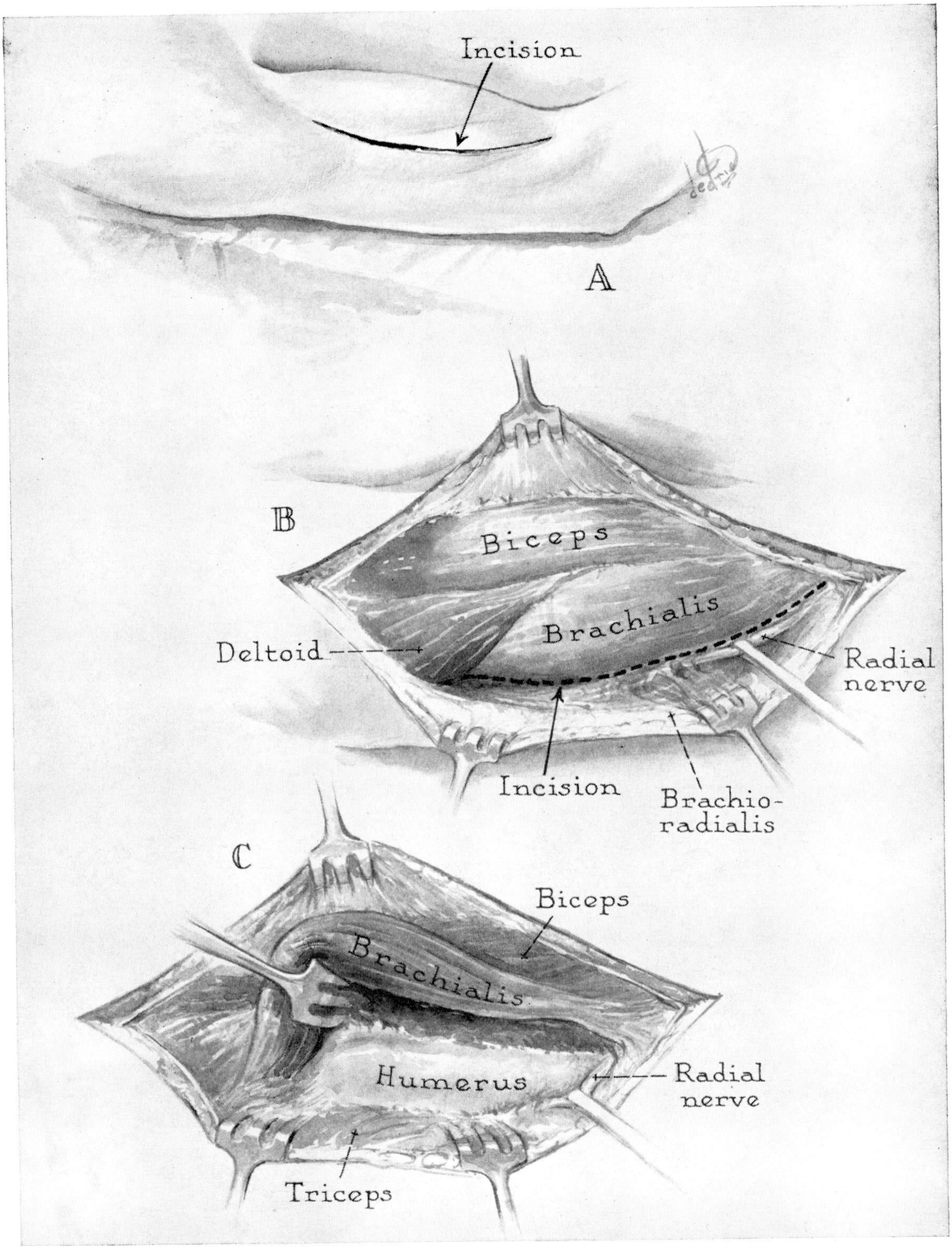

Exposure of the middle third of the humerus through a lateral incision

EXPOSURE OF THE JUNCTION OF THE MIDDLE AND DISTAL THIRDS OF THE SHAFT OF THE HUMERUS THROUGH AN ANTERO-LATERAL INCISION

Indications: 1. Open Reduction of Recent Fractures of the Humerus

2. Treatment of Non-union of Fractures of the Humerus

3. Resection of Benign and Malignant Tumors

4. Partial Ostectomy for Osteomyelitis

Plate 33: Description of Procedure

A The skin incision, approximately 4 inches long, begins just proximal to the flexion crease of the elbow over the groove between the biceps and brachioradialis muscle; it then curves laterally upward between these two muscles and terminates at the required distance.

B The deep fascia is incised and the interval between the brachioradialis and biceps distally, and the brachioradialis and brachialis proximally, is developed so as to separate these muscles. The biceps and brachialis muscles are retracted toward the midline, and the brachioradialis is reflected laterally.

C The radial nerve, in its course from above downward, is located deep in the wound along the lateral and anterior aspects of the humerus. Branches of the nerve pass into the brachioradialis muscle. The nerve can either be left undisturbed, or be mobilized and retracted laterally out of the wound as an additional safeguard from injury.

D The lateral margin of the brachialis muscle is separated from the radial nerve and retracted medially to uncover the underlying bone. The periosteum is incised near the margin of the brachialis muscle and the humerus is exposed subperiosteally for the desired distance. The wound may be extended proximally along the shaft of the humerus, or distally into the elbow joint.

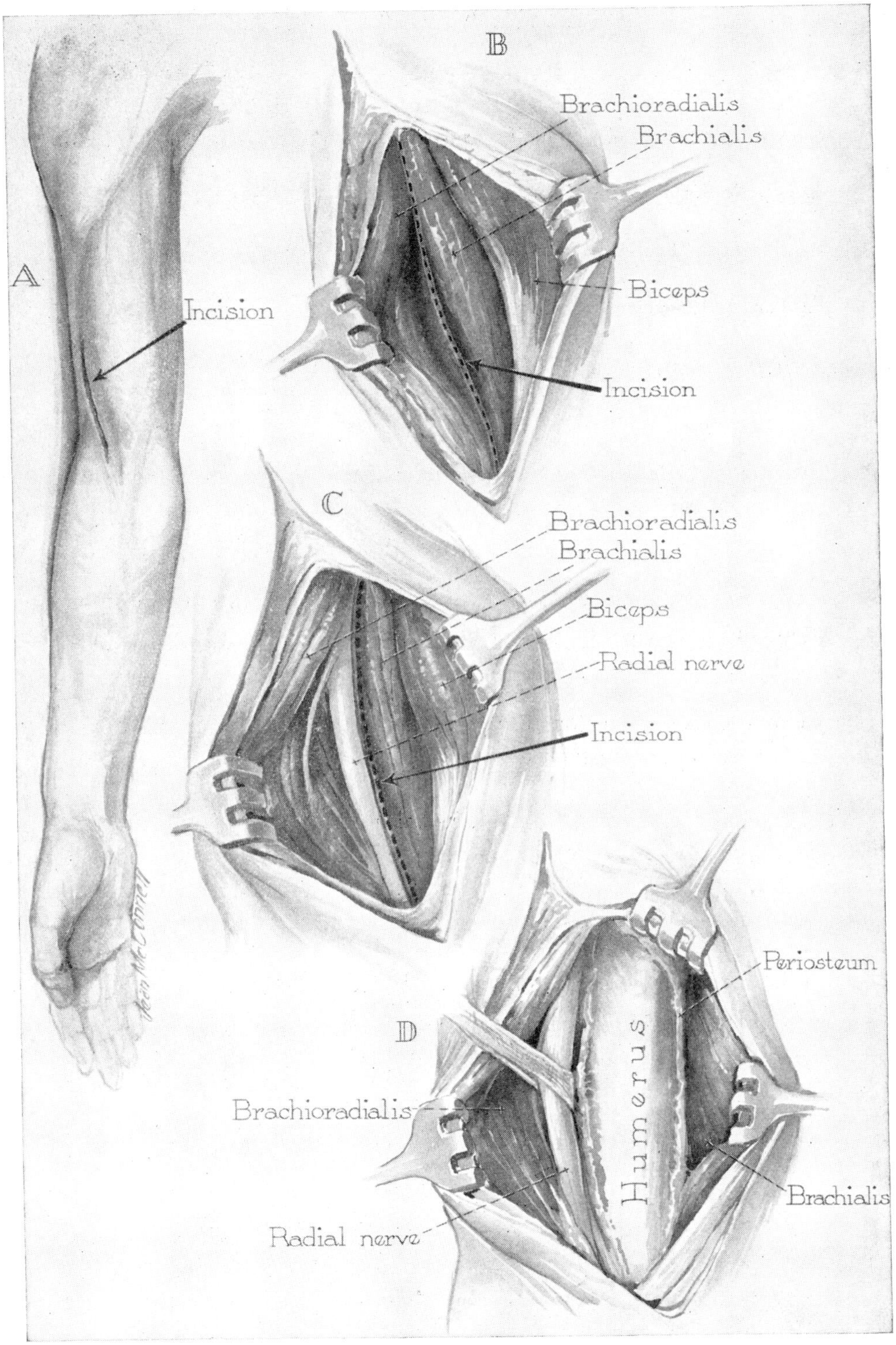

Exposure of the junction of the middle and distal thirds of the shaft of the humerus through an anterolateral incision

EXPOSURE OF THE DISTAL FOUR INCHES OF THE SHAFT OF THE HUMERUS THROUGH A LATERAL EPICONDYLAR INCISION

Indications: 1. Open Reduction of Certain Types of Recent Fractures

2. Applications of Bone Graft for Un-united Fractures

3. Excision of Benign Tumors

4. Partial Ostectomy for Osteomyelitis

Plate 34: Description of Procedure

A The skin incision is made starting from the lateral epicondyle of the humerus and extending upward in a straight line for 4 inches.

B The skin is retracted and the deep fascia is opened along the entire incision. The lateral margin of the brachioradialis muscle is lifted off the bone.

C The periosteum then is incised along the epicondylar ridge and the side of the humerus, thereby exposing the latter subperiosteally.

The radial nerve, after emerging from the radial groove posteriorly, passes distally along the lateral aspect of the humerus before it reaches the sulcus between the proximal portion of the brachioradialis muscle laterally, and the lateral fibers of the brachialis medially. This nerve must not be injured when reflecting the muscles forward and medially.

The deep head of the triceps muscle is next reflected from the humerus and retracted posteriorly. It is necessary to denude the medial surface of the humerus subperiosteally, because it eliminates the danger of damaging the ulnar nerve.

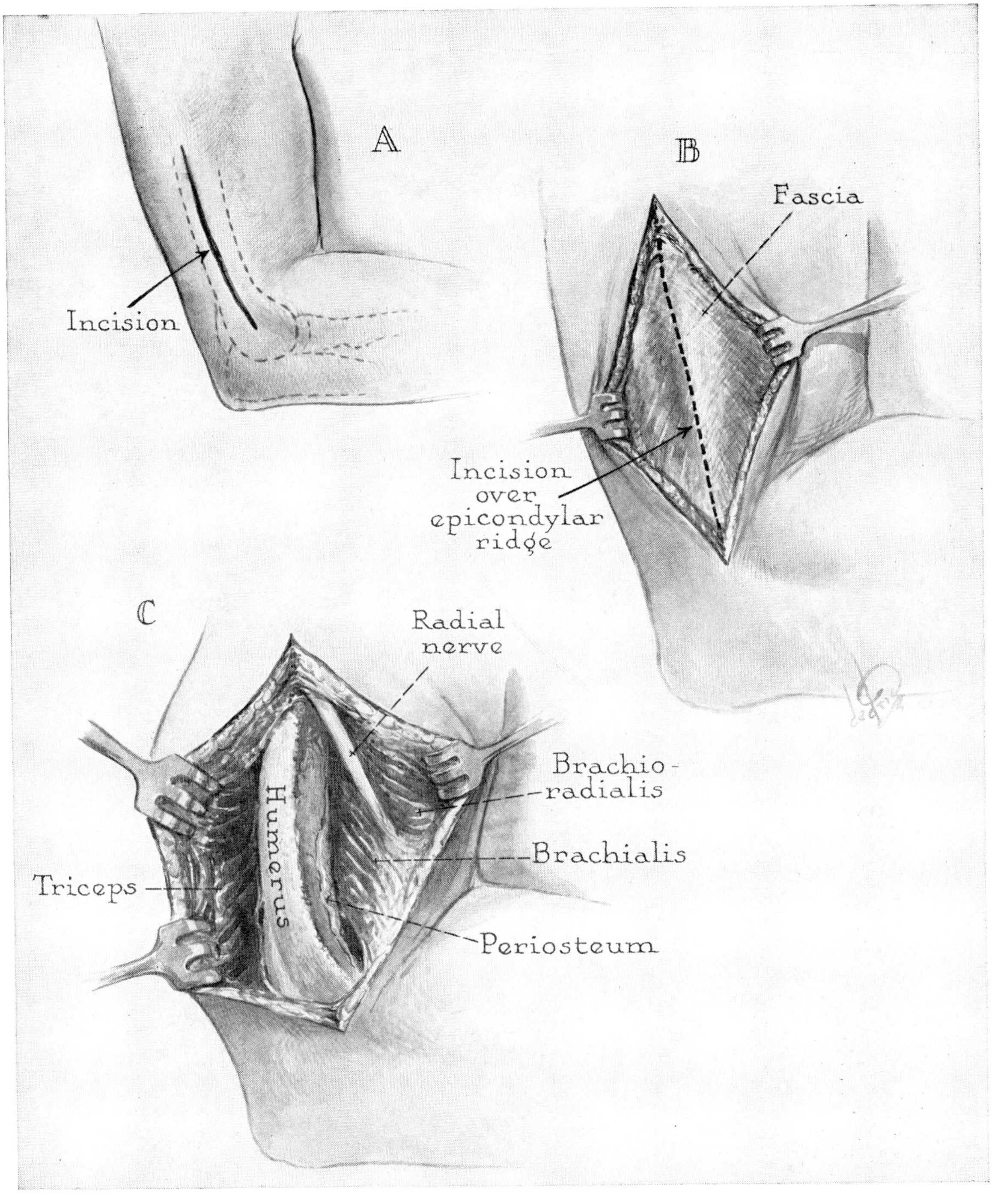

Exposure of the distal four inches of the shaft of the humerus through a lateral epicondylar incision

EXPOSURE OF THE SUPRACONDYLAR REGION OF THE HUMERUS THROUGH A LATERAL EPICONDYLAR INCISION

Indications: 1. Supracondylar Osteotomy of the Humerus

2. Partial Ostectomy for Osteomyelitis

3. Removal of Benign Tumors

Plate 35: Description of Procedure

A The skin incision, about 2 inches long, starts over the lateral epicondyle of the humerus and extends upward in line with the epicondylar ridge.

B The fascia is opened and the flaps are undermined. An incision then is made down to the epicondylar ridge of the humerus, by cutting through the fibers of attachment of the brachioradialis muscle anteriorly, and of the triceps muscle posteriorly.

C The subjacent portion of the humerus is exposed subperiosteally. The brachioradialis at its origin and the distal portion of the brachialis are lifted from the bone anteriorly, while the extensor muscles at their common origin together with the deep head of the triceps are similarly raised posteriorly. Great care must be exercised in lifting the soft tissues from the medial surface of the humerus, and can best be accomplished by inserting a curved elevator subperiosteally from the lateral side of the wound. The ulnar nerve as well as the brachial artery and the median nerve will not be injured in performing a supracondylar osteotomy, if curved periosteal elevators are placed along the front and back of the humerus in such a way that they overlap at the medial surface of the bone.

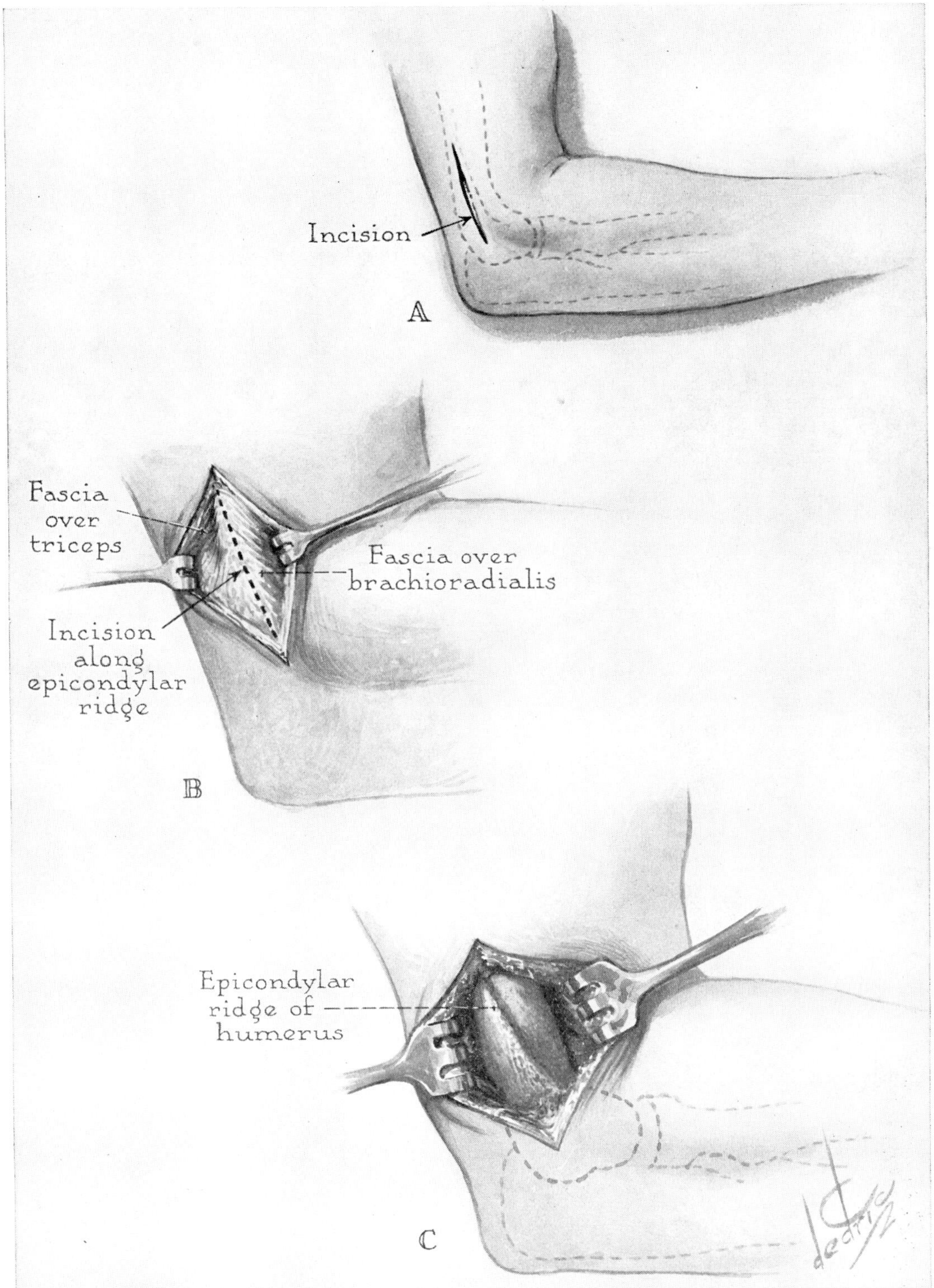

Exposure of the supracondylar region of the humerus through a lateral epicondylar incision

EXPOSURE OF THE MIDDLE TWO-THIRDS OF THE POSTERIOR SURFACE OF THE HUMERUS THROUGH A MIDLINE TRANS-TRICEPS INCISION

Indications: 1. Excision of Benign Tumors Which Cannot Be Removed by a Lateral or a Posterior Medial Incision

2. Local Resection of Malignant Tumors Which Are Best Approached Posteriorly

Plate 36: Description of Procedure

A The skin incision begins at the olecranon fossa and extends proximally in the midline of the arm until it reaches the posterior margin of the deltoid muscle.

B The deep fascia is then incised along the entire distance of the wound. The interval is found by palpating the space between the long and the lateral heads of the triceps muscle. These heads are next separated by an incision which at the same time splits the tendon longitudinally down to the end of the wound. (Procedure continued on Plate 37.)

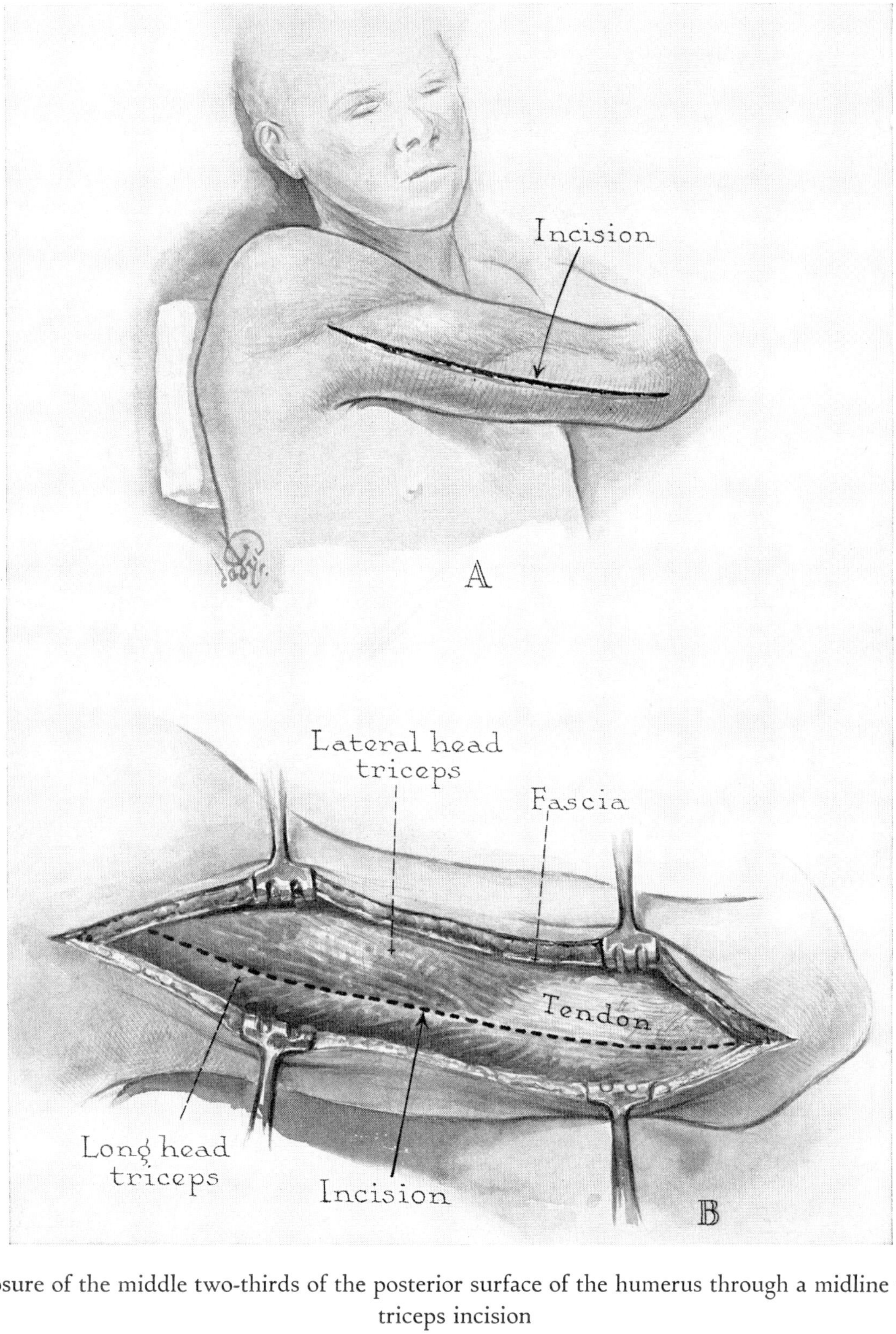

Exposure of the middle two-thirds of the posterior surface of the humerus through a midline trans-triceps incision

EXPOSURE OF THE MIDDLE TWO-THIRDS OF THE POSTERIOR SURFACE OF THE HUMERUS THROUGH A MIDLINE TRANS-TRICEPS INCISION *(Continued)*

Plate 37: Description of Procedure

C The loose areolar tissue below the long and lateral heads of the triceps is separated by blunt dissection to expose the radial nerve and the profunda brachial artery. Both nerve and artery course obliquely downward across the upper third of the field, from the medial corner, and disappear laterally beneath the lateral head of the triceps. The deep (medial) head of the triceps occupies the floor of the wound.

D Access to the bone is afforded by splitting the deep head longitudinally down to the humerus, and exposing the latter subperiosteally. This incision will not damage the nerve supply of the triceps. The ulnar nerve, it may be noted, lies beneath the long head of the triceps muscle and need not be disturbed.

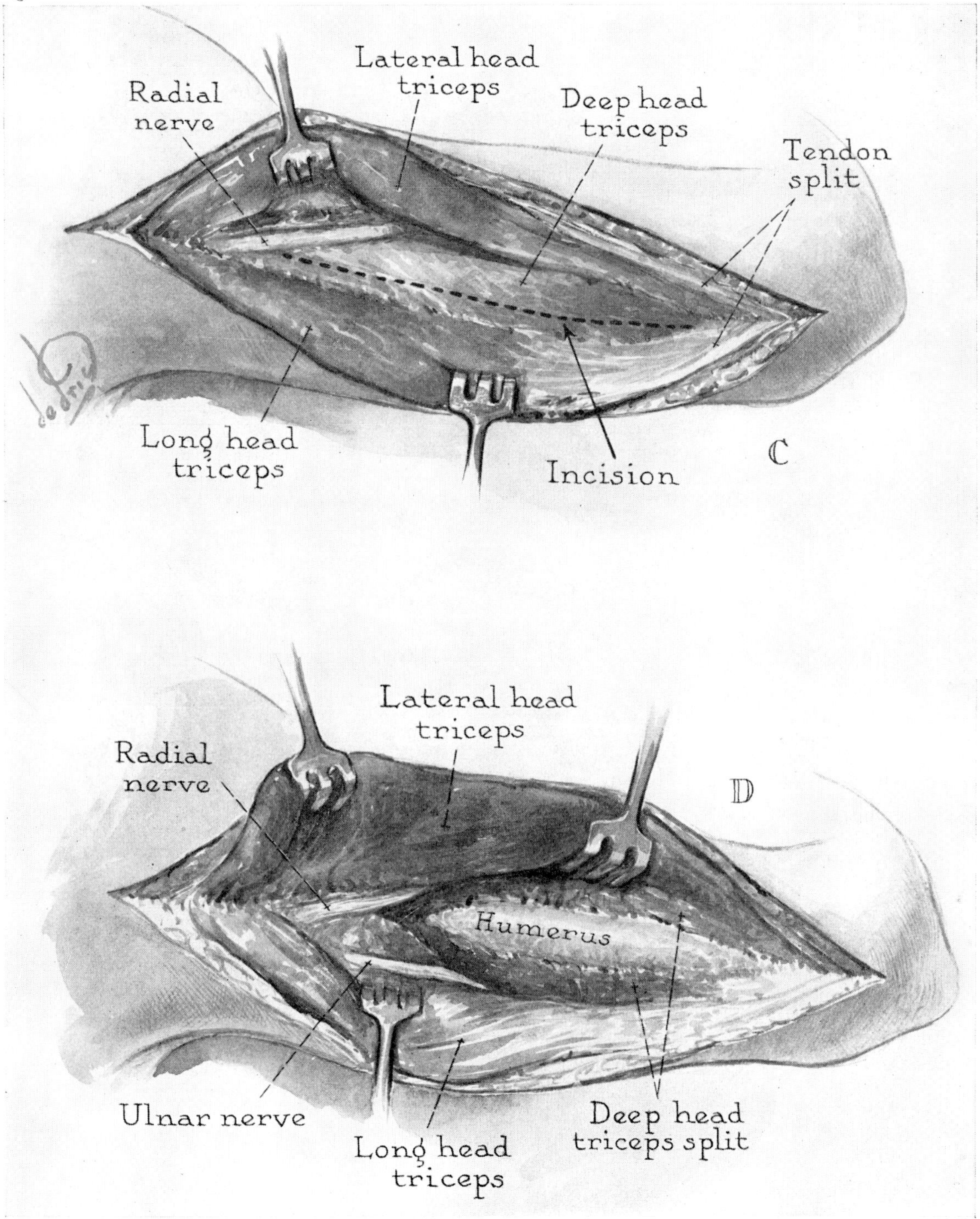

Exposure of the middle two-thirds of the posterior surface of the humerus through a midline trans-triceps incision

EXPOSURE OF THE DISTAL THIRD OF THE POSTERIOR SURFACE OF THE HUMERUS THROUGH A LONGITUDINAL INCISION WITH TENOTOMY OF THE TRICEPS TENDON

Indication: 1. Open Reduction of Comminuted Fractures Involving the Distal End of the Humerus

Plate 38: Description of Procedure

A For this operation the patient's arm is placed across the chest, with the elbow in flexion. The skin incision begins at the tip of the olecranon process and extends upward along the midline for approximately 5 1/2 inches.

B The skin flaps are undermined and the fascia is opened to expose the entire tendon of the triceps muscle.

C The ulnar nerve is isolated directly above the ulnar groove, and then is dissected upward and retracted posteriorly and downward to protect it from injury. The lateral margin of the triceps tendon is separated from the posterior aspect of the lateral intermuscular septum. (Procedure continued on Plate 39.)

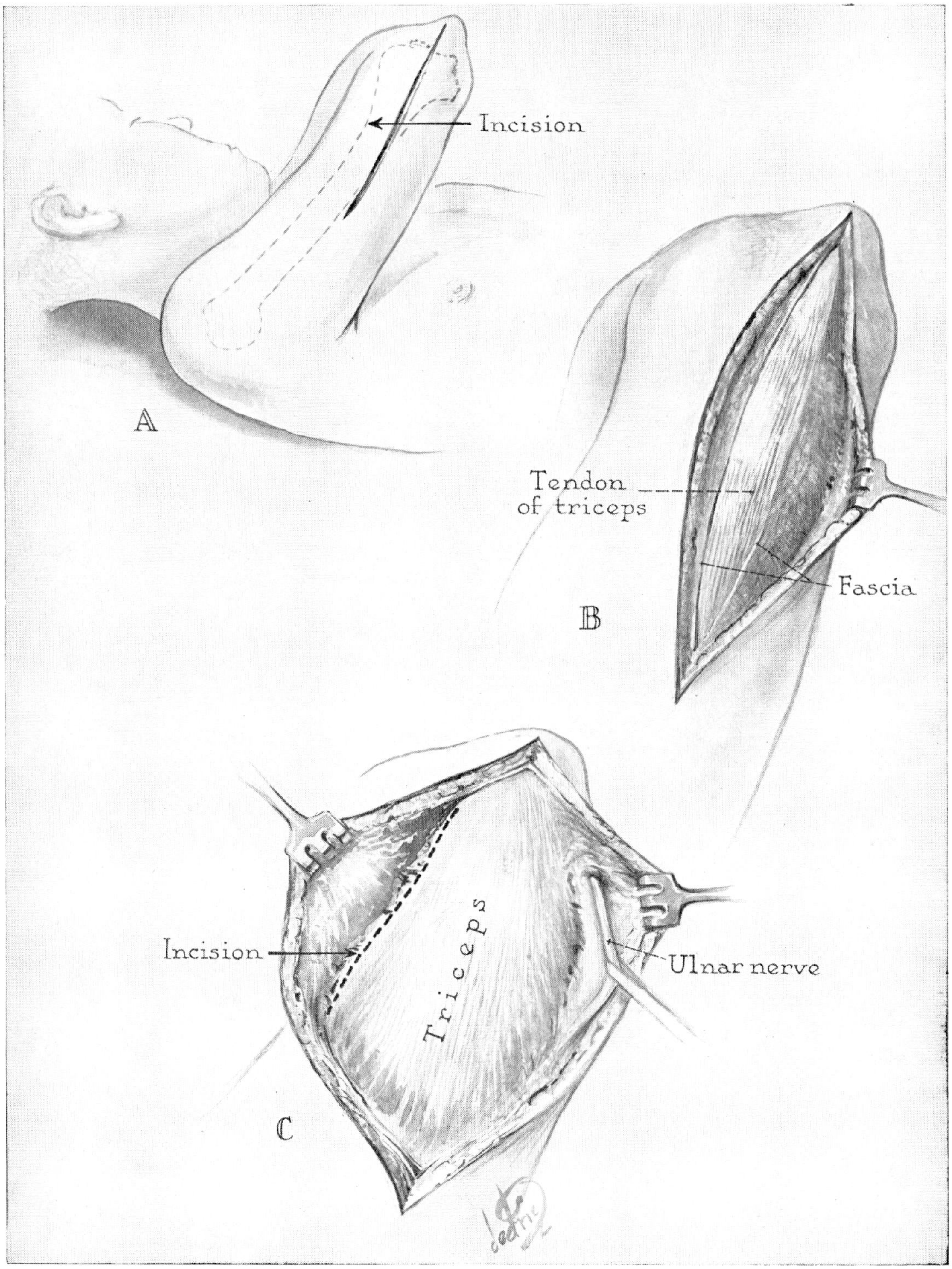

Exposure of the distal third of the posterior surface of the humerus through a longitudinal incision with tenotomy of the triceps tendon

EXPOSURE OF THE DISTAL THIRD OF THE POSTERIOR SURFACE OF THE HUMERUS THROUGH A LONGITUDINAL INCISION WITH TENOTOMY OF THE TRICEPS TENDON (*Continued*)

Plate 39: Description of Procedure

D The tendon and underlying muscle fibers of the deep head of the triceps are separated from the posterior surface of the humerus with the aid of a periosteal elevator. The opposite margin then is separated from the posterior aspect of the medial intermuscular septum.

E The triceps tendon and muscle fibers are transected by a chevron-shaped incision, and the tendon is reflected downward to expose the underlying posterior aspect of the distal third of the humerus.

NOTE: The radial nerve will not be injured provided the site of the tenotomy is not higher than the junction of the middle and distal thirds of the humerus. The triceps tendon must be accurately resutured when the wound is closed, and the ulnar nerve must either be placed in a protective pad of muscle tissue or be transplanted into the subcutaneous tissues anterior to the medial condyle of the humerus.

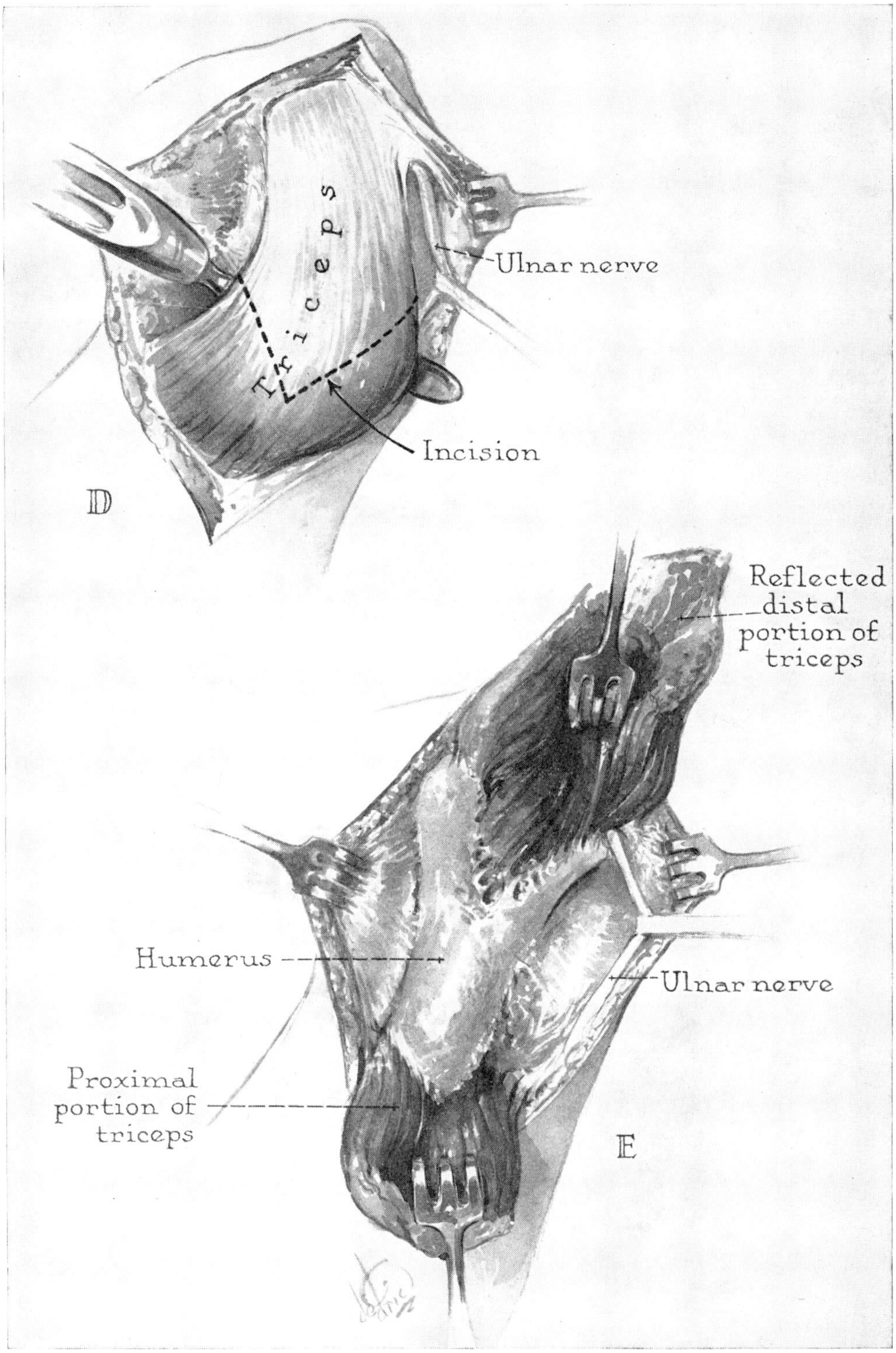

Exposure of the distal third of the posterior surface of the humerus through a longitudinal incision with tenotomy of the triceps tendon

EXPOSURE OF THE SHAFT OF THE HUMERUS THROUGH A POSTERIOR MEDIAL LONGITUDINAL INCISION

Indications: 1. Removal of Benign Tumors

2. Treatment of Chronic Infections Which Cannot Be Reached through a Lateral Incision

Plate 40: Description of Procedure

A The longitudinal incision begins behind the medial epicondyle of the humerus and then continues upward, directly posterior to the medial intermuscular septum, for the desired distance.

B The fascia is opened. The ulnar nerve is freed from the triceps muscle and retracted medially out of the way of possible injury.

C The triceps muscle is separated from the posterior surface of the medial intermuscular septum and the adjacent portion of the humerus, and pulled outward. The periosteum of the humerus is now exposed. (Procedure continued on Plate 41.)

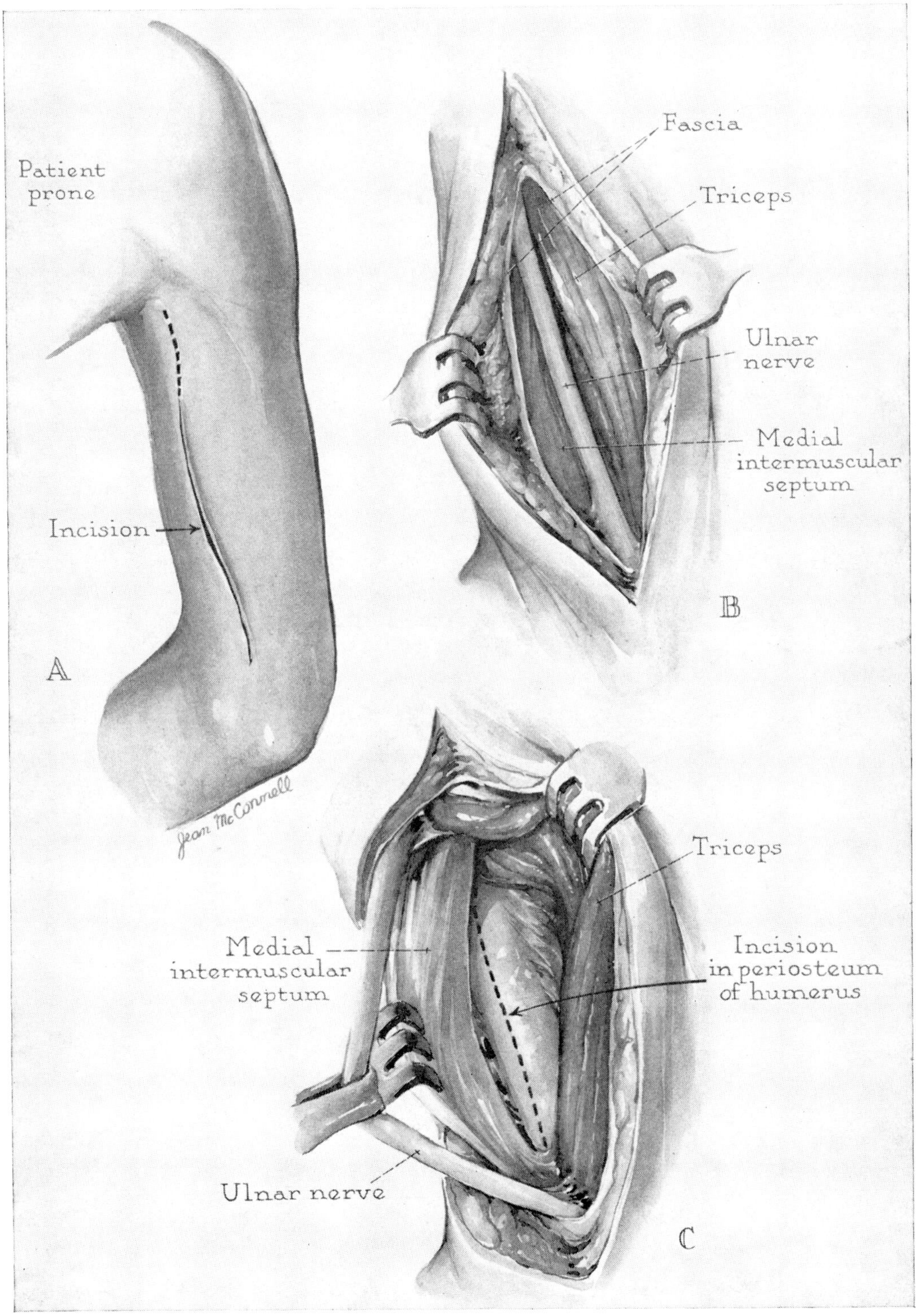

Exposure of the shaft of the humerus through a posterior medial longitudinal incision

EXPOSURE OF THE SHAFT OF THE HUMERUS THROUGH A POSTERIOR MEDIAL LONGITUDINAL INCISION *(Continued)*

Plate 41: Description of Procedure

D The periosteum is incised the length of the wound and reflected so as to expose the humerus. This dissection may be carried completely around the bone.

E It may be necessary, occasionally, to lengthen this incision proximally. This longer incision may be required primarily for adequate exposure of some lesions. The incision may thus be extended upward to the inferior margin of the deltoid muscle. The ulnar nerve is retracted medially out of the wound, while the long head of the triceps muscle is pulled laterally. The radial nerve and the deep branch of the brachial artery are located beneath the proximal fourth of the long head of the triceps muscle and, while they need not be isolated, they must be preserved from injury. The periosteum is cut and reflected from the humerus.

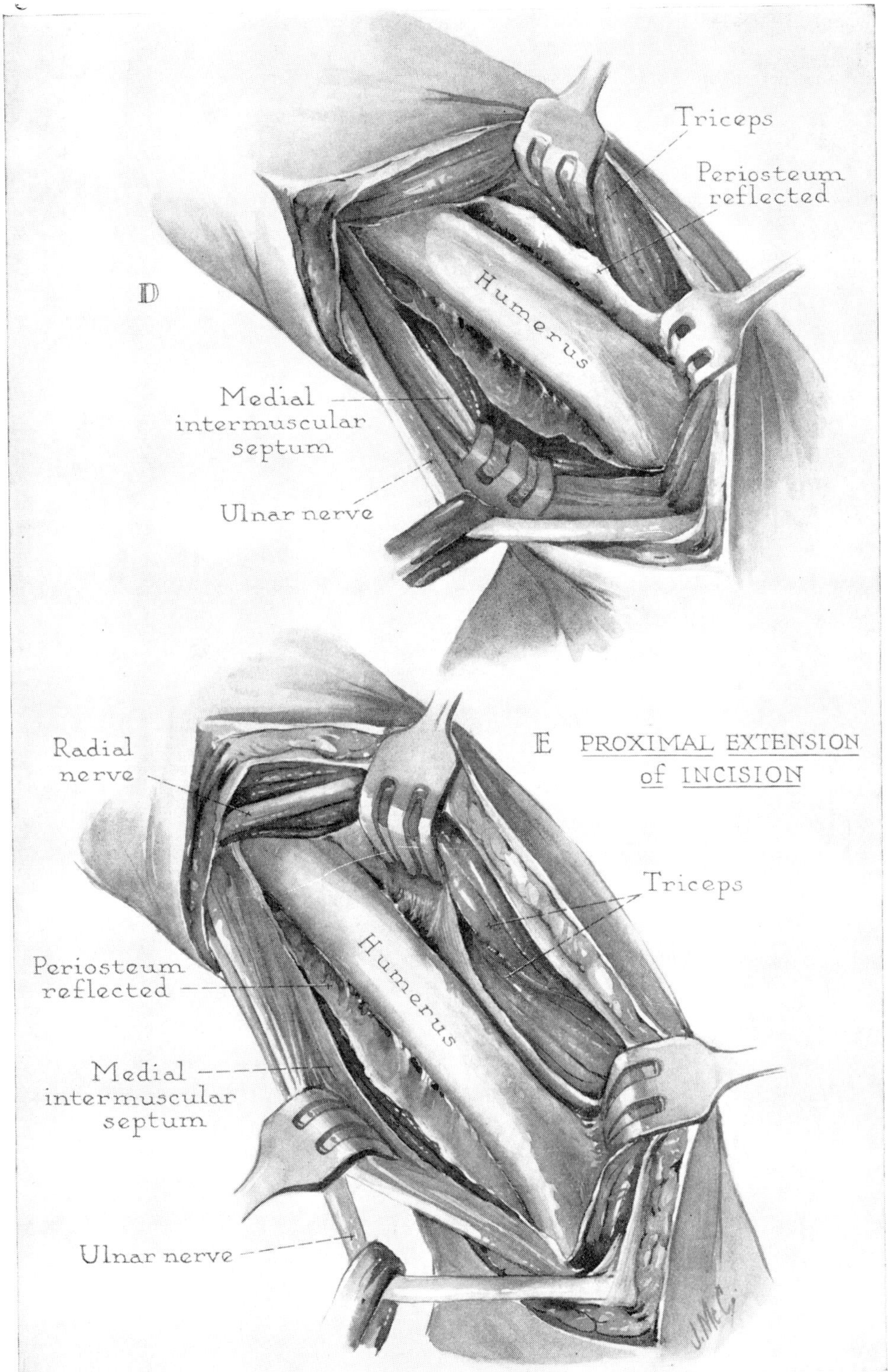

Exposure of the shaft of the humerus through a posterior medial longitudinal incision

EXPOSURE OF THE MEDIAN NERVE IN THE ARM THROUGH AN ANTERIOR MEDIAL LONGITUDINAL INCISION

Indication: 1. Suture or Neurolysis of the Median Nerve

Plate 42: Description of Procedure

A The patient is in a recumbent position on the table with the extremity abducted and externally rotated on an arm board. The posterior medial margin of the biceps muscle serves as the landmark for the location of the skin incision. The incision, approximately 7 inches long, begins at the anterior axillary fold and extends distally over the anterior medial aspect of the arm to end in front of the medial epicondyle of the humerus.

B The deep fascia is opened and the medial margin of the biceps is dissected out while the lateral flap of skin and fascia is being retracted.

C The median nerve is isolated in the proximal portion of the wound and mobilized for the desired distance. The medial nerve lies lateral to the brachial artery and its accompanying veins in the proximal half of the wound. The nerve crosses over the artery and veins and assumes a position medially to these structures, in the lower half of the wound. The vein which crosses superficially to the midportion of the nerve may be ligated. The ulnar nerve is positioned posteriorly to the medial intermuscular septum similar to the way the median nerve is placed anteriorly to the septum.

NOTE: The portion of the median nerve in front of the elbow can be exposed by further elongation of the wound. The type of incision required for this purpose is described elsewhere in this Atlas under the heading of: "Exposure of the Median Nerve Anterior to the Elbow Joint and in the Proximal Portion of the Forearm" (see page 135).

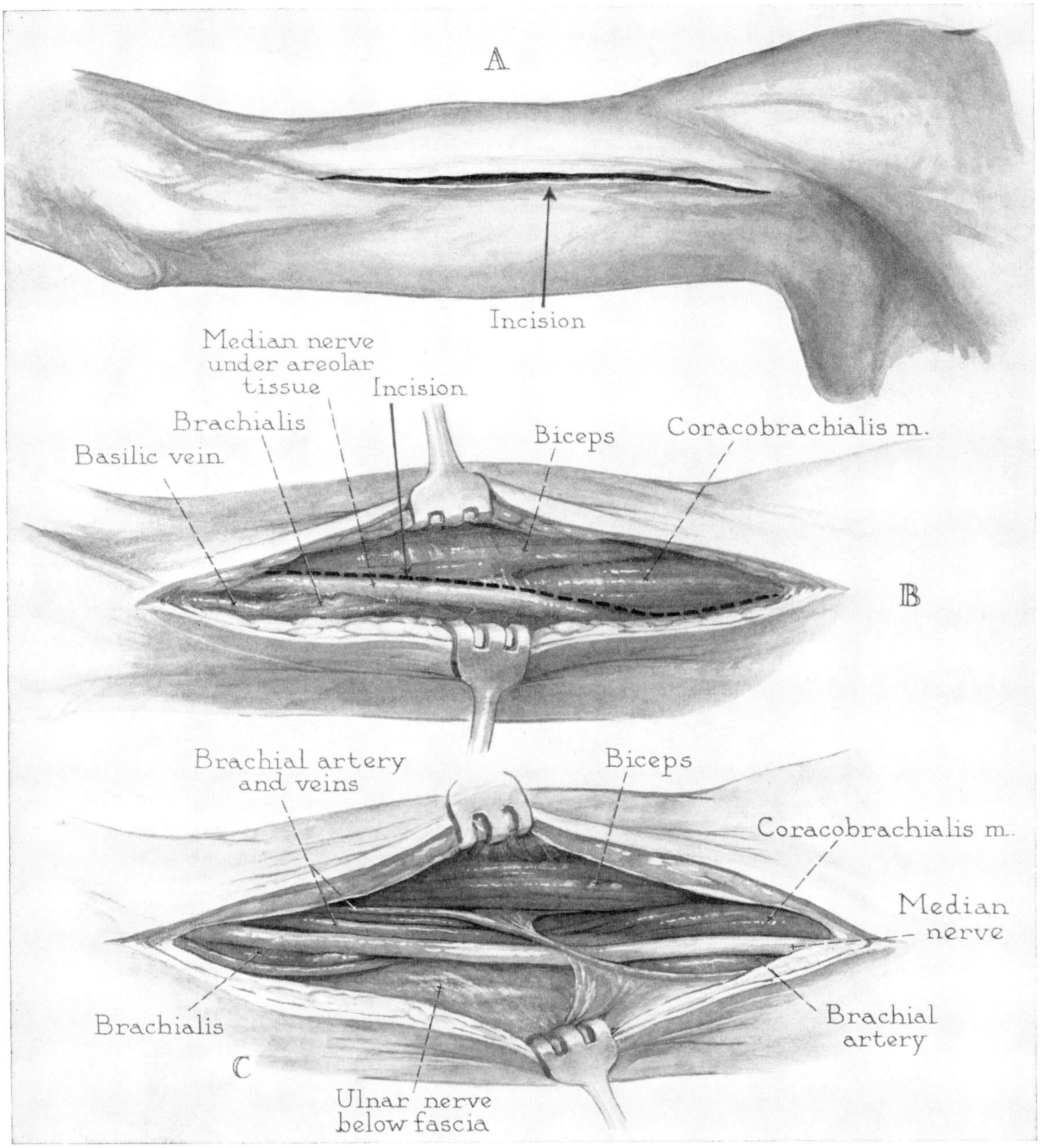

Exposure of the median nerve in the arm through an anterior medial longitudinal incision

EXPOSURE OF THE RADIAL NERVE POSTERIORLY TO THE HUMERUS THROUGH A CURVED POSTERIOR INCISION

Indication: 1. Suture or Neurolysis of the Radial Nerve

Plate 43: Description of Procedure

A The skin incision, approximately 11 inches in length, starts at the posterior margin of the deltoid muscle and extends halfway down the arm in the midline, from whence it curves laterally and forward until its termination at the interval between the brachioradialis and brachialis muscles. The incision follows the groove formed by the long and the lateral heads of the triceps, which landmark can easily be identified by palpation.

B The skin flaps are then undermined and retracted, and the deep fascia is incised in line with the skin incision. The interval between the long and lateral heads of the humerus is enlarged sufficiently to permit isolation of these two components of the triceps muscle.

C The muscles are next retracted to their respective sides of the wound, and the radial nerve and accompanying deep brachial artery and vein are exposed. The radial nerve is isolated down to the point where it passes below the lateral head of the triceps muscle. (Procedure continued on Plate 44.)

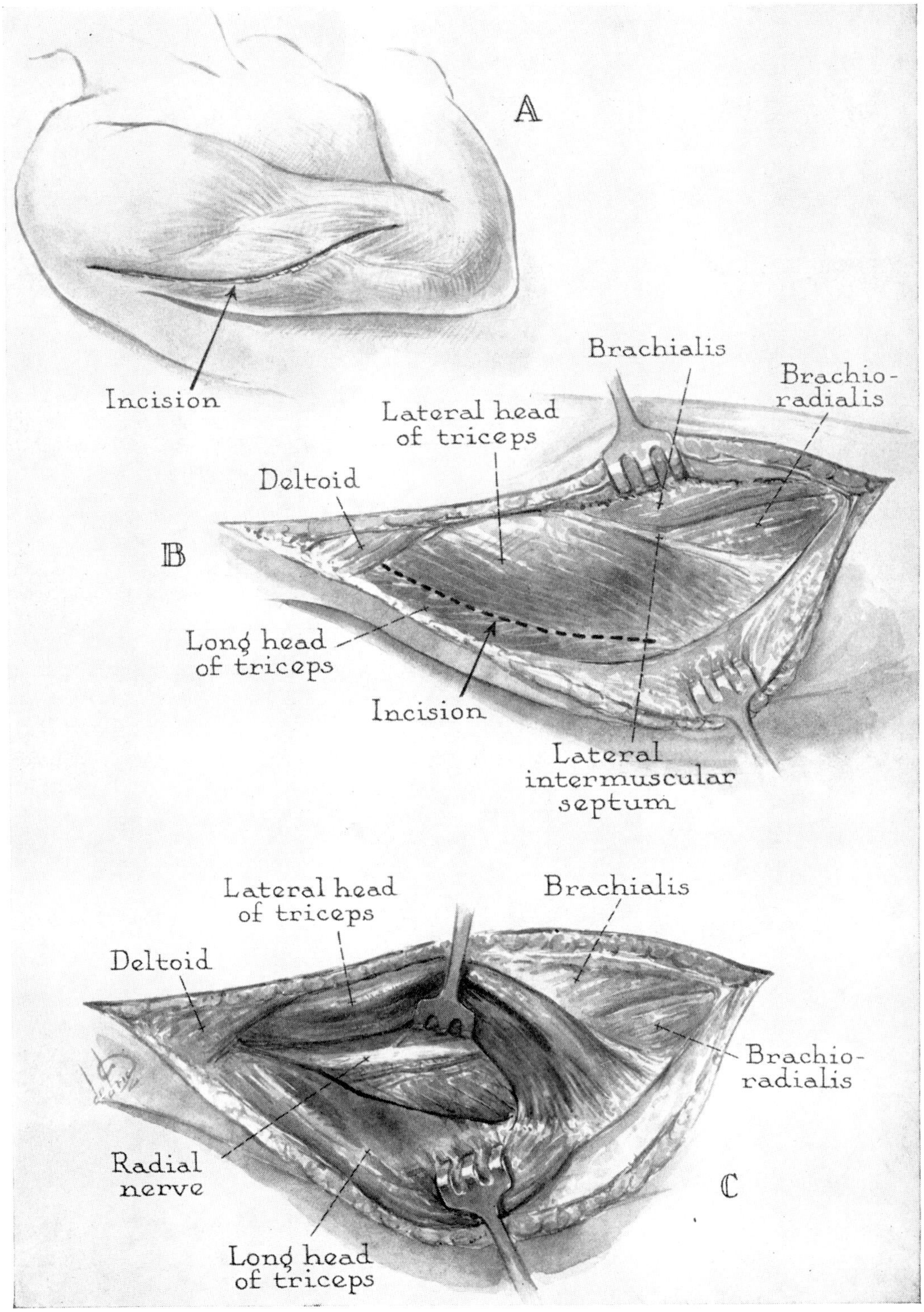

Exposure of the radial nerve posteriorly to the humerus through a curved posterior incision

EXPOSURE OF THE RADIAL NERVE POSTERIORLY TO THE HUMERUS THROUGH A CURVED POSTERIOR INCISION *(Continued)*

Plate 44: Description of Procedure

D The arm is next slightly rotated externally and the space between the upper end of the brachioradialis and brachialis muscles is opened to free the radial nerve along the anterolateral surface of the humerus.

E The lateral head of the triceps may be separated from the humerus, as illustrated, in order to gain a greater degree of mobility for this portion of the triceps muscle and to facilitate isolation of that section of the radial nerve which lies deep under it.

F Care must moreover be exercised when retracting the long head of the triceps that no injury is done to the ulnar nerve, which extends distally in the arm underneath this muscle.

NOTE: The operation may be performed in the supine position with the patient's arm across his chest, or in the prone position with the extremity resting on an arm board in abduction.

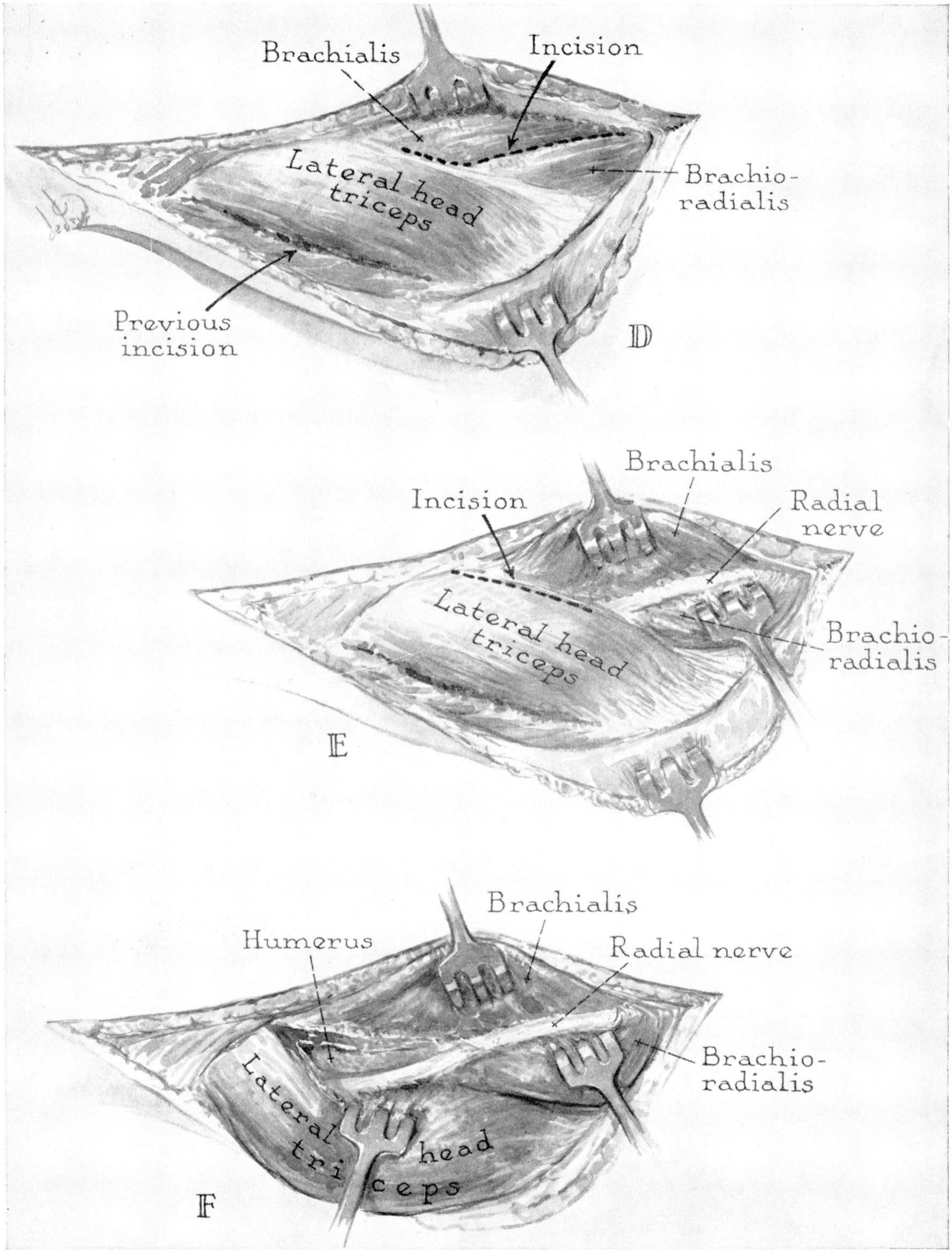

Exposure of the radial nerve posteriorly to the humerus through a curved posterior incision

EXPOSURE OF THE ULNAR NERVE IN THE ARM THROUGH A POSTERIOR MEDIAL LONGITUDINAL INCISION

Indication: 1. Neurolysis or Suture of the Ulnar Nerve

Plate 45: Description of Procedure

A This operation may be performed with the arm of the patient lying across his chest, or externally rotated on an arm board. First the medial epicondyle of the humerus is identified, and then an incision is made which starts posteriorly to it and extends upward in a straight line for the desired distance.

B The fascia then is opened carefully, to avoid injury to the ulnar nerve which lies just below it.

C The ulnar nerve is easily located posteriorly to the medial intermuscular septum, in a groove in the triceps muscle. It is accompanied by the superior ulnar collateral artery.

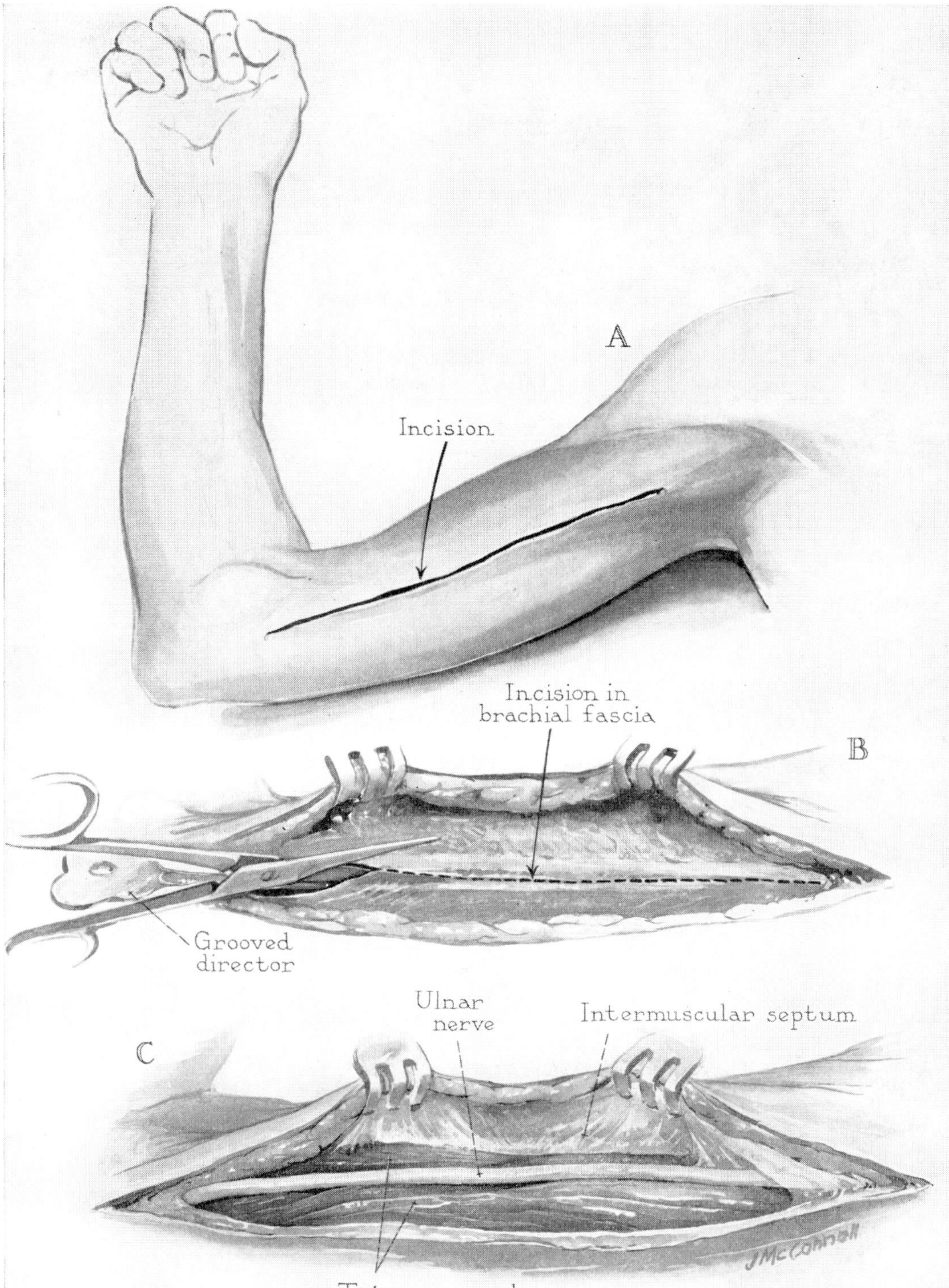

Exposure of the ulnar nerve in the arm through a posterior medial longitudinal incision

EXPOSURE OF THE TENDON OF THE BICEPS MUSCLE THROUGH A CURVED ANTECUBITAL INCISION

Indication: 1. Repair of Avulsions and Ruptures of the Tendon of the Biceps Muscle

Plate 46: Description of Procedure

A The incision begins at the medial side of the biceps muscle about 2 inches above the elbow joint. The cut extends distally to the flexion crease, which it follows transversely to the margin of the brachioradialis muscle; it then turns gracefully into the forearm for several inches. The skin flaps are mobilized and retracted widely. The branches of the lateral antibrachial cutaneous nerve are looked for and protected.

B The fascia is opened, as illustrated, and the lacertus fibrosus is cut.

C The biceps muscle is separated from the surrounding structures. The musculocutaneous nerve emerges laterally from between the biceps and the brachialis muscles. The radial nerve is located between the brachialis and the brachioradialis muscles. The nerve need not be exposed above the level of the elbow, as shown in the illustration; it must, however, be isolated in the distal half of the wound. The brachial artery and median nerve, which flank the medial margin of the biceps tendon, must not be severed.

D The dissection then is continued close to the biceps tendon and down to the posterior aspect of the inner surface of the radial tuberosity where the tendon is attached posteriorly. The supinator muscle is pulled downward and radially, and the forearm is placed in a position of supination in order to facilitate the exposure of the biceps attachment. A bursa is present between the tendon and the radius.

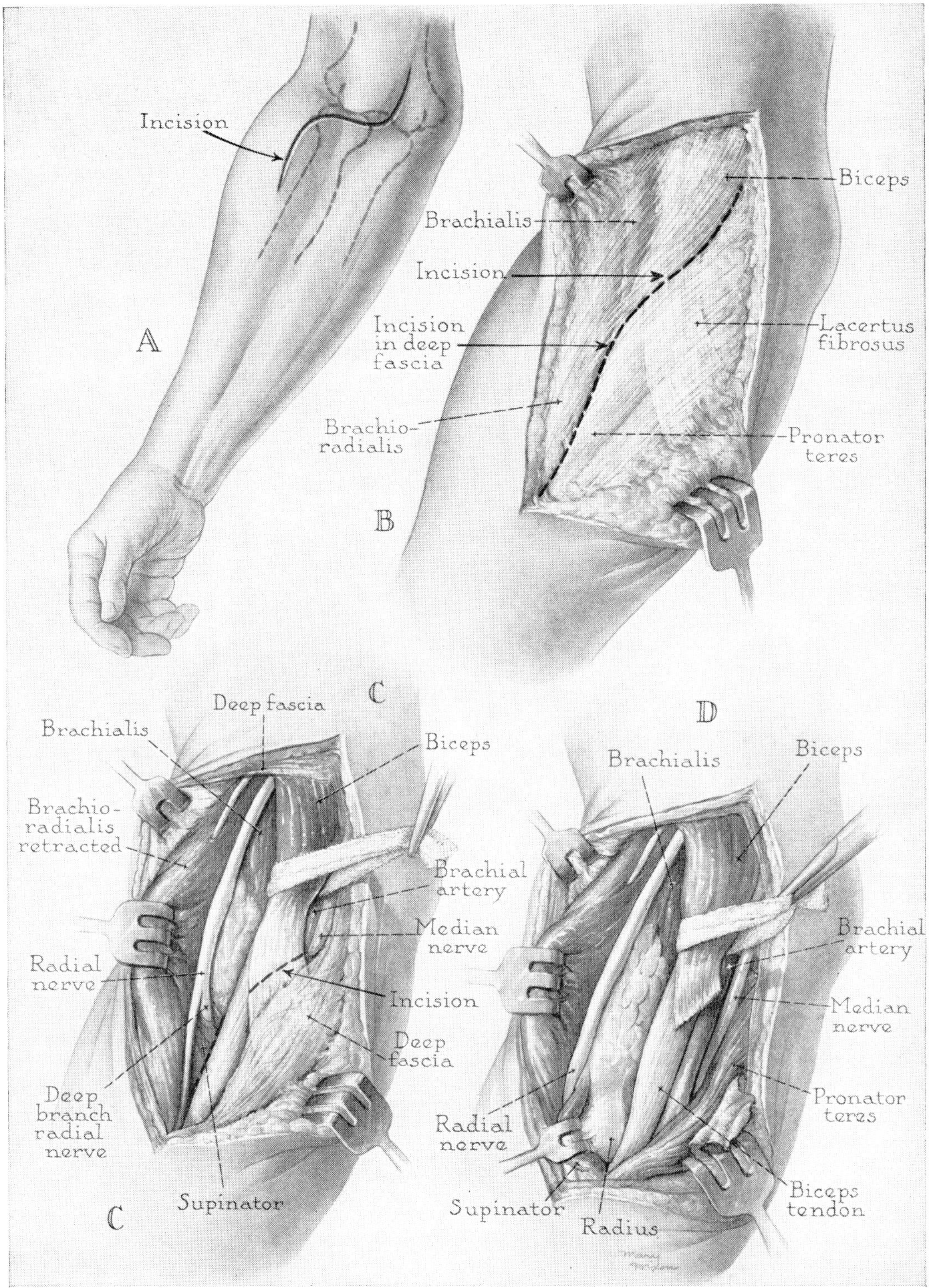

Exposure of the tendon of the biceps muscle through a curved antecubital incision

Section IV

Region of the Elbow Joint

EXPOSURE OF THE ANTERIOR COMPARTMENT OF THE ELBOW JOINT AND OF THE ANTERIOR SURFACE OF THE SUPRACONDYLAR REGION OF THE HUMERUS THROUGH AN ANTERIOR LATERAL INCISION

Indications: 1. Removal of Loose Bodies

2. Repair of Fractures of the Lateral Condyle and Capitellum of the Humerus

Plate 47: Description of Procedure

A The anterior margin of the brachioradialis muscle serves as the landmark for the skin incision. The incision begins about 2 inches above the lateral epicondyle of the humerus and extends distally for a total length of approximately 4 inches, by curving around the flexion crease, as shown in the illustration.

B The skin flaps are mobilized and retracted, and the fascia is opened the length of the incision. The superficial veins which cross the operative field may be ligated or mobilized and retracted.

C The anterior margins of the brachioradialis muscle laterally and of the biceps medially are identified. The dissection is continued in the loose areolar tissue between these two muscles and carried down to the humerus. The brachioradialis muscle is retracted outward and the biceps medially. (Procedure continued on Plate 48.)

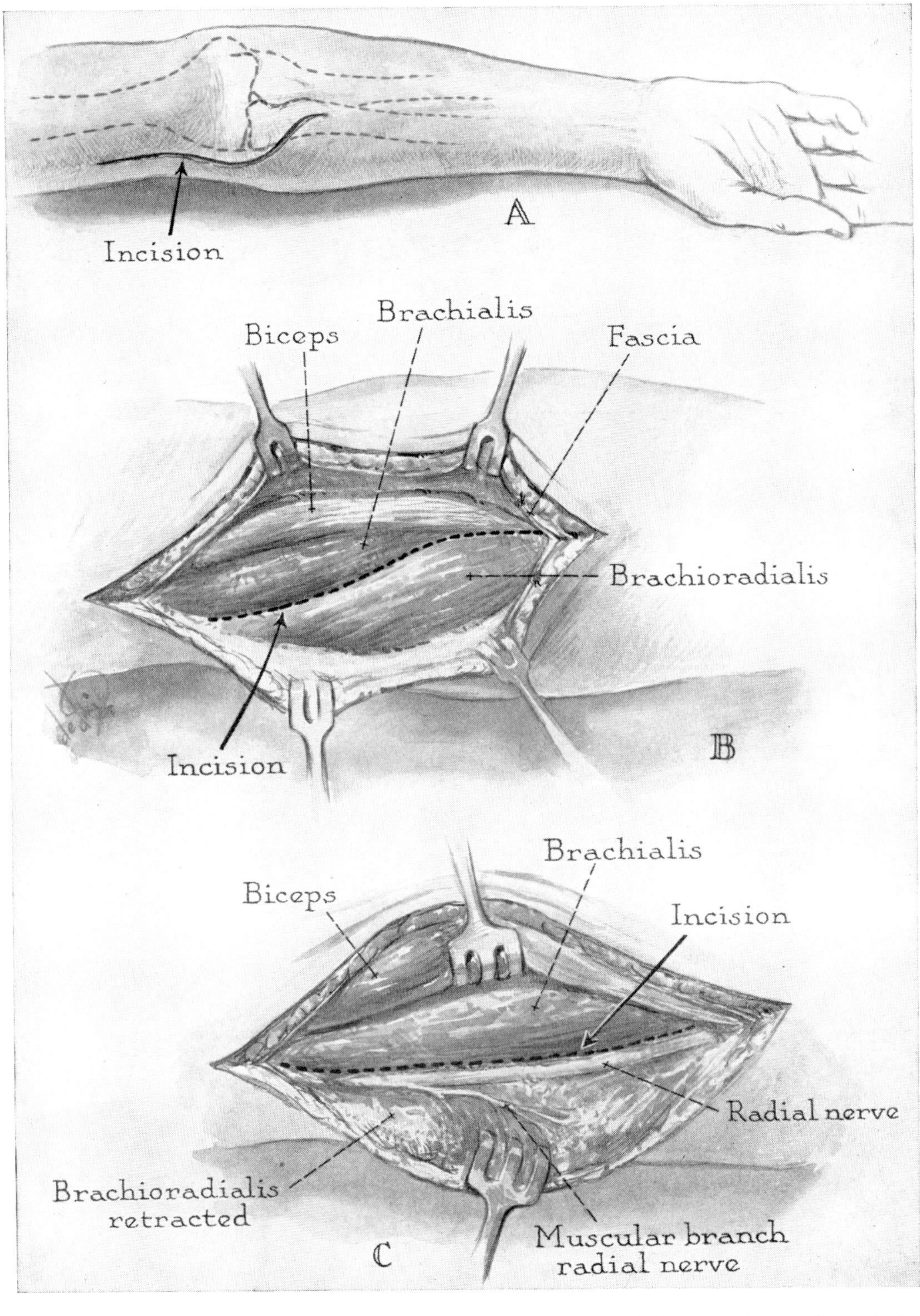

Exposure of the anterior compartment of the elbow joint and of the anterior surface of the supracondylar region of the humerus through an anterior lateral incision

EXPOSURE OF THE ANTERIOR COMPARTMENT OF THE ELBOW JOINT AND OF THE ANTERIOR SURFACE OF THE SUPRA-CONDYLAR REGION OF THE HUMERUS THROUGH AN ANTERIOR LATERAL INCISION (*Continued*)

Plate 48: Description of Procedure

D The radial nerve is located at the bottom of the wound and is gently retracted by means of a hernia tape. The retraction medially of the biceps muscle has brought into view the lateral portion of the brachialis muscle beneath it. The musculocutaneous nerve descends between these two muscles and then emerges laterally to the biceps tendon; it must not be injured. The lateral antibrachial cutaneous nerves supply the skin of the anterior and lateral surfaces of the forearm.

E The periosteum is incised along the interrupted line shown in the illustration, and the brachiali muscle is raised from the front of the lower end of the humerus subperiosteally, and reflected toward the midline. The anterior lateral capsule of the elbow joint is now exposed in tne wound, and an incision through it brings to view the components of the lateral half of the elbow joint. By placing a retractor beneath the medial capsule as it is elevated from the front of the humerus, one can obtain a clear view of the distal articular surface of the humerus and of the head of the radius.

NOTE: No important structures are encountered in this exposure, aside trom the radial nerve. This nerve will not suffer damage if it is isolated and kept under scrutiny.

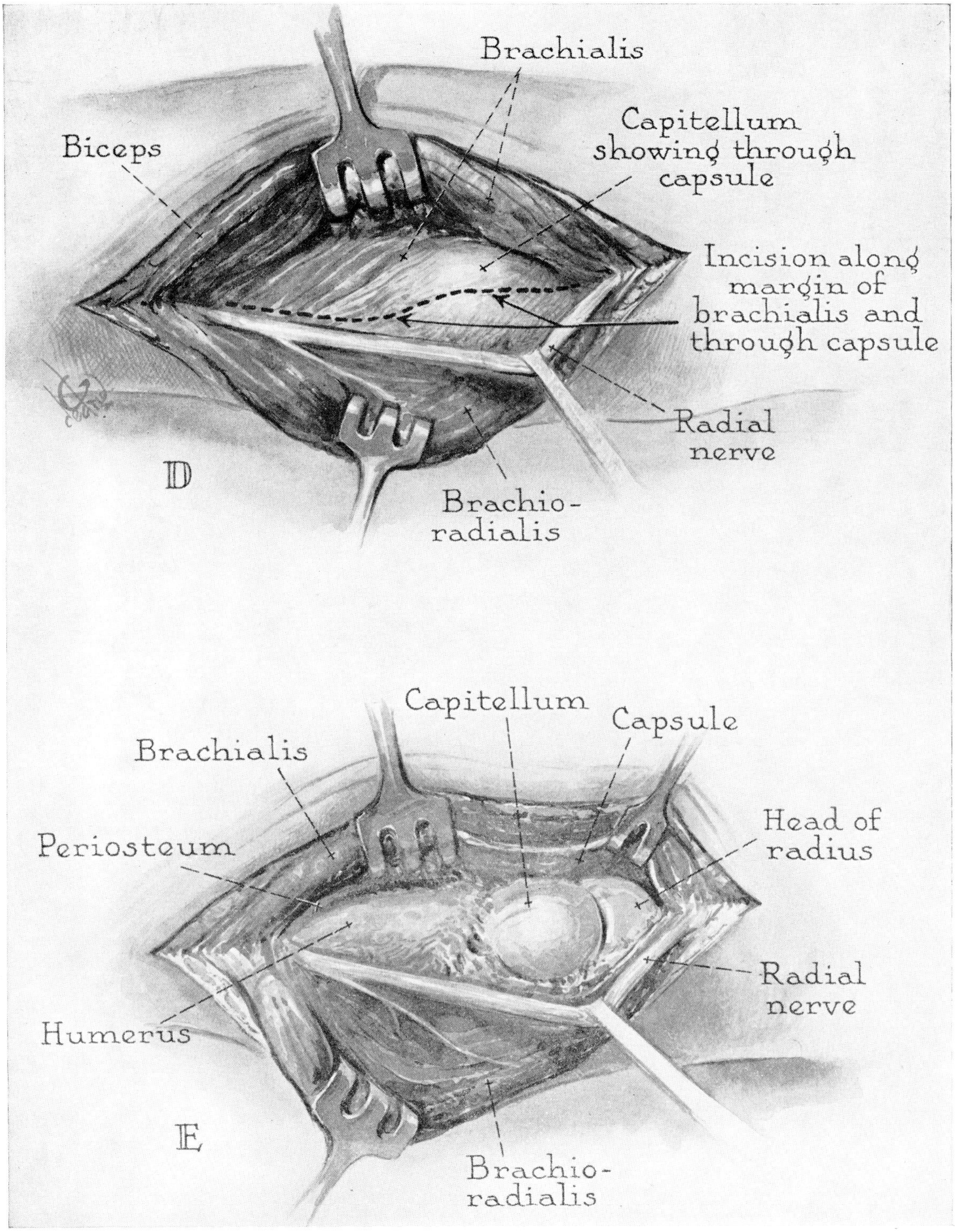

Exposure of the anterior compartment of the elbow joint and of the anterior surface of the supracondylar region of the humerus through an anterior lateral incision

EXPOSURE OF THE ELBOW JOINT AND THE ANTERIOR ASPECT OF THE PROXIMAL THIRD OF THE RADIUS THROUGH AN ANTERIOR LATERAL INCISION

Indications: 1. Open Reduction of Fractures of the Radius

2. Treatment of Non-unions of Fractures

3. Excision of Tumors

Plate 49: Description of Procedure

A A skin incision is made, beginning 2 inches above the flexion crease of the elbow joint and extending downward along the anterior margin of the brachioradialis muscle. At the level of the elbow joint the incision curves gently laterally to avoid crossing the flexion crease because of the danger of keloid formation and secondary flexion contracture.

B The deep fascia is opened, and the radial nerve which, in this region, passes in front of the humerus, is brought into view. The landmark for locating this nerve is the interval between the brachioradialis laterally, and the biceps and brachialis muscles medially.

C The nerve is then isolated and traced downward along the inner aspect of the brachioradialis muscle to the point where it divides into its superficial sensory branch and its deep motor (dorsal interosseus) branch. The sensory branch continues along the forearm under protection of the deep surface of the brachioradialis and must not be compressed by retractors. The dorsal interosseus nerve enters the supinator muscle and then continues to the dorsum of the forearm. At the level of the insertion of the biceps tendon into the radial tuberosity, the recurrent radial artery crosses the incision from the medial to the lateral side, and must be ligated.

The radial artery passes distally in the forearm over the pronator teres muscle at this level and must be identified and protected.

The lateral antibrachial cutaneous nerve emerges between the biceps tendon and brachialis muscle and then passes downward laterally to the biceps tendon into the subcutaneous tissue of the anterolateral aspect of the forearm. This nerve must be identified and kept intact. It is retracted with the medial skin flap. (Procedure continued on Plate 50.)

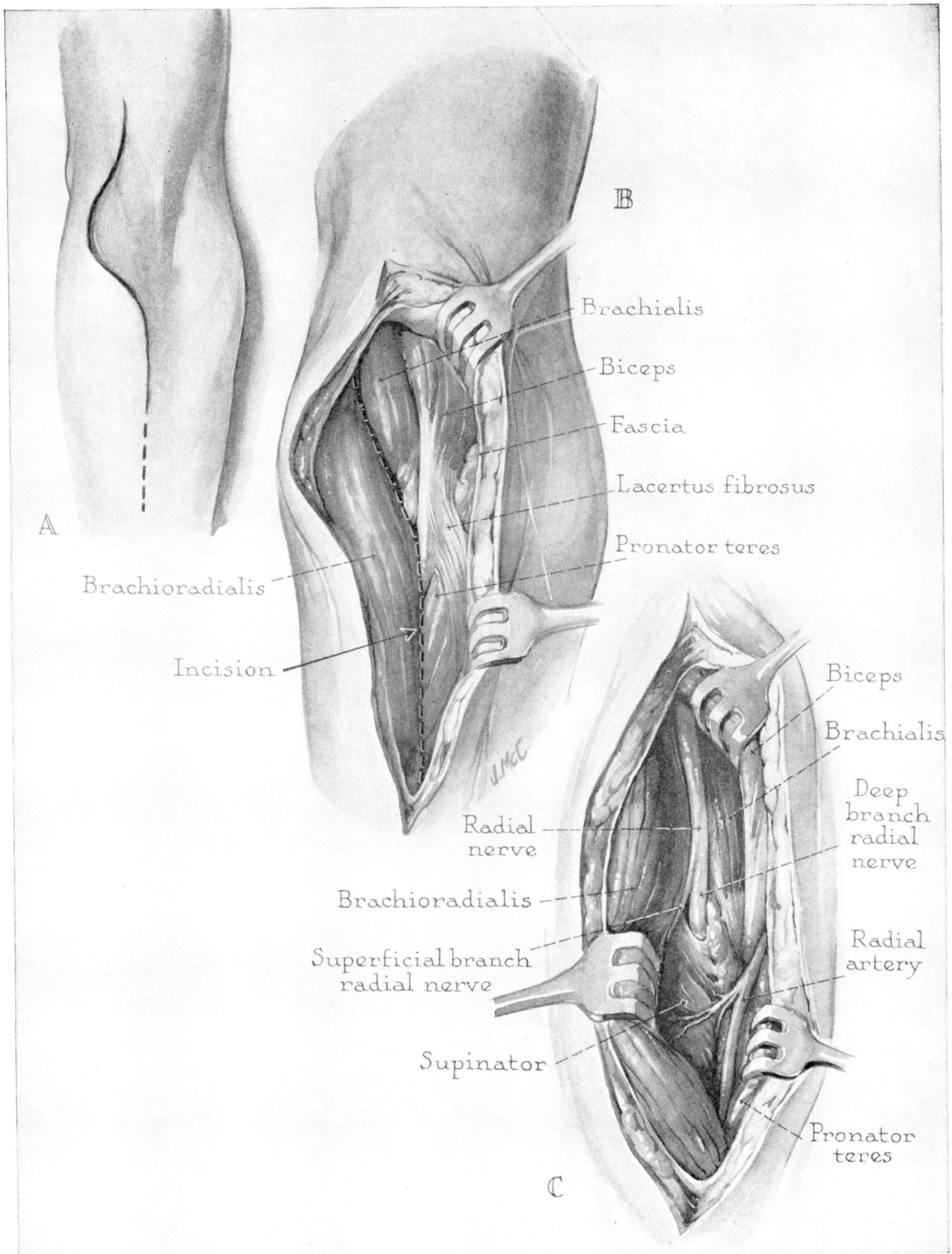

Exposure of the elbow joint and the anterior aspect of the proximal third of the radius through an anterior lateral incision

EXPOSURE OF THE ELBOW JOINT AND THE ANTERIOR ASPECT OF THE PROXIMAL THIRD OF THE RADIUS THROUGH AN ANTERIOR LATERAL INCISION *(Continued)*

Plate 50: Description of Procedure

D The dissection continues in the distal half of the wound to expose the supinator muscle which lies deep under the brachioradialis muscle and covers the radius. Attached to the anteromedial surface of the radius, distal to the supinator, are the tendon of the pronator teres and a portion of the origins of the flexor digitorum sublimis and flexor pollicis longus muscles.

E The hand is firmly supinated, and an incision is made in the periosteum of the radius medially to the attachment of the supinator muscle and laterally to the attachment of the pronator teres. The radius is freed subperiosteally. The incision may be extended into the elbow joint proximally and also distally along the radius if desired for additional exposure.

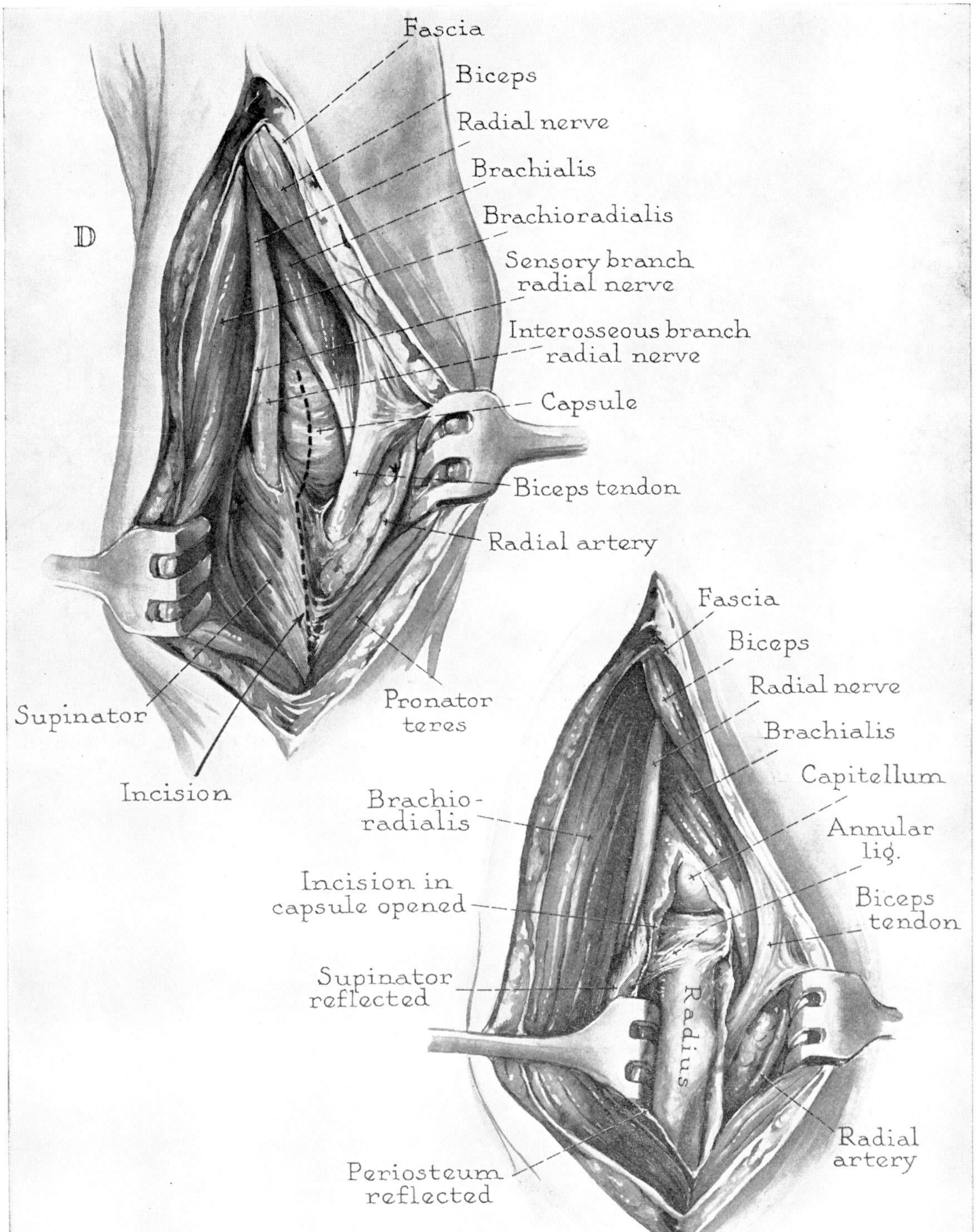

Exposure of the elbow joint and the anterior aspect of the proximal third of the radius through an anterior lateral incision

EXPOSURE OF THE ELBOW JOINT THROUGH A MEDIAL INCISION WITH OSTEOTOMY OF THE MEDIAL EPICONDYLE OF THE HUMERUS

Indications: 1. Removal of Loose Bodies from the Elbow Joint

2. Open Reduction of Certain Fractures of the Medial Condyle of the Humerus

3. Open Reduction of Certain Fractures of the Coronoid Process of the Ulna

Plate 51: Description of Procedure

A A curved skin incision, approximately 4 inches long, is made over the medial aspect of the elbow joint centering on the medial epicondyle of the humerus.

B The fascia is incised and the flaps are retracted. The ulnar nerve is isolated in its groove posterior to the medial condyle, and a piece of hernia tape is used to facilitate its handling. The anterior flap is retracted to expose the proximal ends of the flexor muscles as they pass from the medial epicondyle of the humerus downward, forward and laterally into the forearm.

C A retractor is placed on the superior margin of the pronator teres muscle to lift it from the underlying structures. Care must be taken not to injure the brachial artery and accompanying veins as well as the median nerve lying near the midline. The branches of the median nerve to the pronator teres muscle must be identified and protected. (Procedure continued on Plate 52.)

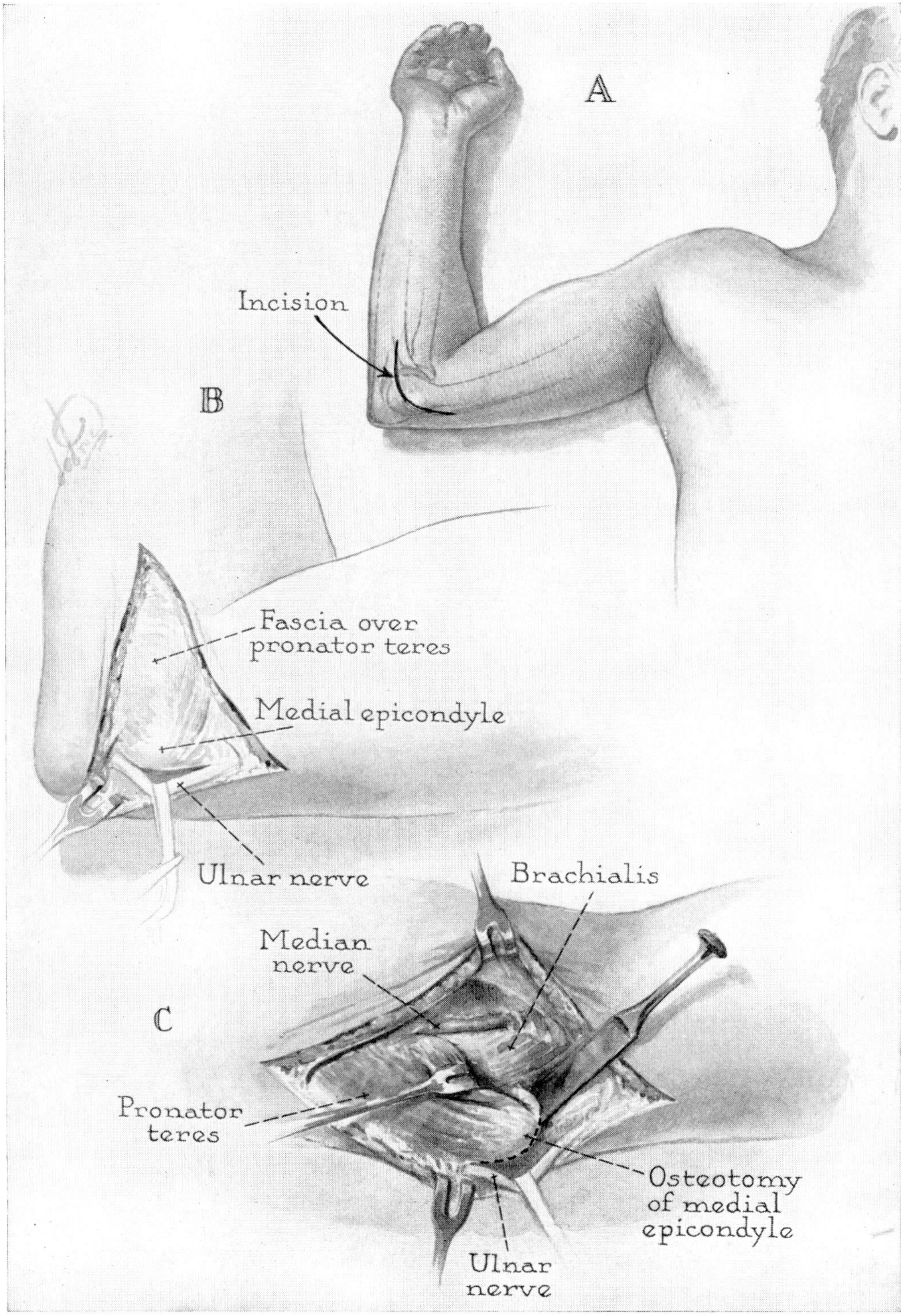

Exposure of the elbow joint through a medial incision with osteotomy of the medial epicondyle of the humerus

EXPOSURE OF THE ELBOW JOINT THROUGH A MEDIAL INCISION WITH OSTEOTOMY OF THE MEDIAL EPICONDYLE OF THE HUMERUS (*Continued*)

Plate 52: Description of Procedure

D The ulnar nerve is retracted out of the way, and the medial epicondyle is osteotomized so that it and the attached muscles can be reflected downward and forward, thereby affording a clear view of the muscular branches of the median nerve as they enter the under surface of the pronator teres muscle.

E The medial condyle of the humerus and the adjacent portion of the ulna are visible through the thin capsule of the elbow joint which is now exposed. Entrance into the capsule is made by a longitudinal incision, although the amount of exposure thus obtained is not ample. It can be increased, however, by subperiosteal reflection of the brachialis muscle and the capsule from the distal anterior surface of the humerus, and by abducting the forearm so as to wedge the joint. A constant awareness of the location of important arteries and nerves in the area exposed by the incision and its vicinity is necessary.

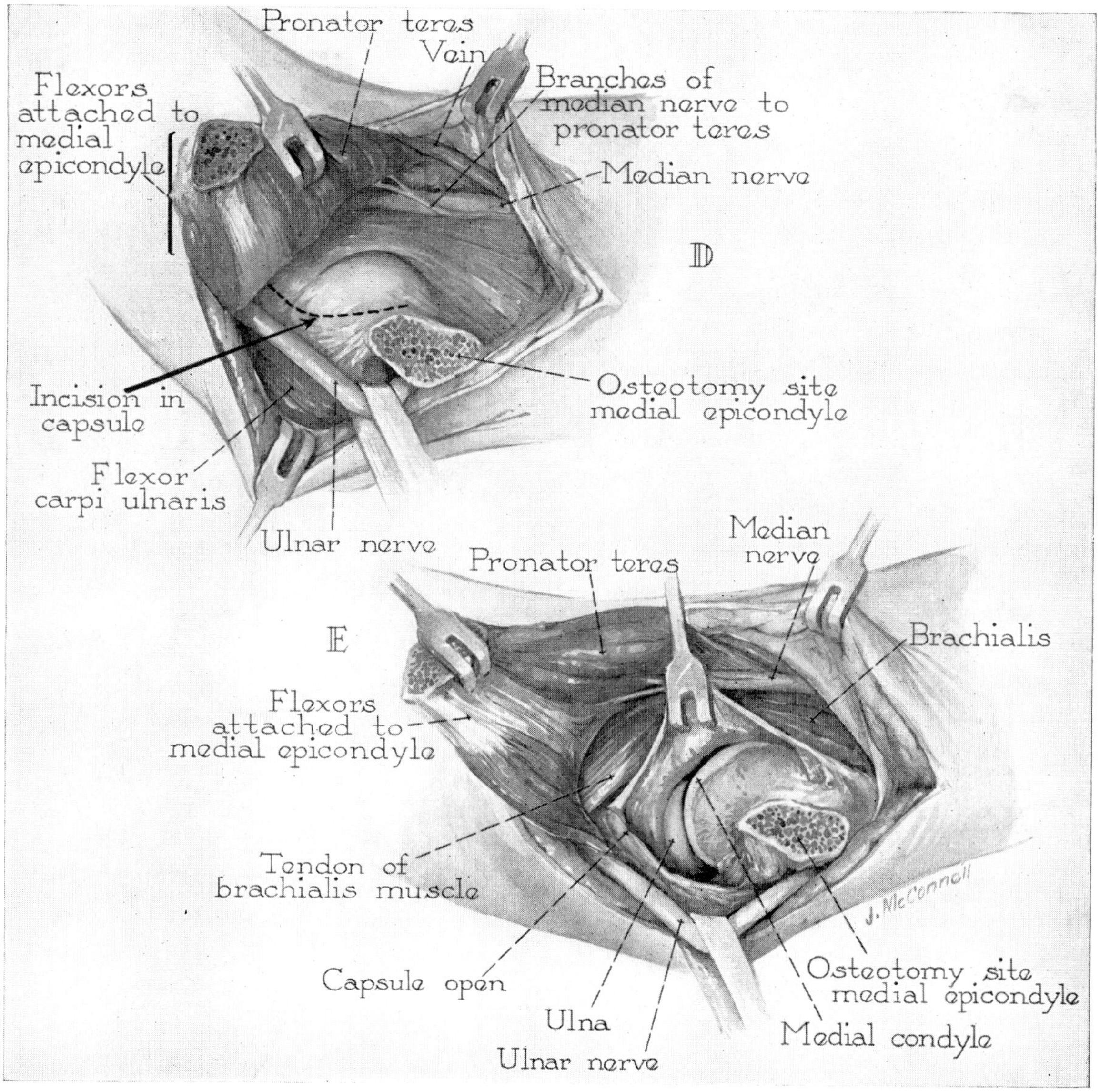

Exposure of the elbow joint through a medial incision with osteotomy of the medial epicondyle of the humerus

EXPOSURE OF THE ELBOW JOINT THROUGH A POSTERIOR MEDIAL INCISION

Indications: 1. Removal of Loose Bodies from the Posterior Medial Compartment of the Elbow Joint

Plate 53: Description of Procedure

A An incision, about 2 1/2 inches long, is centered over the posterior medial aspect of the elbow joint about midway between the medial epicondyle of the humerus and the olecranon process of the ulna. The deep fascia is incised and, on the medial side, the flap is undermined as far as the medial epicondyle and, on the lateral side, as far as the edge of the olecranon.

B The ulnar nerve is identified in the ulnar groove behind the medial epicondyle of the humerus. The roof of the fascial canal is opened so the nerve can be kept under direct vision during the remainder of the procedure. This part of the operation can be omitted, provided the exact location of the nerve is known and it is not injured by the capsular incision.

C The capsule of the elbow joint is opened by an incision placed lateral to the ulnar groove. The dissection is continued proximally so as to separate the fibers of the adjacent portion of the triceps muscle and tendon. The proximal fibers of the flexor carpi ulnaris muscle are seen distally in the wound and are retracted away from the ulna. The joint cavity is exposed by opening the synovia.

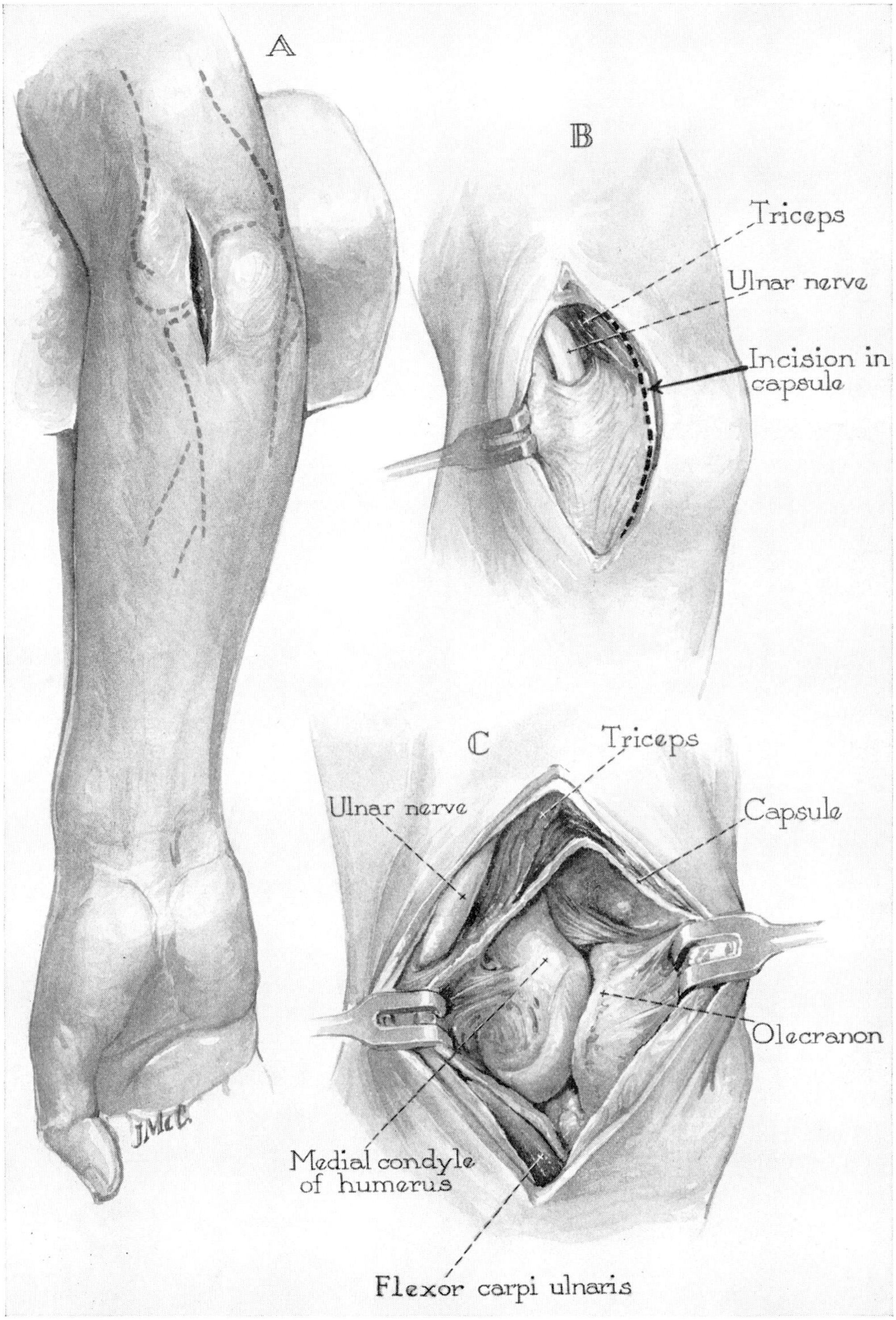

Exposure of the elbow joint through a posterior medial incision

EXPOSURE OF THE POSTERIOR LATERAL COMPARTMENT OF THE ELBOW JOINT THROUGH A POSTERIOR LATERAL INCISION

Indications: 1. Removal of Loose Bodies

2. Biopsy of the Synovia of the Elbow Joint

Plate 54: Description of Procedure

A The incision begins 1/2 inch below the head of the radius and extends upward for 3 inches, midway between the olecranon and the lateral epicondyle of the humerus.

B The lower portion of the triceps tendon, which is exposed in the wound, is cut as illustrated The fascia over the anconeus is sectioned distally, and the muscle is retracted downward.

C The capsule of the elbow joint is opened, thus bringing into view the lateral portion of the articular surface of the olecranon, the posterior aspect of the lateral condyle of the humerus, and the head of the radius.

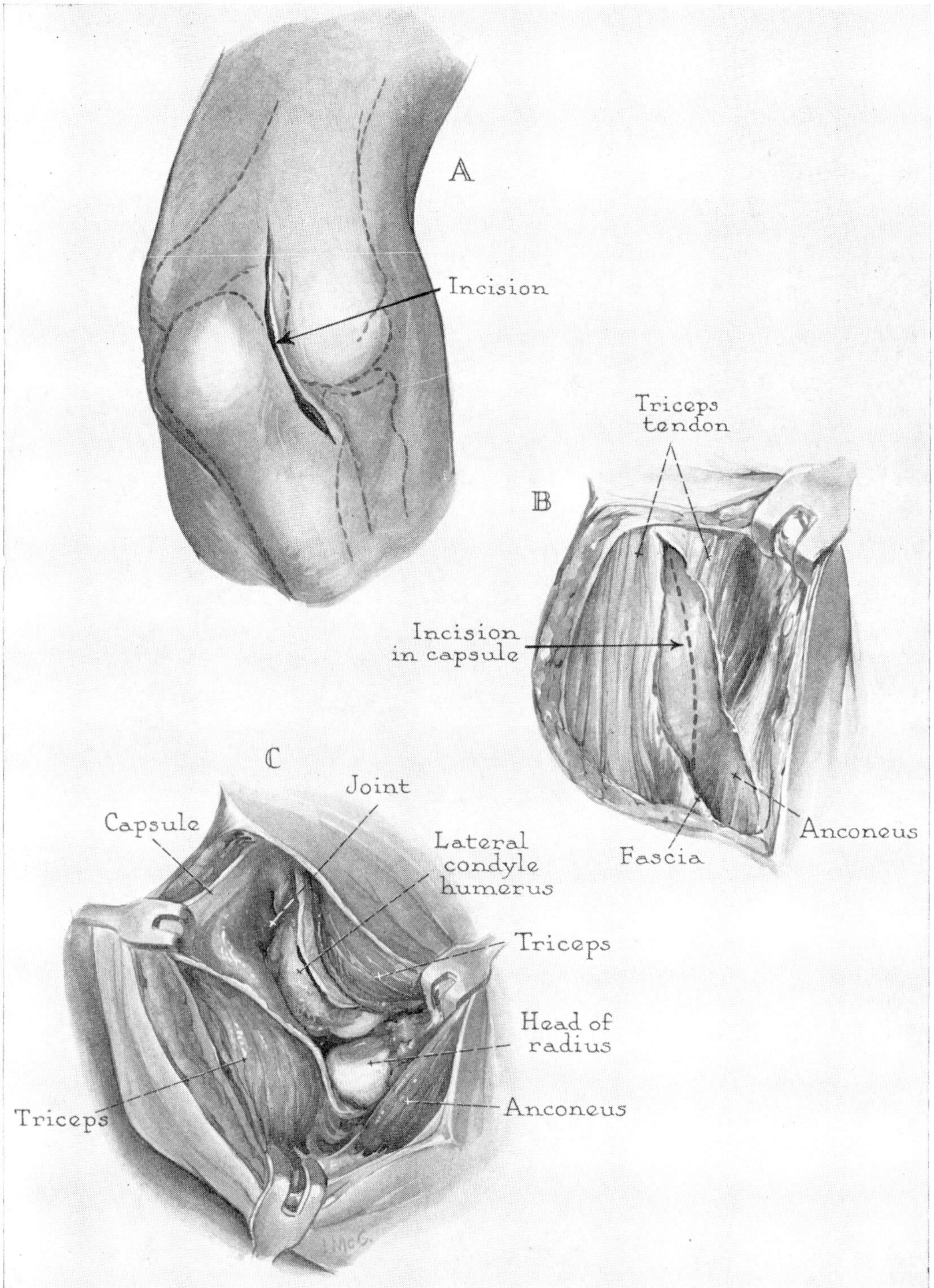

Exposure of the posterior lateral compartment of the elbow joint through a posterior lateral incision

EXPOSURE OF THE ELBOW JOINT AND THE HEAD OF THE RADIUS THROUGH AN INCISION BETWEEN THE ANCONEUS AND THE EXTENSOR CARPI ULNARIS MUSCLES

Indication: 1. Excision of the Head of the Radius

2. Excison of Loose Bodies

Plate 55: Description of Procedure

A The skin incision starts at the lateral epicondyle of the humerus and extends obliquely downward over the interval between the anconeus and the extensor carpi ulnaris muscles, terminating near the ulna.

B The skin margins are retracted, the fascia is opened between the anconeus and the extensor carpi ulnaris, and the dissection is extended down to the capsule.

C The muscles are retracted to their respective sides of the incision. The tendon of the anconeus is sectioned to obtain more room and permit wider retraction of this muscle.

D A longitudinal incision is made into the capsule to expose the head of the radius and the adjacent portion of the capitellum.

NOTE: No important nerves are encountered in this incision. The anconeus receives its nerve supply at its superior margin; the extensor carpi ulnaris is supplied by the dorsal interosseus nerve which lies distal and lateral to the incision.

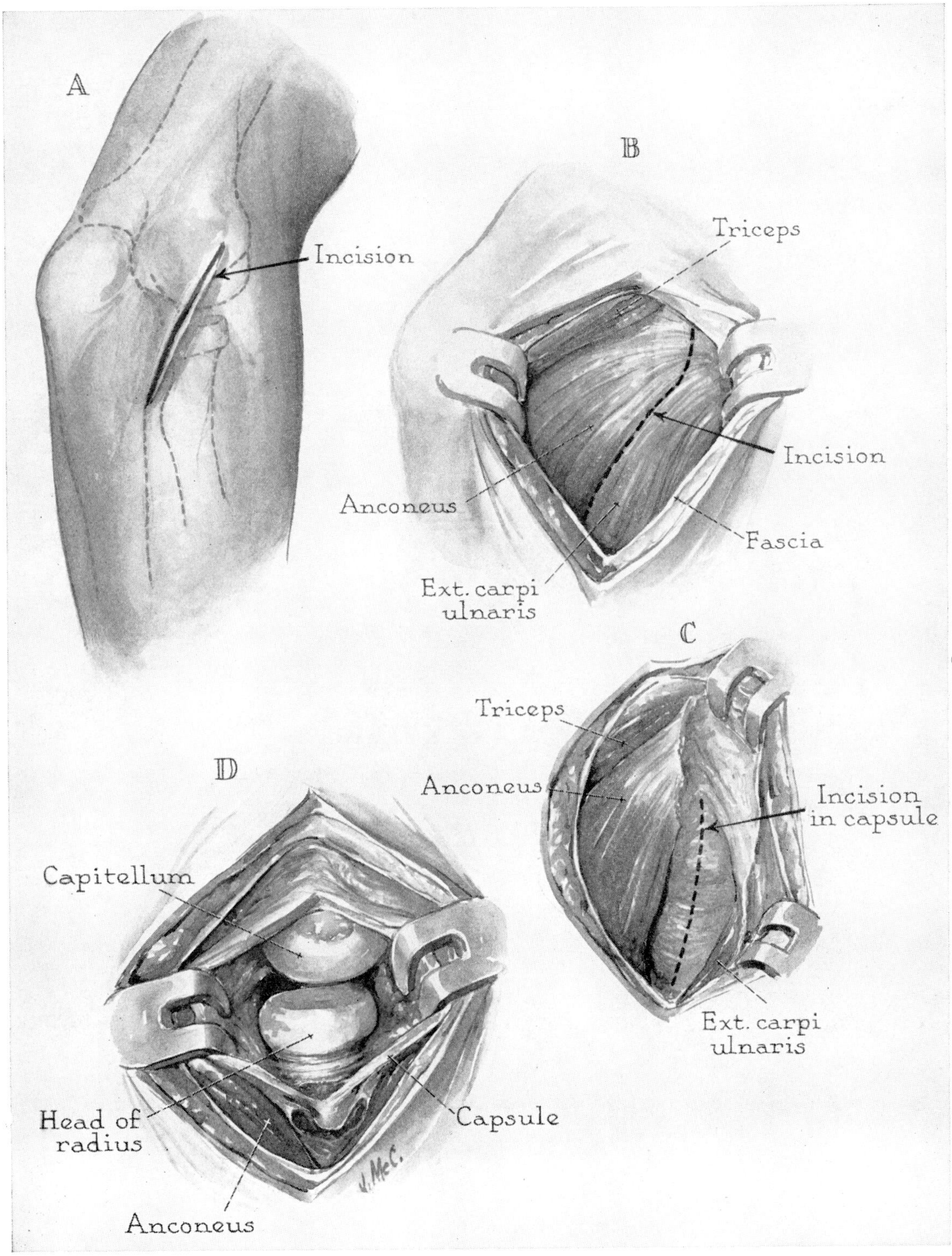

Exposure of the elbow joint and the head of the radius through an incision between the anconeus and the extensor carpi ulnaris muscles

EXPOSURE OF THE HEAD OF THE RADIUS AND THE ELBOW JOINT THROUGH A LATERAL INCISION BETWEEN THE ANCONEUS AND EXTENSOR CARPI ULNARIS MUSCLES, WITH SUBPERIOSTEAL DISSECTION OF THE LATERAL EPICONDYLAR RIDGE

Indications: 1. Resection of the Head of the Radius

2. Removal of Loose Bodies from the Elbow Joint

3. Reduction of a Fracture of the Lateral Condyle of the Humerus

Plate 56: Description of Procedure

A The incision is made along the interval between the anconeus and the extensor carpi ulnaris muscles, extending from the lateral epicondyle of the humerus to the crest of the ulna. It can be continued upward over the lateral epicondylar ridge, if deemed necessary for adequate exposure of the interior of the elbow joint.

B Anconeus and extensor carpi ulnaris muscles are next brought into view by opening and retracting the deep fascia, and the interval between these two muscles is developed down to the capsule of the elbow joint. It will be necessary to cut across the anconeus muscle proximally, as indicated in the illustration.

C The anconeus muscle is then retracted backward and the extensor carpi ulnaris muscle downward and forward. A linear incision is made in the capsule, extending from the lateral epicondyle to the lower end of the wound. (Procedure continued on Plate 57.)

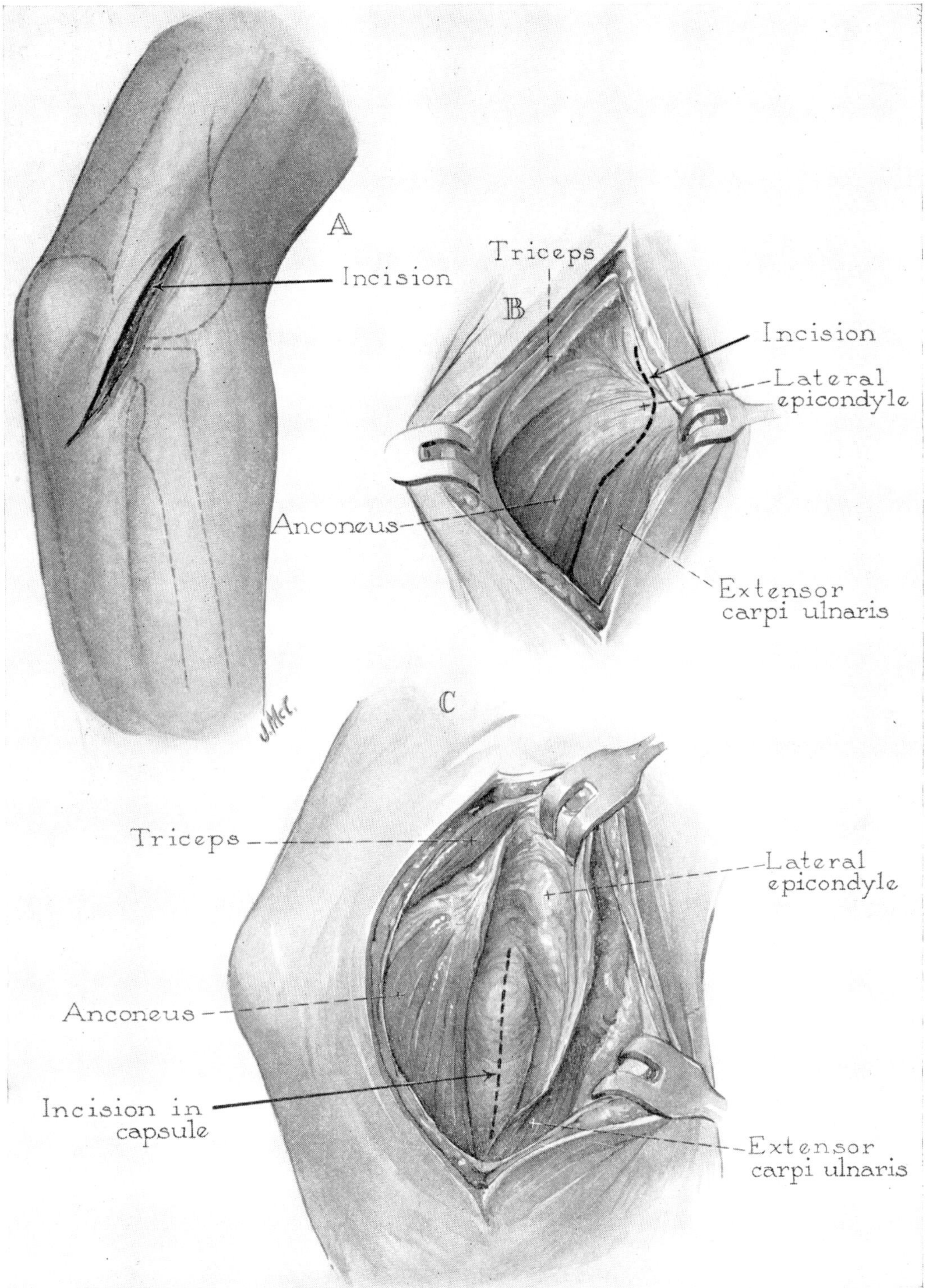

Exposure of the head of the radius and the elbow joint through a lateral incision between the anconeus and extensor carpi ulnaris muscles, with subperiosteal dissection of the lateral epicondylar ridge

EXPOSURE OF THE HEAD OF THE RADIUS AND THE ELBOW JOINT THROUGH A LATERAL INCISION BETWEEN THE ANCONEUS AND EXTENSOR CARPI ULNARIS MUSCLES, WITH SUBPERIOSTEAL DISSECTION OF THE LATERAL EPICONDYLAR RIDGE *(Continued)*

Plate 57: Description of Procedure

D The head of the radius, the capitellum and the annular ligament are exposed in the wound. This exposure will permit excision of the head of the radius, treatment of fractured fragments or other pathological lesions of the capitellum, and removal of loose bodies from the joint. This exposure does not suffice for the removal of loose bodies from the most medial and superior aspects of the joint, or for the repair of fractures involving the lateral condyle of the humerus. For these the incision must be extended upward, as shown in the illustrations. The soft tissues and the lateral collateral ligament of the elbow joint are raised from the lateral epicondyle and epicondylar ridge.

E The dissection is then continued subperiosteally in front and back of the humerus to obtain the desired exposure of the lower end of this bone as well as of the interior of the joint, the coronoid process and the head of the radius. In closing the wound, the soft tissues are sutured in layers without attempting to reattach them to bone.

NOTE: No important nerves or vessels are encountered in the wound. The radial nerve courses below the brachioradialis muscle and along the front of the anterior lateral portion of the capsule; it must not be injured.

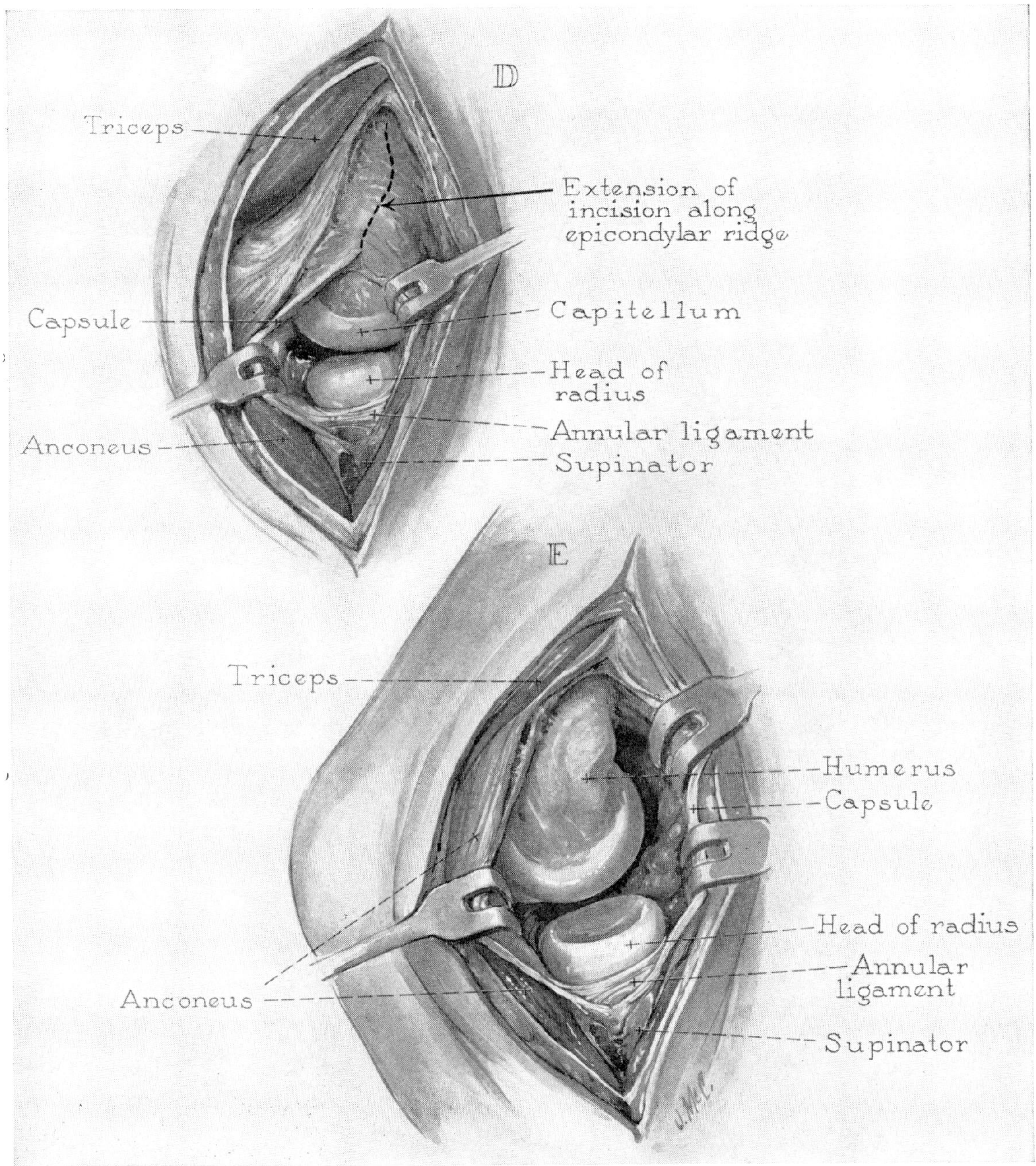

Exposure of the head of the radius and the elbow joint through a lateral incision between the anconeus and extensor carpi ulnaris muscles, with subperiosteal dissection of the lateral epicondylar ridge

EXPOSURE OF THE ELBOW JOINT THROUGH A LATERAL INCISION BETWEEN THE ANCONEUS AND EXTENSOR CARPI ULNARIS MUSCLES, WITH SUBPERIOSTEAL DISSECTION OF THE EPICONDYLAR RIDGE AND ADJACENT PORTION OF THE HUMERUS, RADIUS AND ULNA

Indications: 1. Resection of the Elbow Joint

2. Arthroplasty of the Elbow Joint

3. Arthrodesis of the Elbow Joint

Plate 58: Description of Procedure

A The incision begins over the lateral aspect of the distal third of the humerus and then extends downward over the epicondylar ridge, the epicondyle and the capsule of the elbow joint; it next continues along the interval between the anconeus and the extensor carpi ulnaris muscles and ends medially to the subcutaneous margin of the ulna.

B The skin is mobilized sufficiently to permit wide retraction. The fascia is opened in line with the skin incision.

C The periosteum is incised along the lateral epicondylar ridge and adjacent humerus. The brachioradialis muscle is seen anteriorly, and the triceps muscle posteriorly. The dissection proceeds distally through the tendon of the anconeus and the extensor carpi ulnaris muscles. The lower fibers of the anconeus muscles are severed as the incision turns posteriorly and crosses the ulna. The supinator now is exposed at the lower end of the wound between the latter two muscles.

D A wide exposure of the distal extremity of the humerus is obtained by reflecting the muscles and periosteum. At the same time, the capsule is detached from the humerus and then is retracted forward together with the lateral collateral ligament, thereby exposing the head of the radius and the interior of the joint. (Procedure continued on Plate 59.)

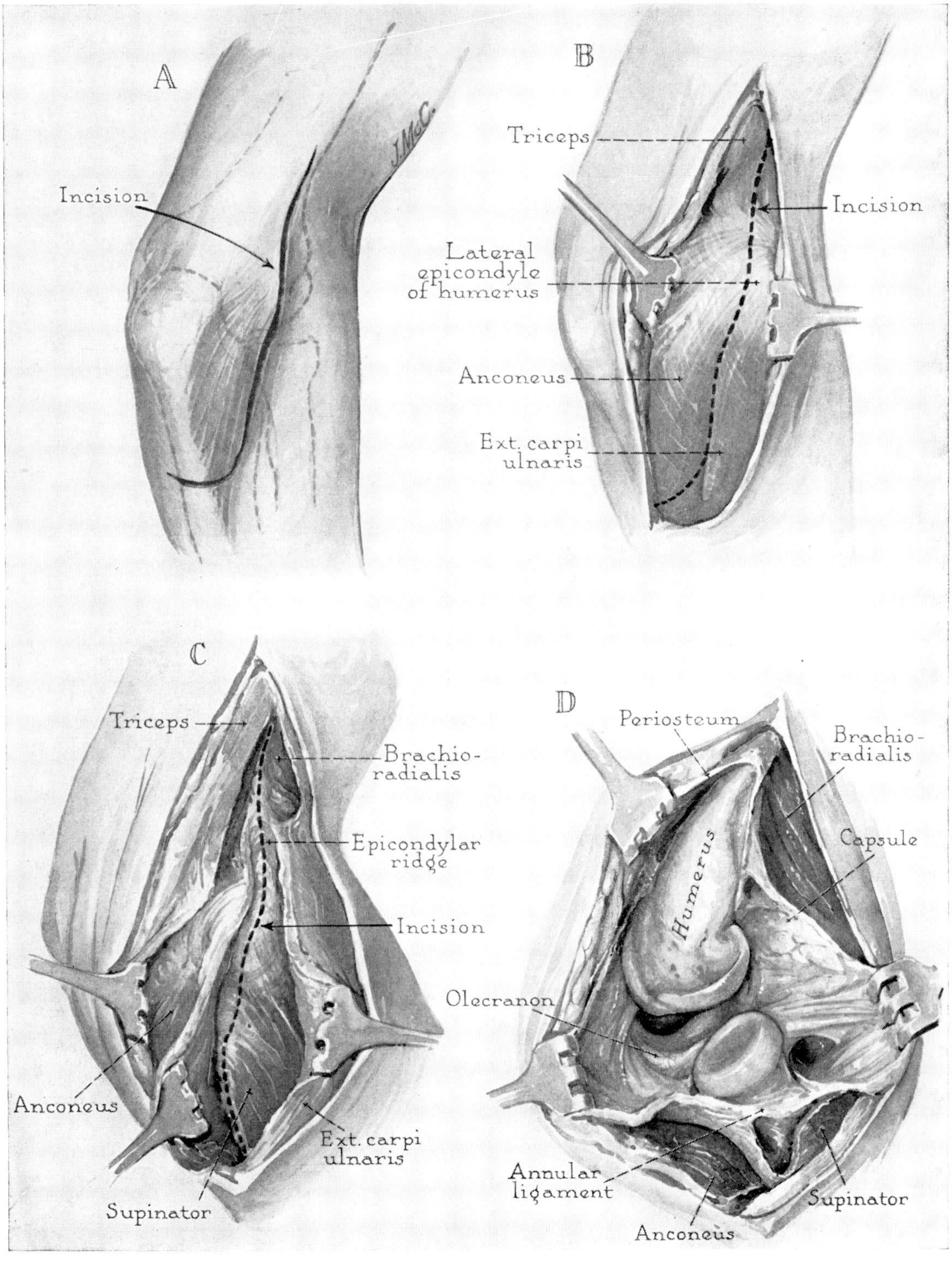

Exposure of the elbow joint through a lateral incision between the anconeus and extensor carpi ulnaris muscles, with subperiosteal dissection of the epicondylar ridge and the adjacent portion of the humerus, radius and ulna

EXPOSURE OF THE ELBOW JOINT THROUGH A LATERAL INCISION BETWEEN THE ANCONEUS AND EXTENSOR CARPI ULNARIS MUSCLES, WITH SUBPERIOSTEAL DISSECTION OF THE EPICONDYLAR RIDGE AND THE ADJACENT PORTION OF THE HUMERUS, RADIUS AND ULNA *(Continued)*

Plate 59: Description of Procedure

E A still wider exposure of the elbow joint and of the adjacent portion of the humerus, the ulna and radius can be obtained by dislocating the elbow joint laterally, as illustrated. The olecranon process is next denuded of soft tissues; the anconeus is raised subperiosteally from the ulna and reflected posteriorly together with the triceps tendon. The supinator muscle is reflected from the side of the ulna and retracted downward and forward. The annular ligament may be cut to uncover the neck of the radius; the adjacent shaft can be exposed subperiosteally. No important nerves are cut by this incision. The radial nerve is located medially to the brachioradialis muscle, and its dorsal interosseous branch runs through and is protected by the supinator muscle. The ulnar nerve courses along the medial aspect of the olecranon and must be isolated if the dissection extends to it. The nerve supply to the anconeus from the radial is not endangered by the incision, since it enters the superior aspect of the muscle. The wound is closed easily by suturing the layers in their respective order. It may be noted that this incision is less popular today than the direct posterior approach with tenotomy of the triceps tendon, or osteotomy of the olecranon process.

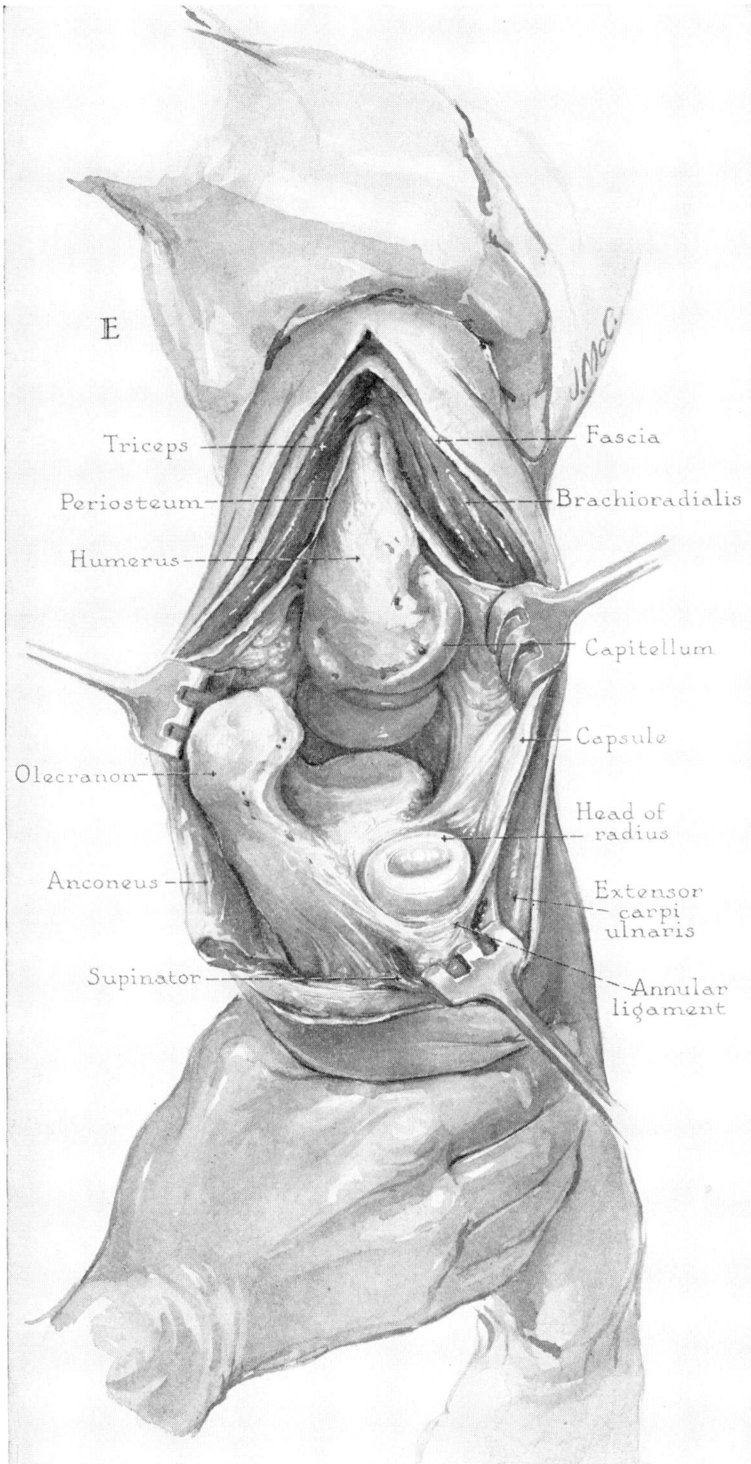

Exposure of the elbow joint through a lateral incision between the anconeus and the extensor carpi ulnaris muscles, with subperiosteal dissection of the epicondylar ridge and the adjacent portion of the humerus, radius and ulna

EXPOSURE OF THE ELBOW JOINT THROUGH A POSTERIOR LONGITUDINAL INCISION WITH OSTEOTOMY OF THE OLECRANON PROCESS

Indications: 1. Arthroplasty of the Elbow Joint

2. Open Reduction of Comminuted Fractures of the Distal End of the Humerus

Plate 60: Description of Procedure

A The incision starts about 3 inches distal to the tip of the olecranon process and then extends upward for the desired distance, while being centered over the dorsal margin of this process and the triceps tendon. The skin and deep fascia are undercut as far as the medial and lateral epicondyles of the humerus.

B The ulnar nerve is located along the medial margin of the triceps muscle, posterior to the medial intermuscular septum. Placing a hernia tape around the nerve will facilitate its careful handling. The nerve then is dissected free from the surrounding tissues for the entire length of the wound. The olecranon process distal to the triceps insertion is exposed subperiosteally.

C The olecranon is osteotomized 1 inch distal to its tip, and the proximal fragment is lifted upward to expose the interior of the joint.

D The next incision is made along the lateral margin of the triceps tendon, up to the lateral epicondyle. The tendon is thus separated from the anconeus muscle radially, and then the capsule and synovia are opened, as shown in the illustration. A similar incision is made along the medial margin of the triceps tendon, up to the medial epicondyle, followed by the cutting of the capsule and synovia of this portion of the joint. The interior of the elbow joint is thus made completely accessible. The posterior surface of the distal fourth of the humerus can be exposed to view similarly by raising the triceps muscle subperiosteally and retracting it upward. On closing the wound, it is of the utmost importance that the olecranon process be restored accurately and that the ulnar nerve be transplanted anteriorly to the elbow. If the osteotomized portion of the olecranon is small, it may be excised and the triceps tendon reattached to the proximal end of the remaining part of the process.

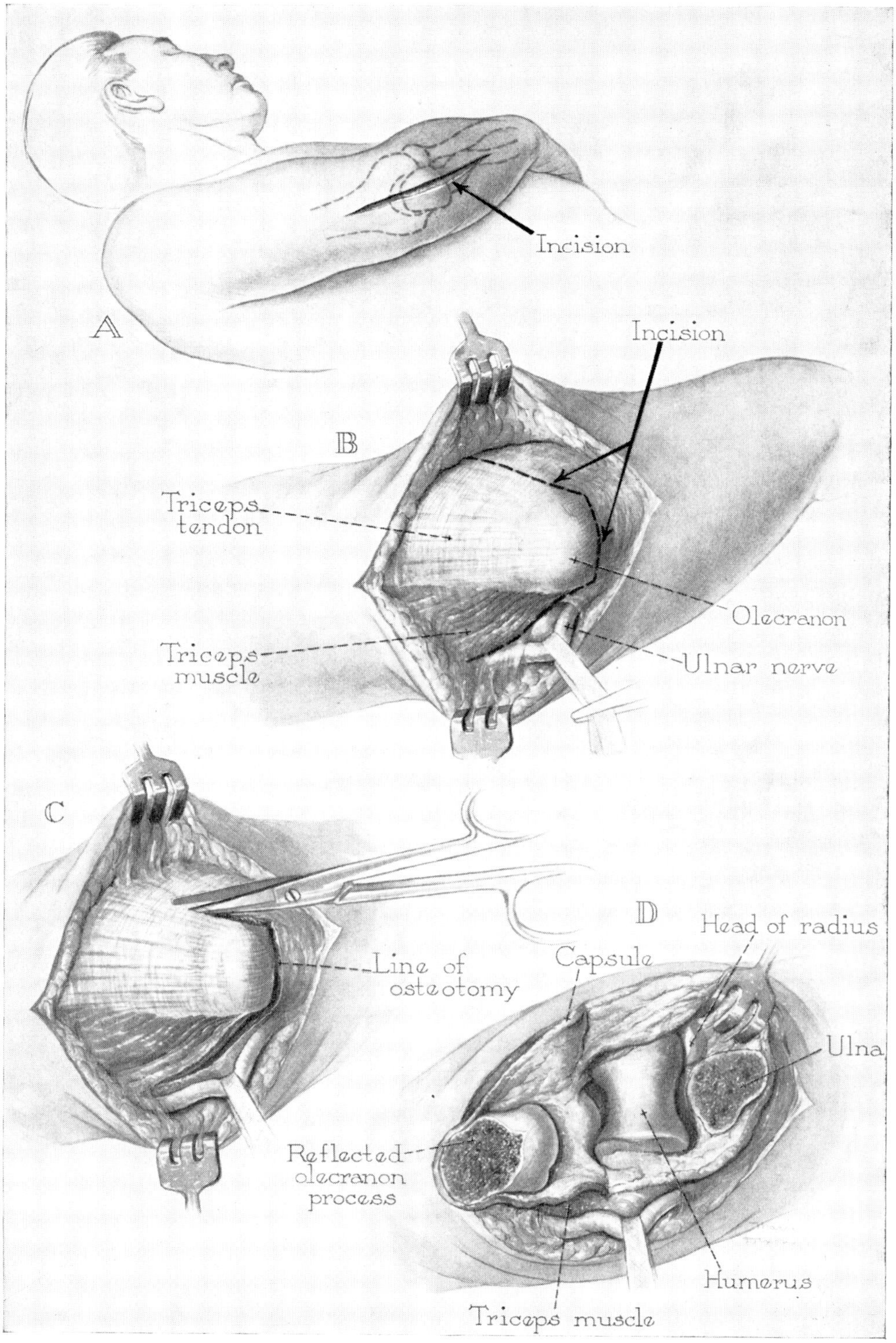

Exposure of the elbow joint through a posterior longitudinal incision with osteotomy of the olecranon process

EXPOSURE OF THE ELBOW JOINT THROUGH A POSTERIOR ULNAR INCISION WITH LATERAL REFLECTION OF THE ANCONEUS AND THE SUPINATOR MUSCLES

Indication: 1. Excision of the Head of the Radius

Plate 61: Description of Procedure

A The incision centers over the subcutaneous dorsal margin of the ulna and extends from the olecranon process to a point 3 inches distal to it.

B The fascia is incised, and the radial skin and fascial flap are widely mobilized to expose the anconeus muscle.

C This muscle together with the supinator which lies beneath it is separated from the side of the ulna and interosseous membrane so that they can be retracted far radialward.

D The posterior capsule of the elbow joint is identified and incised along the line shown in Illustration C, to expose the head of the radius and the articular surface of the capitellum. The neck and adjacent portion of the radius may be bared by mobilizing the anconeus and supinator muscles in the distal part of the wound. The dorsal interosseous nerve transverses the supinator muscle and must not be injured.

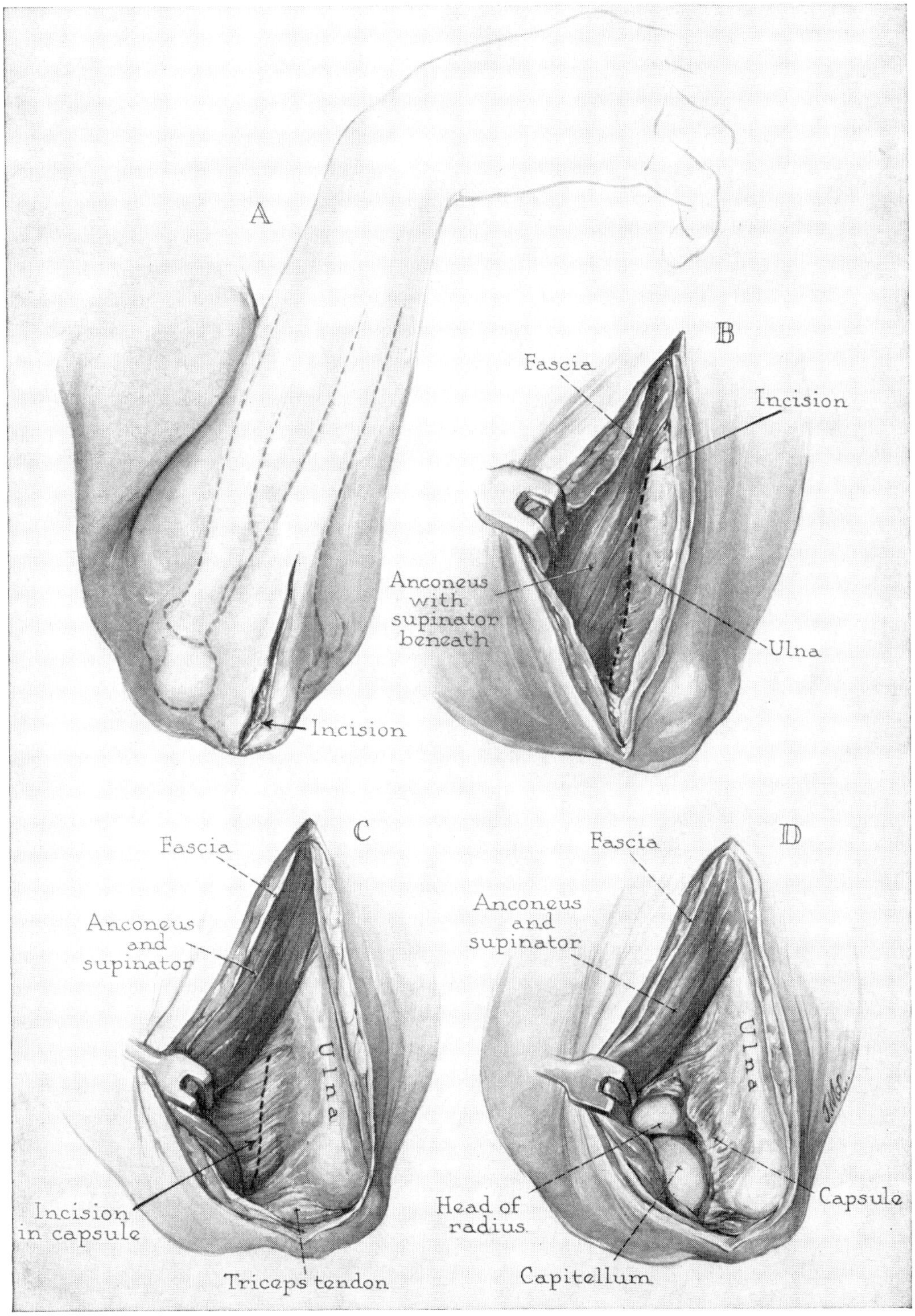

Exposure of the elbow joint through a posterior ulnar incision with lateral reflection of the anconeus and supinator muscles

EXPOSURE OF THE PROXIMAL END OF THE RADIUS, INCLUDING THE ELBOW JOINT AND THE UPPER THIRD OF THE ULNA, THROUGH A POSTERIOR ULNAR INCISION

Indications: 1. Treatment of Recent Fractures ot the Ulna with Dislocation of the Radius, or a Fracture of the Head of the Radıus

2. Treatment of a Pseudo-arthrosis of the Ulna with An Associated Chronic Dislocation of the Radius

Plate 62: Description of Procedure

A An incision, extending from the olecranon process to a point approximately 4 inches distal to it, is made along the crest of the ulna. The skin margins are undercut and retracted.

B The next incision is along the subcutaneous margin of the ulna and reaches to the bone by cutting through the fascia and the periosteum.

C The flexor carpi ulnaris muscle is retracted medially while the corresponding surface of the shaft of the ulna and the olecranon process are exposed subperiosteally. The anconeus and supinator muscle are reflected laterally as far as possible from the surface of the ulna and the interosseous membrane, to permit exposure of the posterior surface of the elbow joint. A longitudinal opening is made in the capsule to bring into view the head of the radius, the annular liament and the capitellum.

NOTE: The ulnar nerve is located just medial to the olecranon process and must not be injured when it is retracted with the flexor carpi ulnaris muscle which protects it

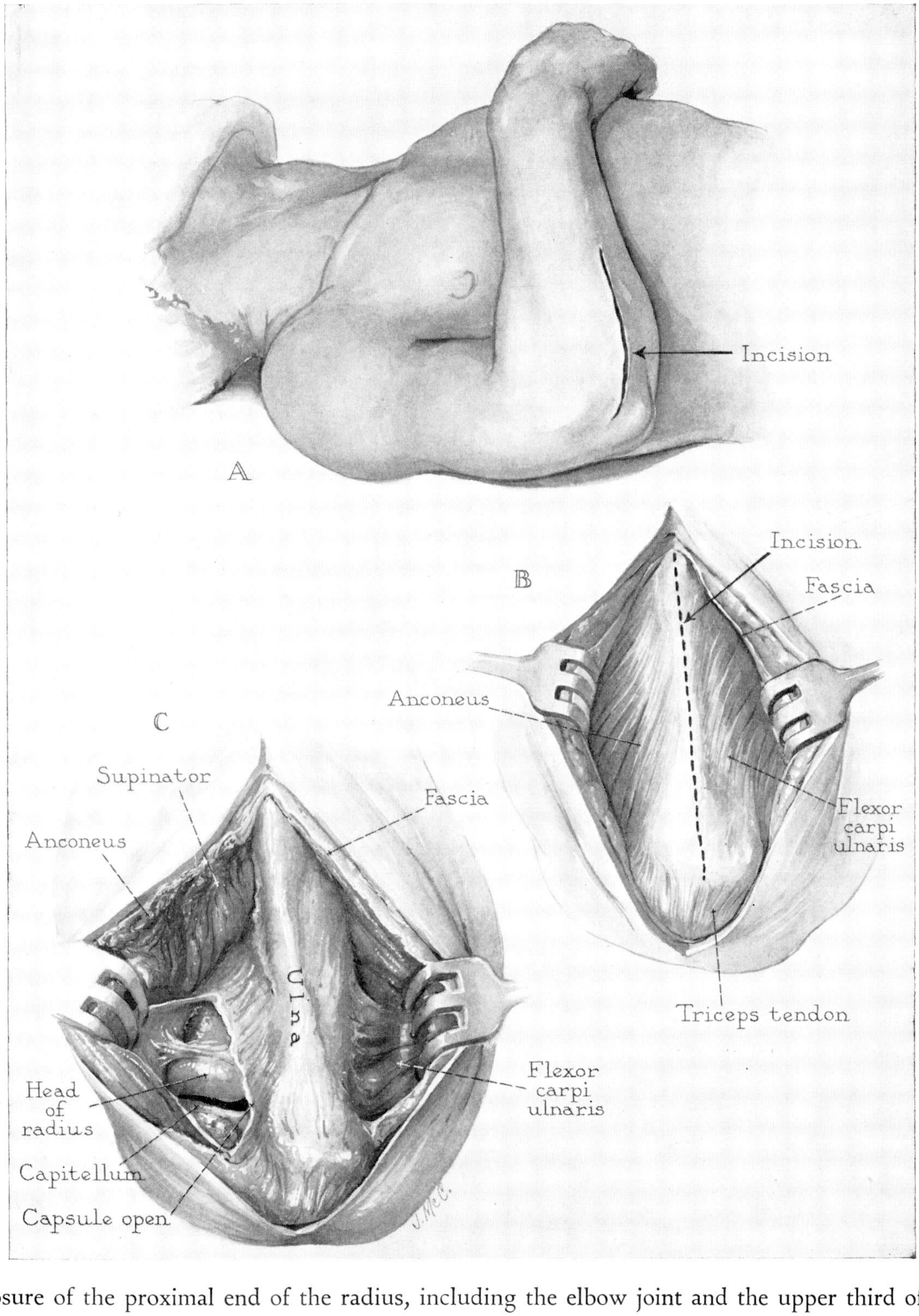

Exposure of the proximal end of the radius, including the elbow joint and the upper third of the ulna, through a posterior ulnar incision

EXPOSURE OF THE RADIAL NERVE AT THE ELBOW JOINT THROUGH AN ANTERIOR LATERAL INCISION

Indication: 1. Neurolysis or Suture of the Radial Nerve

Plate 63: Description of Procedure

A The incision begins 3 inches above the anterolateral aspect of the elbow joint and extends 3 inches distal to the flexion crease, by following along the anterior margin of the brachioradialis muscle. The lateral portion of the flexion crease is avoided as shown in the illustration.

B The fascia is opened above to expose the brachioradialis laterally, and the biceps and brachialis muscles medially. A retractor is placed on the anterior margin of the brachioradialis, and this muscle is lifted laterally away from the biceps. The proximal third of the wound is then developed through the areolar tissue which separates the two muscles, thereby giving access to the anterior surface of the humerus. Distally, the deep approach is made between the biceps tendon and pronator teres muscle medially, and the brachioradialis muscle laterally.

C The radial nerve courses deep in the wound along the inner surface of the brachioradialis muscle, and superficial to the humerus but lateral to the brachialis muscle. Care must be taken not to injure the branches of the radial nerve which enter the brachioradialis muscle. At the level of the supinator muscle, the radial nerve divides into its two terminal branches, one sensory and one motor. The sensory branch proceeds distally beneath the brachioradialis muscle and emerges on the dorsum of the wrist to supply a portion of the skin. The motor, or dorsal interosseous, branch passes through the supinator muscle and then reaches the dorsum of the forearm where it supplies the extensors of the wrist, fingers and thumb. The muscular branches of the radial artery which cross the field may be ligated. The recurrent radial artery passes upward and posteriorly (as illustrated), and can be spared.

NOTE: The lateral antibrachial cutaneous nerve which emerges from below and laterally to the biceps tendon is not illustrated; it must not, however, be injured.

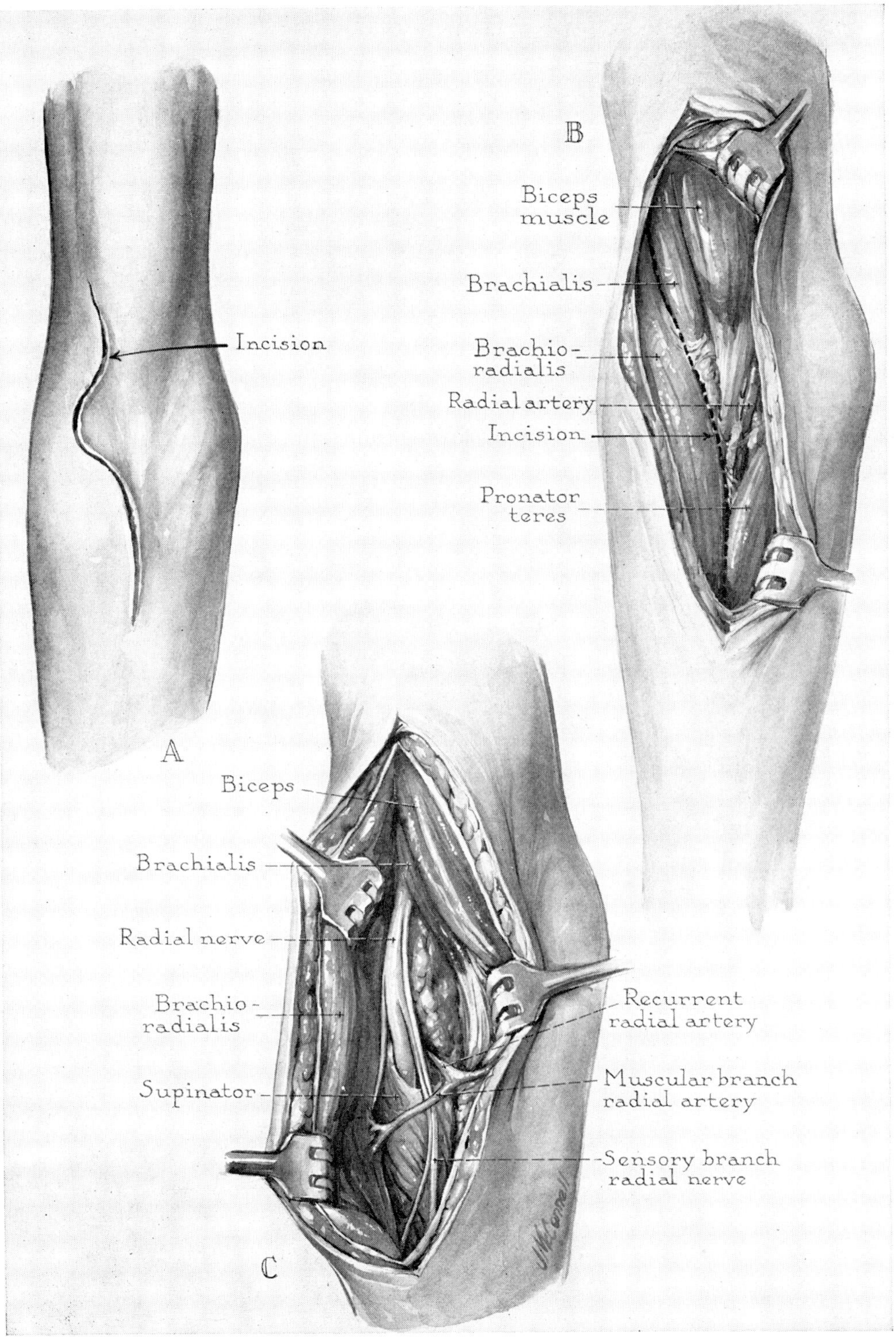

Exposure of the radial nerve at the elbow joint through an anterior lateral incision

EXPOSURE OF THE MEDIAN NERVE ANTERIOR TO THE ELBOW JOINT AND IN THE PROXIMAL PORTION OF THE FOREARM

Indication: 1. Repair of Lacerations of the Median Nerve, Recent and Old

Plate 64: Description of Procedure

A The incision begins approximately 1 1/2 inches above the flexion crease of the elbow joint, over the interval between the biceps tendon and the pronator teres muscle. It then turns laterally at the joint level and continues, along a prominent skin crease, to the brachioradialis muscle where it is gently directed downward along the medial margin of this muscle, for a distance of approximately 2 1/2 inches. Straight-line incisions across the joint must be avoided because they give rise to flexion contractures.

B The skin flaps are widely mobilized and the fascia is cut in line with the skin incision. The lateral antibrachial cutaneous nerve emerges from beneath the biceps tendon and then is distributed to the skin over the radial half of the forearm; it must be preserved from injury. Next, the lacertus fibrosus is cut near the biceps tendon and the fascia is retracted with the skin. The interval between the biceps and pronator teres muscles is developed. The brachial artery with its accompanying veins, and also the median nerve, are identified. The nerve is dissected free of the surrounding structures as it is being exposed distally. The branches of the median nerve to the pronator teres muscle must be looked for but not cut. (Procedure continued on Plate 65.)

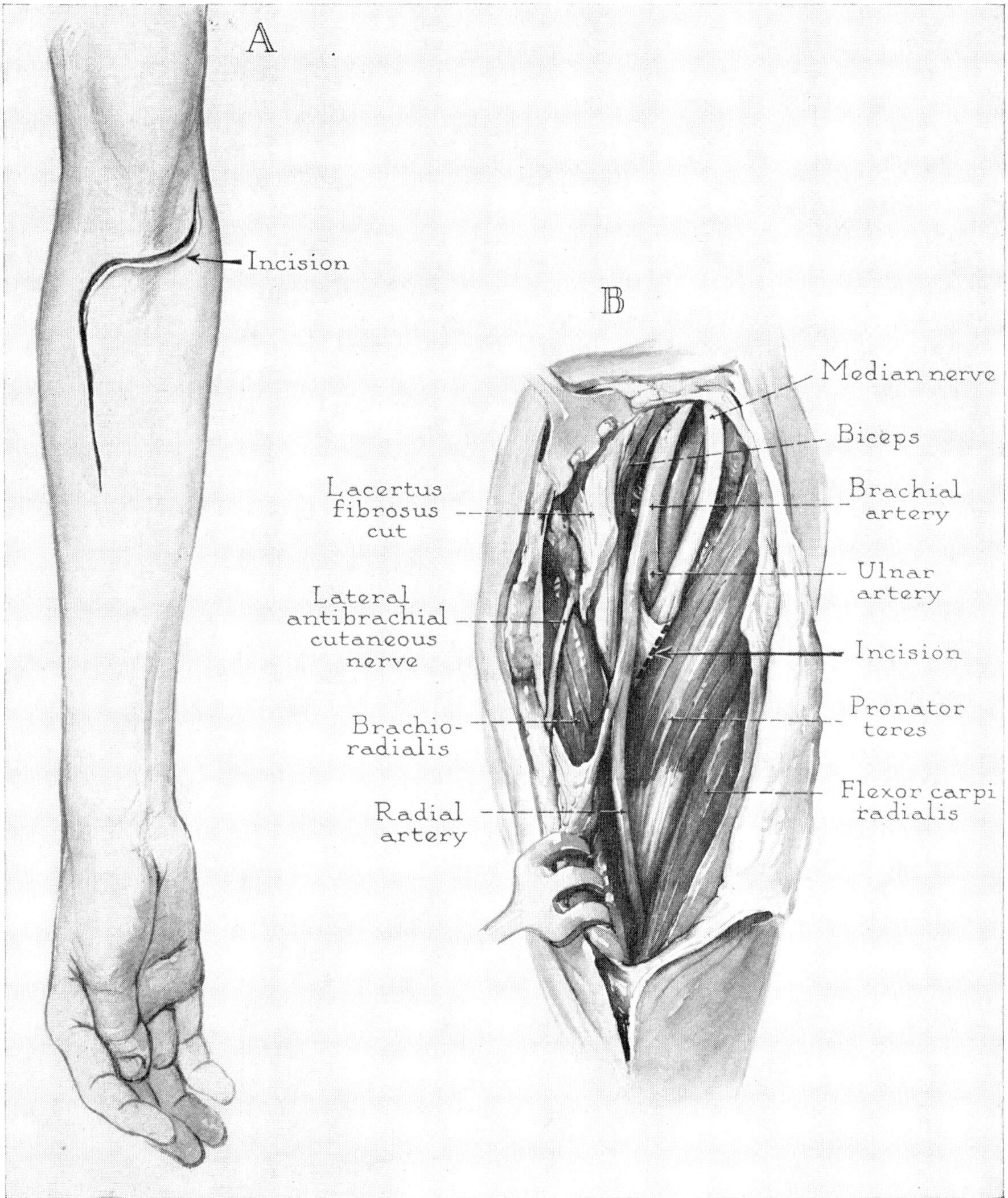

Exposure of the median nerve anterior to the elbow joint and in the proximal portion of the forearm

EXPOSURE OF THE MEDIAN NERVE ANTERIOR TO THE ELBOW JOINT AND IN THE PROXIMAL PORTION OF THE FOREARM (*Continued*)

Plate 65: Description of Procedure

C It should be noted that the median nerve disappears beneath the superior margin of the pronator teres near the midline. The brachial artery gives rise to the radial artery which passes distally and laterally to cross the pronator teres, and then enters the interval between the brachioradialis laterally and the flexor carpi radialis medially.

D The ulnar artery passes distally beneath the ulnar head of the pronator teres muscle. The two heads (ulnar and humeral) of the pronator teres are separated distally for a short distance, as shown in the illustration, in order to expose that portion of the median nerve which is located behind the junction of the two heads. Still more distally, the inferior margin of the pronator teres is separated from the flexor carpi radialis muscle, to afford additional exposure of the median nerve. This exposure of the nerve can, moreover, be continued distally beneath the flexor carpi radialis muscle and then deep to the flexor digitorum sublimis, for the length of the forearm.

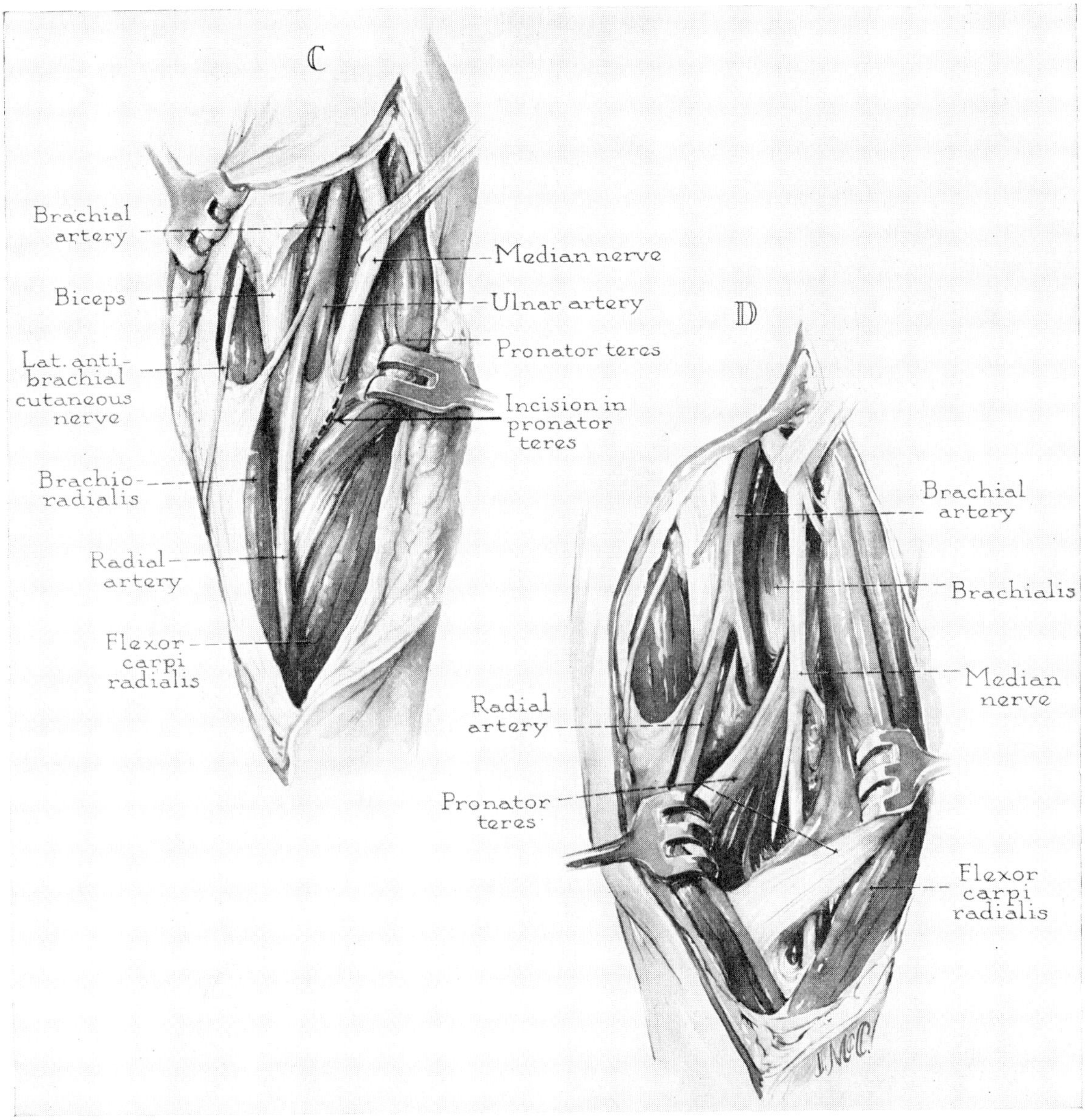

Exposure of the median nerve anterior to the elbow joint and in the proximal portion of the forearm

EXPOSURE OF THE ULNAR NERVE IN THE REGION OF THE ELBOW JOINT THROUGH A POSTERIOR MEDIAL INCISION

Indications: 1. Neurolysis of the Ulnar Nerve

2. Transplantation of the Ulnar Nerve

3. Suture of Lacerations of the Ulnar Nerve

Plate 66: Description of Procedure

A First, the ulnar groove is located between the posterior aspect of the medial epicondyle of the humerus and the olecranon process of the ulna. An incision some 4 inches long is centered over this groove.

B The skin margins are retracted and the deep fascia in the proximal end of the wound is opened in line with the skin incision. The ulnar nerve can be found in a longitudinal groove of the triceps muscle, just posteriorly to the medial intermuscular septum. A piece of tape is placed around this nerve to facilitate its careful handling. The fascia in the lower third of the wound is then opened over a grooved director.

C The sectioning of this fascial roof over the ulnar nerve must be done under direct vision, so that the nerve may be exposed without suffering injury. The dissection then continues distally between the two heads of the flexor carpi ulnaris muscle to a point where the nerve passes to the front of the forearm. Branches of the nerve are given off to the two portions of the flexor carpi ulnaris muscle exposed in the wound, and these must not be cut.

NOTE: The recurrent ulnar artery accompanies the ulnar nerve and may be sacrificed if necessary, although the nerve can usually be isolated without doing so.

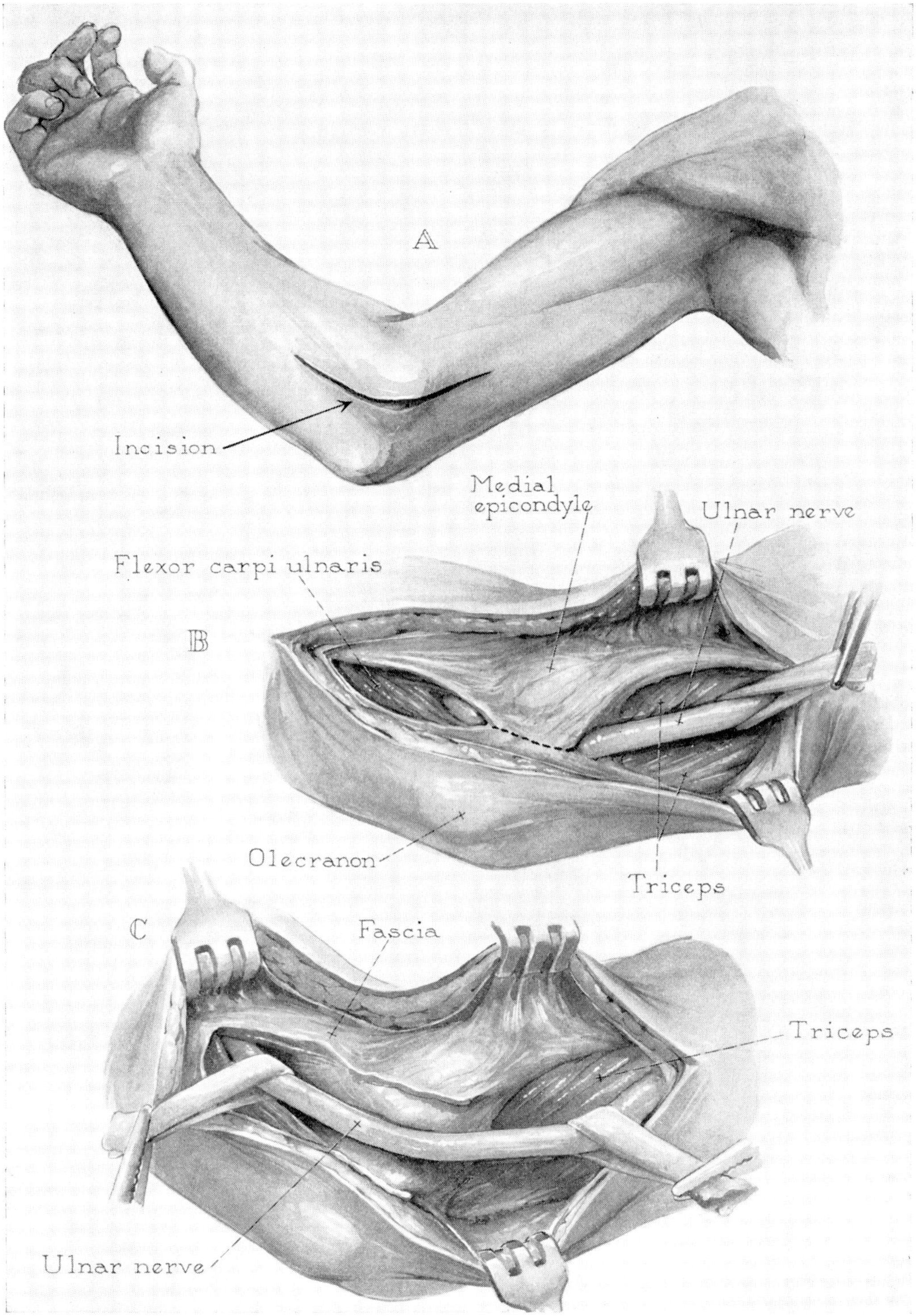

Exposure of the ulnar nerve in the region of the elbow joint through a posterior medial incision

EXPOSURE OF THE BRACHIAL ARTERY IN THE ANTECUBITAL FOSSA

Indications: 1. Ligation of the Brachial Artery

2. Embolectomy of the Brachial Artery

Sling Control of the Brachial Artery

Plate 67: Description of Procedure

A The S-shaped skin incision begins at the medial side of the biceps muscle and extends distally to the flexion crease of the elbow, which it follows before it extends distally for the desired distance. The incision is carried through the superficial fascia. Superficial veins may be ligated.

B The wound flaps are retracted and the tendon of the biceps muscle is identified. The next incision is made through the deep fascia along the medial aspect of the biceps muscle and the lacertus fibrosus.

C The brachial artery is located below the incised fascia and runs along the medial side of the biceps muscle. It is usually accompanied closely by two small veins, which must be separated from the artery and ligated if necessary. The median nerve lies medially to the artery. The artery can be retracted easily after it is separated from the surrounding structures.

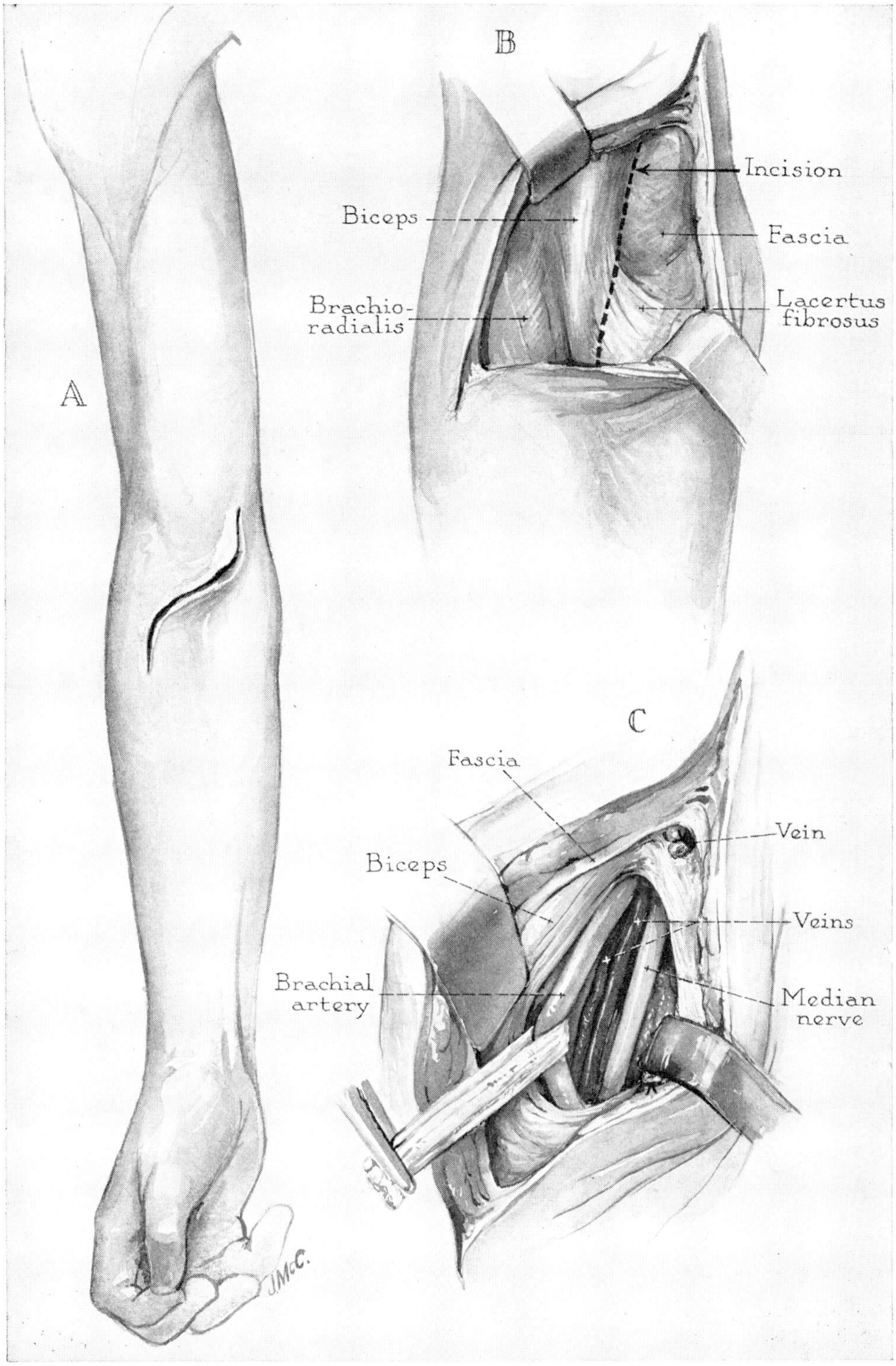

Exposure of the brachial artery in the antecubital fossa

Section V

Region of the Radius and Ulna

EXPOSURE OF THE PROXIMAL AND MIDDLE THIRDS OF THE RADIUS THROUGH AN ANTERIOR LATERAL INCISION

Indications: 1. Open Reduction of Fractures

2. Treatment of Un-united Fractures

3. Resection of Benign Tumors

4. Osteotomy of the Radius for Angular Deformity

Plate 68: Description of Procedure

A The skin incision begins directly distal to the flexion crease of the elbow and extends downward along the anterior margin of the brachioradialis muscle for a distance of approximately 7 inches.

B The fascia is opened and the anterior margin of the brachioradialis muscle is identified. The fascia over this muscle is incised the whole length of the wound, and the muscle is mobilized and retracted laterally. The superficial branch of the radial nerve lies beneath this muscle; it must be identified and protected.

C The pronator teres and the flexor carpi radialis muscles form the medial wall of the incision. Before retracting these muscles inward, it is necessary to identify and protect the radial artery which courses superficially along the margin of the medial flap. When the lateral side of the wound is retracted, the supinator muscle can be located in front of the radius and the proximal lateral aspect of the wound. The tendon of the pronator teres muscle is seen medial to it.

D An incision is made into the periosteum along the line of junction of the supinator and pronator teres muscles, and the bone is exposed by subperiosteal dissection. An effort should be made to preserve the insertion of the pronator teres muscle. If necessary, it can be raised from the radius, and replaced at the end of the operation.

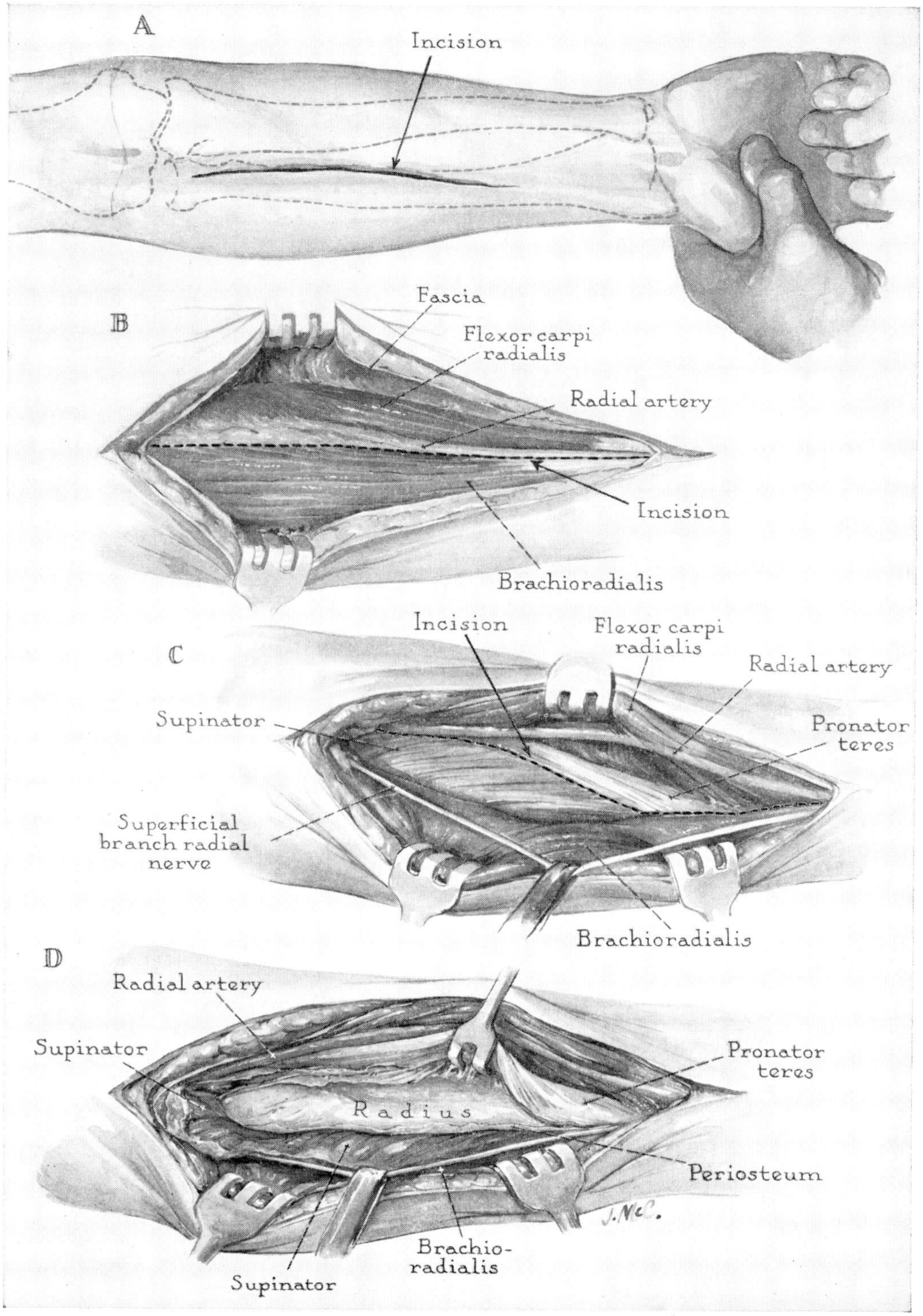

Exposure of the proximal and middle thirds of the radius through an anterior lateral incision

EXPOSURE OF THE DISTAL THIRD OF THE RADIUS THROUGH AN ANTERIOR LATERAL INCISION

Indications: 1. Open Reduction of Recent Fractures

2. Treatment of Non-union of the Radius

3. Repair of Partial and Complete Defects in the Radius

4. Partial Ostectomy for Osteomyelitis

5. Resection of Benign or Malignant Tumors

Plate 69: Description of Procedure

A The incision, about 5 1/2 inches long, begins in front of the radial styloid process, and extends upward in a straight line along the anterior margin of the brachioradialis muscle for the required distance. The fascia is incised in line with the incision and the flaps are mobilized and retracted. The tendon of the brachioradialis can be seen within its fascial sheath. The radial artery courses between this tendon and that of the flexor carpi radialis muscle medially, and must be identified.

B The radial artery is protected from injury by cutting the deep fascia along a line medial to the brachioradialis muscle over a grooved director. The tendon is retracted outward. The sensory branch of the radial nerve is beneath the brachioradialis muscle and must be kept uninjured. Radially to it is the tendon of the extensor carpi radialis longus muscle.

C The radial artery and vein and the flexor carpi radialis tendon are carefully mobilized and then retracted together medially, as illustrated. The flexor digitorum sublimis, the flexor pollicis longus and the pronator quadratus muscles are now exposed at the bottom of the wound. (Procedure continued on Plate 70.)

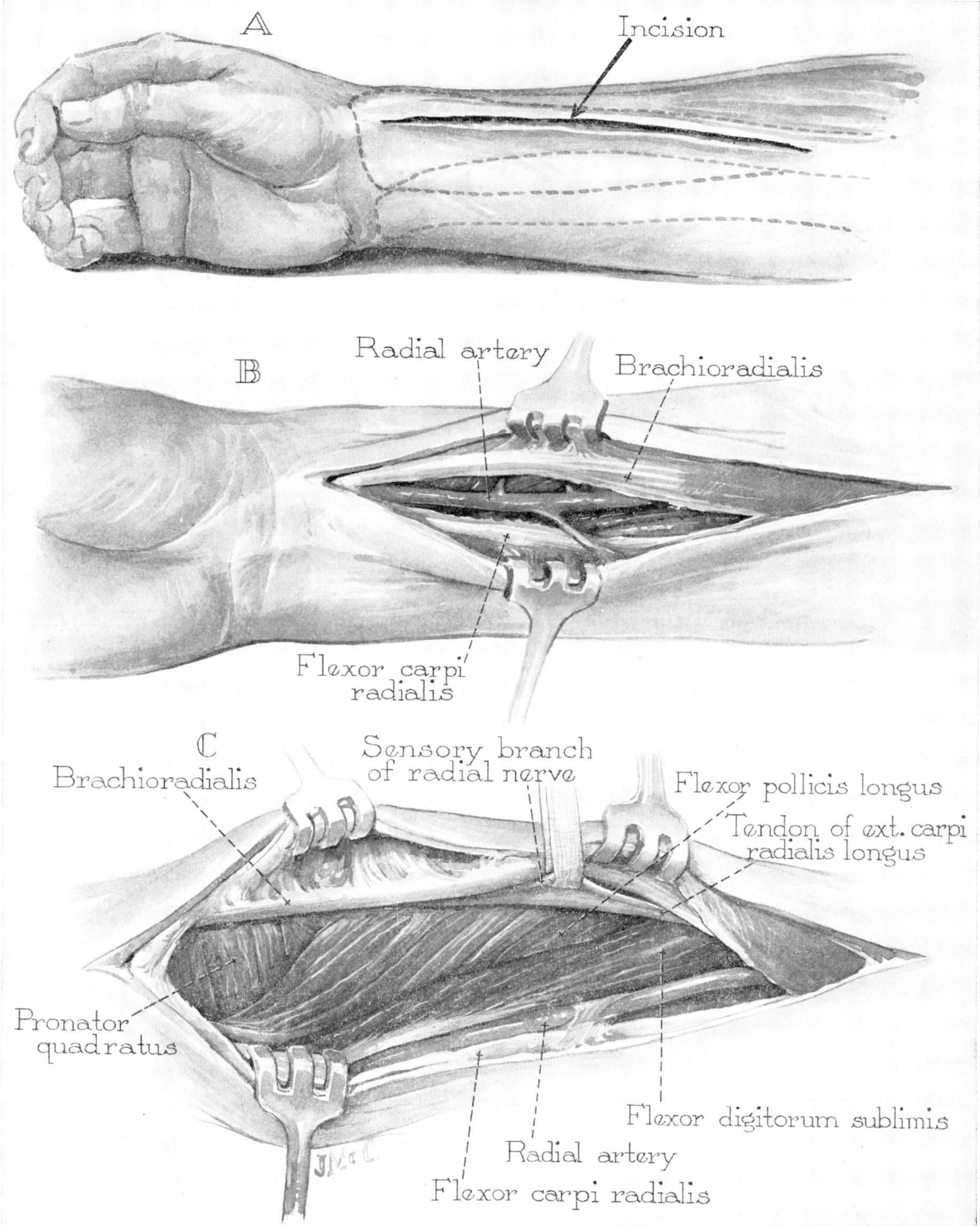

Exposure of the distal third of the radius through an anterior lateral incision

EXPOSURE OF THE DISTAL THIRD OF THE RADIUS THROUGH AN ANTERIOR LATERAL INCISION *(Continued)*

Plate 70: Description of Procedure

D The position of the forearm is changed from that of supination to pronation in order to bring that portion of the radius just lateral to the pronator quadratus and flexor pollicis longus muscles into the wound.

E The brachioradialis and the sensory branch of the radial nerve are retracted outward. A longitudinal incision is made into the periosteum of the radius along the interval between the line of origin of the pronator quadratus and the flexor pollicis longus muscles medially, and the extensor carpi radialis longus tendon laterally.

F The radius is exposed subperiosteally. A considerable portion of the bone can be brought successively into the operating field by alternate pronation and supination of the forearm.

NOTE: Closure of the incision is not easy, for great care must be taken not to injure the nerve and not to put excessive tension on the radial artery when suturing the fascia.

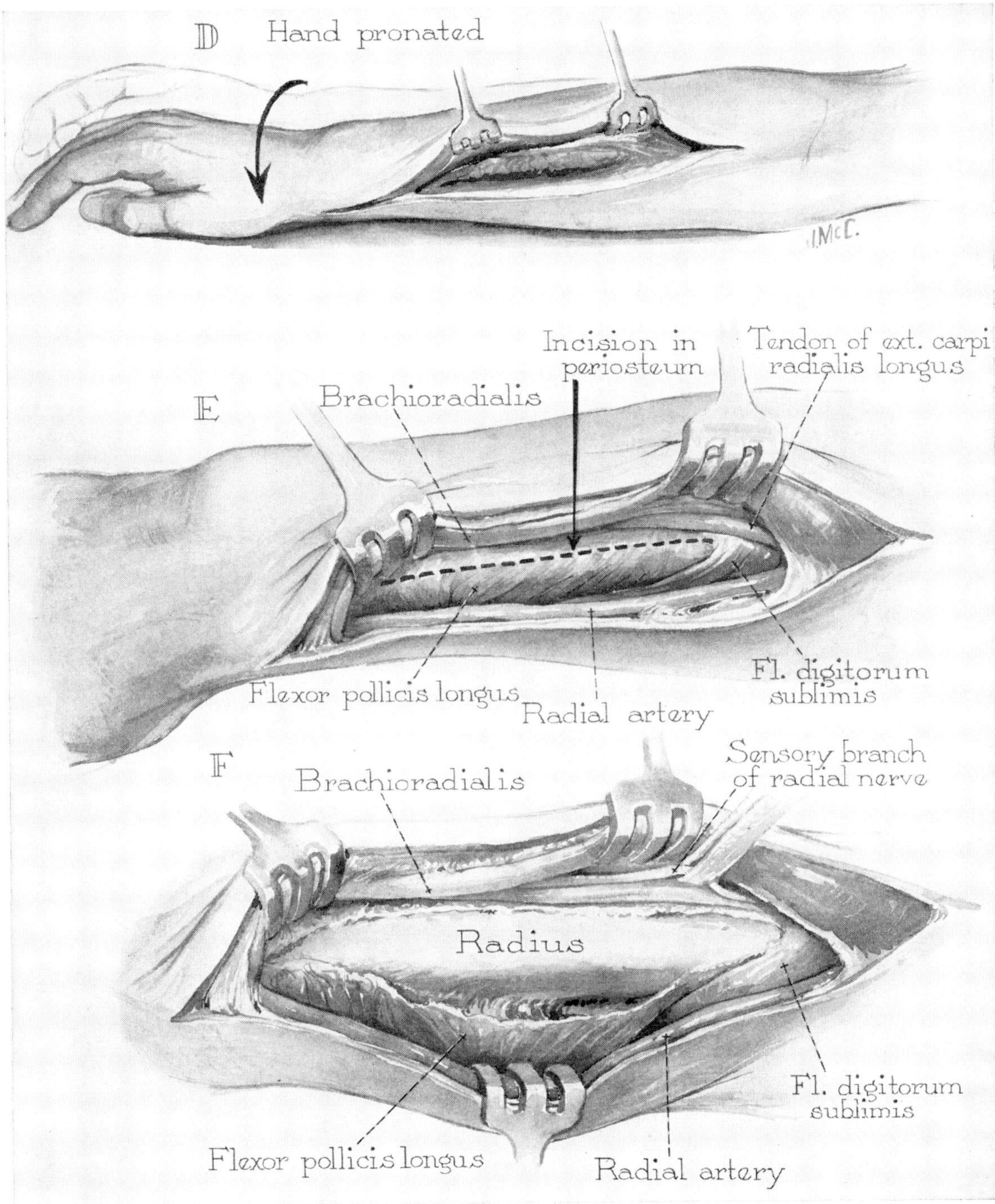

Exposure of the distal third of the radius through an anterior lateral incision

EXPOSURE OF THE PROXIMAL THIRD OF THE ULNA THROUGH AN ANTERIOR MEDIAL INCISION

Indication: 1. Resection of Benign Tumors or Other Lesions Which Cannot Be Exposed Adequately through a Posterior Incision

Plate 71: Description of Procedure

A The skin incision starts at the flexion crease of the elbow and then extends distally, for approximately 5 inches, over the anterior margin of the flexor carpi ulnaris muscle. More precisely, the incision is made in the area just described along a line drawn from the medial epicondyle of the humerus to the inner aspect of the styloid process of the ulna. The medial skin flap is retracted, which may bring into view branches of the medial antibrachial cutaneous nerve.

B The deep fascia is incised, and the interval between the margin of the flexor carpi ulnaris and the flexor digitorum sublimis is opened.

C The latter two muscles are then mobilized and retracted to their respective sides of the wound to expose the ulnar nerve, which has gained entrance to the anterior aspect of the forearm by passing forward through the two heads of the flexor carpi ulnaris muscle from the posterior aspect of the elbow joint. The flexor digitorum profundus muscle, upon which the nerve is located, is identified at the bottom of the wound. (Procedure continued on Plate 72.)

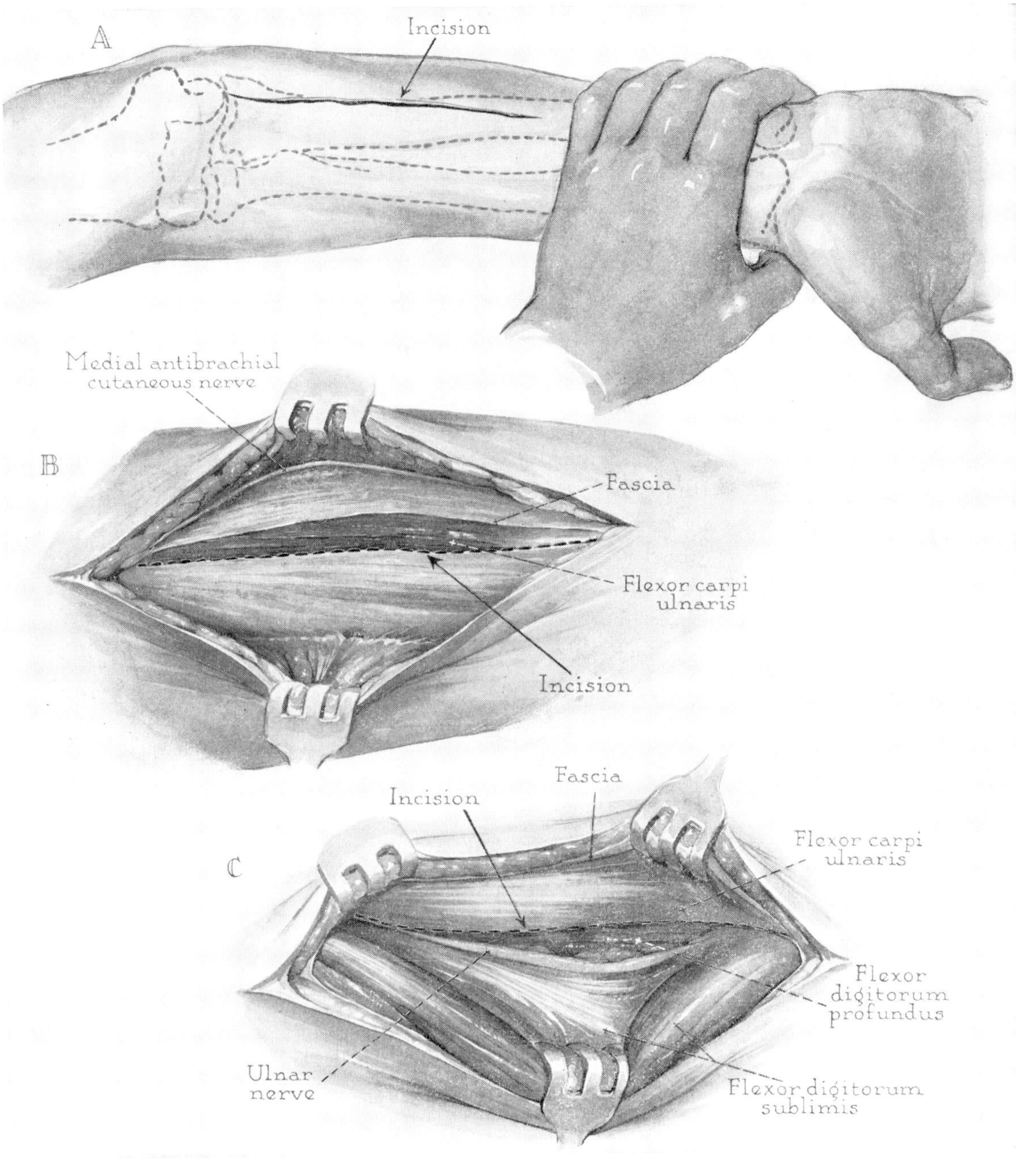

Exposure of the proximal third of the ulna through an anterior medial incision

EXPOSURE OF THE PROXIMAL THIRD OF THE ULNA THROUGH AN ANTERIOR MEDIAL INCISION *(Continued)*

Plate 72: Description of Procedure

D The flexor digitorum profundus is pulled radialward with a rake retractor to expose the junction between its most medial fibers and the adjacent fibers of the flexor carpi ulnaris muscle. The ulnar nerve is protected from injury, and the flexor digitorum sublimis is retracted radially to enlarge the wound. The ulnar artery is not encountered, although the ulnar recurrent artery accompanies the ulnar nerve in the most proximal portion of the exposure.

E An incision is next made into the periosteum directly beyond the margin of the flexor digitorum profundus, as marked in the illustration, and the muscle and periosteum are reflected away from the ulna to expose this bone. The flexor digitorum profundus muscle has a large fleshy belly which is difficult to retract without the use of periosteal elevators placed beneath the margin of the ulna, as shown.

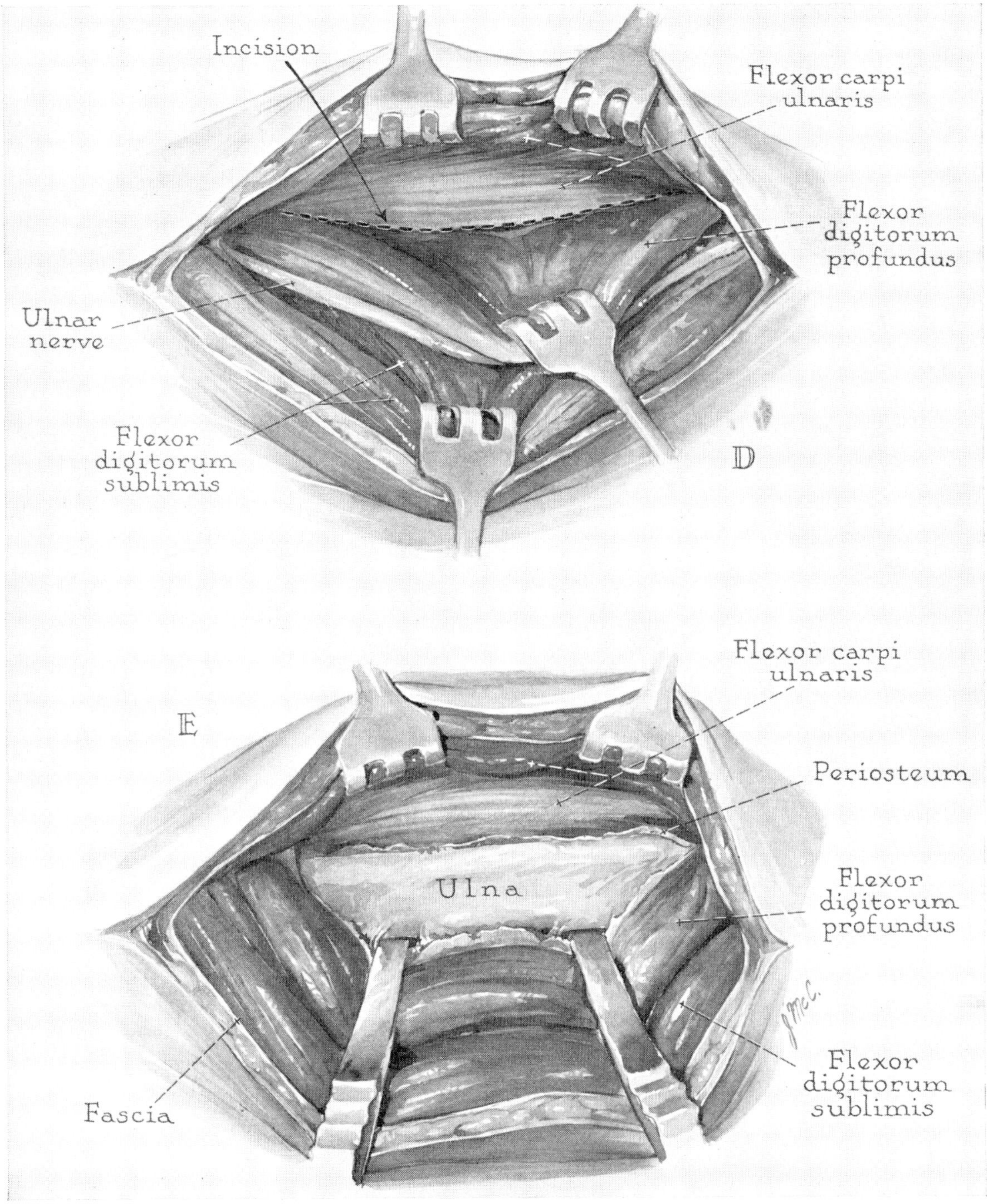

Exposure of the proximal third of the ulna through an anterior medial incision

EXPOSURE OF THE MIDDLE THIRD OF THE ULNA THROUGH AN ANTERIOR MEDIAL INCISION

Indication: 1. Excision of Benign Tumors of the Anterior Surface of the Ulna

Plate 73: Description of Procedure

A An incision approximately 5 inches long is made over the anterior medial aspect of the middle two-thirds of the forearm. The incision follows the anterior margin of the flexor carpi ulnaris muscle, which can be palpated easily throughout its entire length. The skin flaps are undermined and retracted.

B The deep fascia is opened in line with the skin incision and the flexor carpi ulnaris muscle is identified.

C The margin of the flexor carpi ulnaris is mobilized and the dissection is deepened between it and the flexor digitorum sublimis muscle, which is located beneath the radial flap of fascia. Care must be taken not to injure the ulnar nerve, which is situated just beneath and medial to the flexor carpi ulnaris muscle belly proximally, and its tendon distally. It is not necessary to disturb the nerve, but it must always be identified and kept under observation during the operation.

D The flexor carpi ulnaris is mobilized as far posteriorly as its attachment to the ulna, and is then lifted upward and retracted medially to expose the muscle belly of the flexor digitorum profundus. The latter muscle covers the anterior surface of the ulna. The bone is uncovered by separating the medial margin of the flexor digitorum profundus from the ulna and retracting it strongly to the radial side of the wound. The periosteum is incised along the midline of the ulna and reflected adequately to the sides.

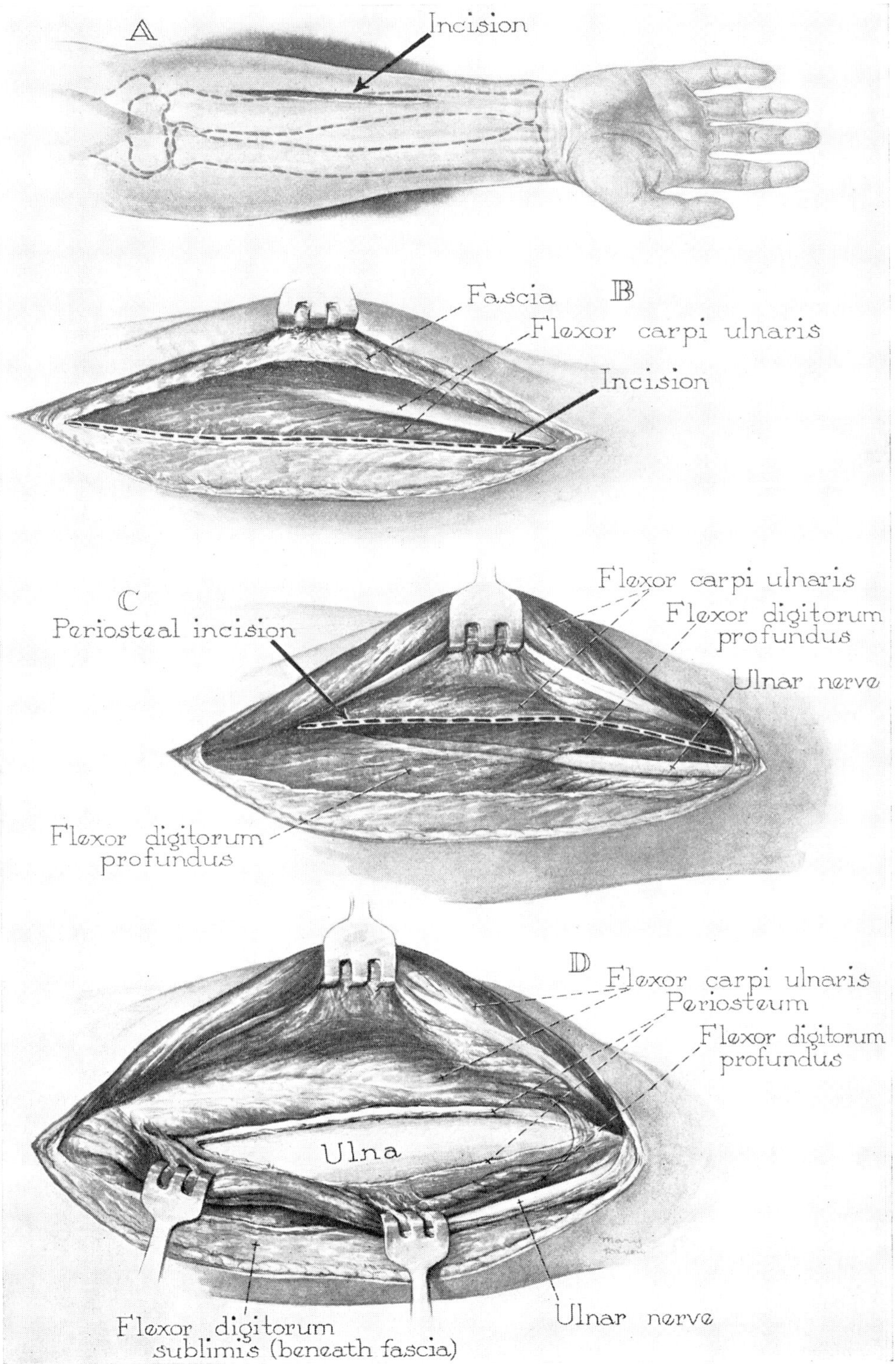

Exposure of the middle third of the ulna through an anterior medial incision

EXPOSURE OF THE ANTERIOR AND MEDIAL SURFACES OF THE MIDDLE THIRD OF THE ULNA THROUGH A POSTERIOR INCISION

Indications: 1. Resection for Benign Tumors

2. Partial Ostectomy for Osteomyelitis

Plate 74: Description of Procedure

A An incision is made along the inner aspect of the posterior subcutaneous border of the ulna and extended distally from the region of the olecranon process for the desired distance.

B The deep fascia is incised and the posterior margin of the flexor carpi ulnaris muscle is identified.

C The latter muscle is separated from the adjacent medial surface of the ulna and retracted anteriorly. The belly of the flexor digitorum profundus is now visible.

D The latter muscle is lifted subperiosteally from the anterior surface of the ulna.

NOTE: The ulnar nerve is not encountered unless the incision is extended so high as to expose the nerve between the two heads of the flexor carpi ulnaris muscle. Retraction of the tight muscle mass is best obtained by means of two periosteal elevators, as shown in the illustration.

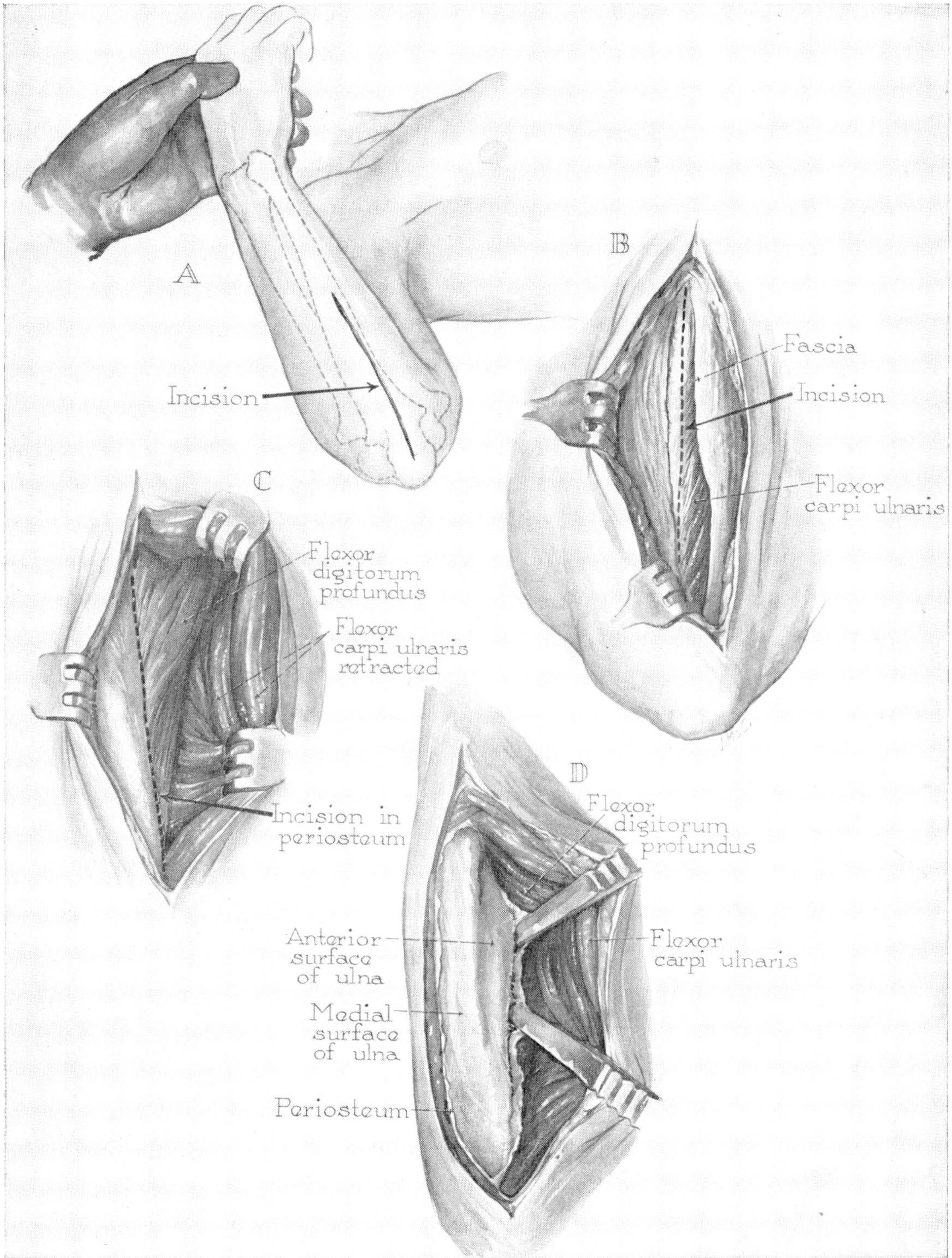

Exposure of the anterior and medial surfaces of the middle third of the ulna through a posterior incision

EXPOSURE OF THE POSTERIOR ASPECT OF THE PROXIMAL THIRD OF THE RADIUS THROUGH A POSTERIOR INCISION

Indications: 1. Treatment of Recent and Un-united Fractures

2. Resection of Benign Tumors

Plate 75: Description of Procedure

A The skin incision begins at a point and level just posterior to the lateral epicondyle of the humerus, and then extends distally between the extensor carpi radialis brevis and the extensor digitorum longus muscles for a distance of approximately 7 inches.

B The deep fascia is opened. The muscle belly of the extensor digitorum communis muscle is identified and then carefully separated from the extensor carpi radialis brevis musce and retracted downward, while the latter muscle is retracted upward.

C The dorsal interosseous nerve is located at its place of emergence from the inferior margin of the supinator muscle. The nerve divides into three main branches which innervate the muscles on the dorsum of the forearm.

D In order to expose the proximal end of the radius, it is necessary to supinate the forearm, and to locate the anterior margin of the supinator muscle. An incision then is made through the muscle attachment and periosteum to permit reflection of the supinator downward and away from the radius. The dorsal interosseous nerve passes obliquely downward through the substance of the muscle and is relatively free from danger. Additional exposure of the radius can be obtained by downward elevation and retraction of the abductor pollicis longus muscle.

NOTE: The exposure is difficult in so far as it is necessary to isolate and protect the dorsal interosseous nerve. Cutting of this nerve will result in loss of dorsiflexion of the wrist and the ability to extend the thumb and metacarpal-phalangeal joints of the fingers.

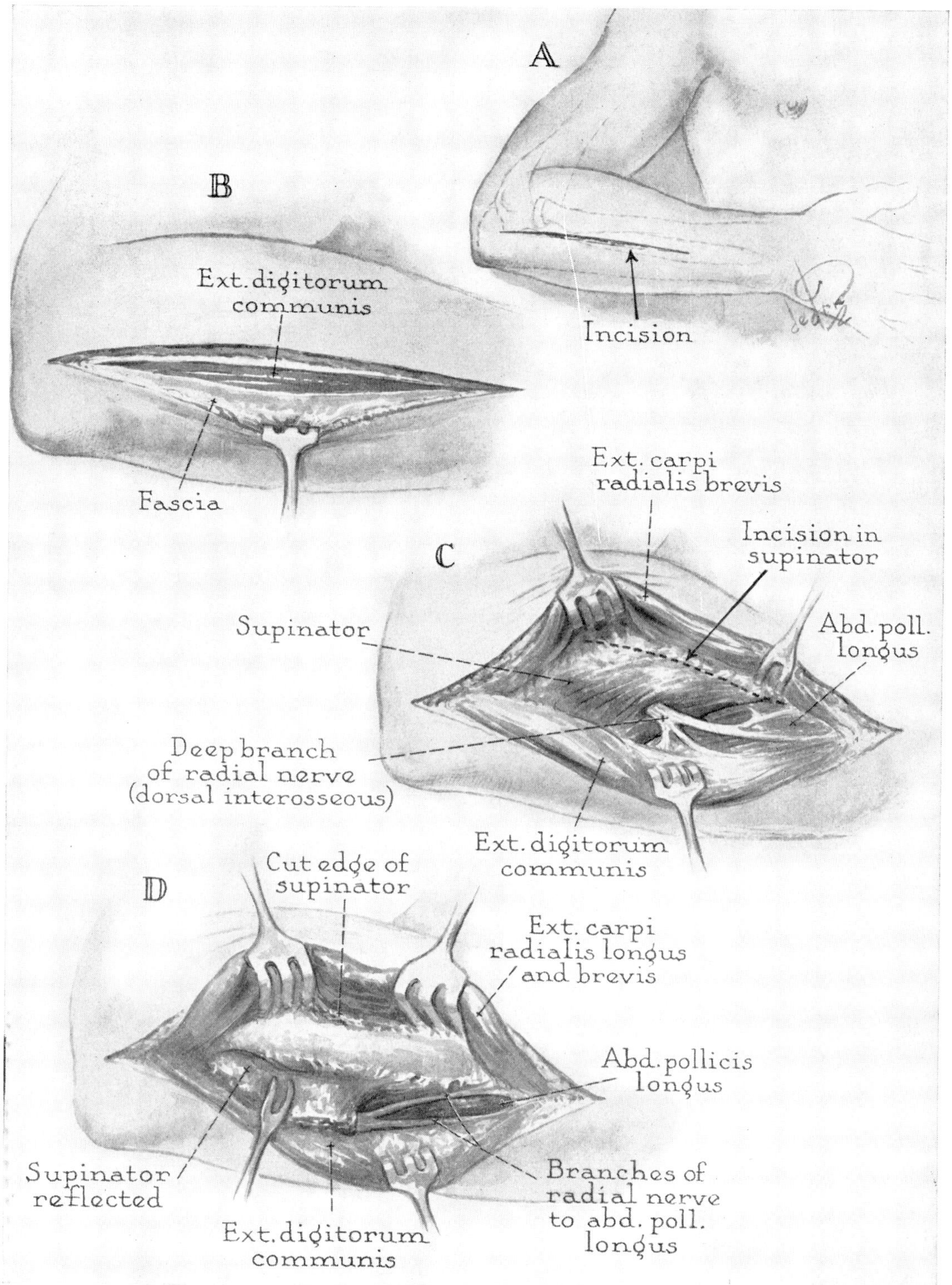

Exposure of the posterior aspect of the proximal third of the radius through a posterior incision

EXPOSURE OF THE POSTERIOR SURFACE OF THE DISTAL HALF OF THE RADIUS THROUGH A POSTERIOR INCISION

Indications: 1. Open Reduction of Recent Fractures

2. Treatment of Non-unions and Defects of the Radius

3. Excision of Benign and Malignant Tumors

4. Correction of Deformities by Osteotomy

Plate 76: Description of Procedure

A In this procedure, the forearm is held in pronation on an armboard which extends from the side of the operating table. The skin incision, approximately 6 inches long, begins at the wrist joint and extends upward, centering on the posterior aspect of the radius.

B The skin flaps are undermined and the veins crossing the field are ligated. The deep fascia is incised, thus bringing into view the abductor pollicis longus and the extensor pollicis brevis muscle bellies which cross the center of the field obliquely downward and radialward. The tendons of the extensor carpi radialis longus and brevis are located proximal to, beneath and distal to the above two muscles.

C The abductor pollicis longus and extensor pollicis brevis muscles are raised dorsally from the underlying radius and the tendons of the extensor carpi radialis longus and brevis muscles, by making an incision along their superior and inferior margins, as illustrated. A hernia tape is placed around the muscles so that they can be retracted out of the surgical field.

The periosteum is incised along the midline of the radius, the whole length of the wound, and is raised to either side. The extensor carpi radialis longus and brevis tendons are retracted radialward, while the extensor digitorum communis and the extensor pollicis longus muscles are retracted ulnaward.

The obliquely placed abductor pollicis longus and extensor pollicis brevis muscles are retracted upward and forward or distally and backward as may be necessary. The wound can be extended in either direction by following the ulnar margin of the extensor carpi radialis brevis. At the same time the supinator must be peeled from the proximal third of the radius, or the extensor pollicis longus must be elevated from the back of the distal extremity of the bone.

NOTE: Care must be exercised in dissecting the ulnar side of the deep portion of the wound, for the nerve supply to the extensor pollicis longus muscle is located on the ulnar side of the obliquely placed muscles and may be injured.

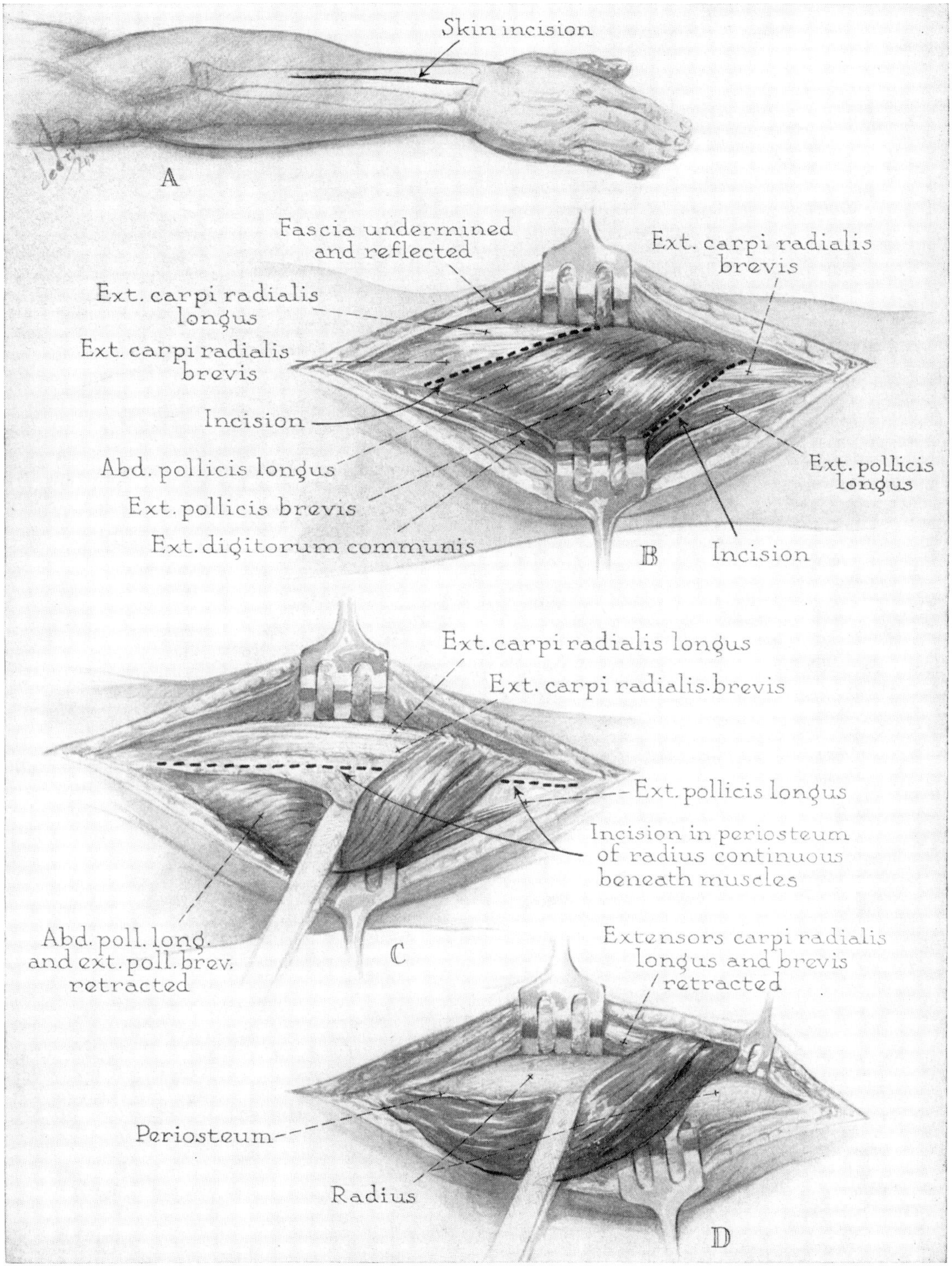

Exposure of the posterior surface of the distal half of the radius through a posterior incision

EXPOSURE OF THE POSTERIOR ASPECT OF THE DISTAL FOURTH OF THE RADIUS THROUGH A POSTERIOR INCISION

Indications: 1. Open Reduction of Recent Fractures of the Radius

2. Treatment of Un-united Fractures of the Radius

3. Resection of Benign and Malignant Tumors

4. Treatment of Chronic Infections

Plate 77: Description of Procedure

A The incision begins at the level of the wrist joint and extends upward in the midline of the dorsal aspect of the radius for 3 1/2 inches.

B The skin flaps are undermined and the deep fascia is opened to expose the abductor pollicis longus and extensor pollicis brevis muscles as well as the tendons of the extensor carpi radialis longus and brevis, which emerge from beneath the distal margin of the extensor pollicis brevis. The tendon of the extensor pollicis longus muscle is located at the ulnar side of the distal portion of the incision. It should be noted that its tendon changes its course in the direction of the thumb as it passes through the fascial tunnel at the distal margin of the radius.

C The bellies of the abductor pollicis longus and extensor pollicis brevis muscles are separated from the underlying tendons and bone and retracted upward.

D Exposure of approximately 2 1/2 inches of the radius is obtained by making a longitudinal incision through the periosteum of the radius, between the extensor carpi radialis brevis and the extensor pollicis longus. The incision can be extended further downward subperiosteally if exposure of the articular end of the radius is desired. The tendon of the extensor pollicis longus muscle can be mobilized from its fascial canal and retracted to either side of the incision, as may be necessary.

NOTE: No important arteries or nerves are encountered in this incision. Care must be taken in the ulnar portion of the proximal end of the wound not to sever the nerve to the extensor pollicis longus muscle.

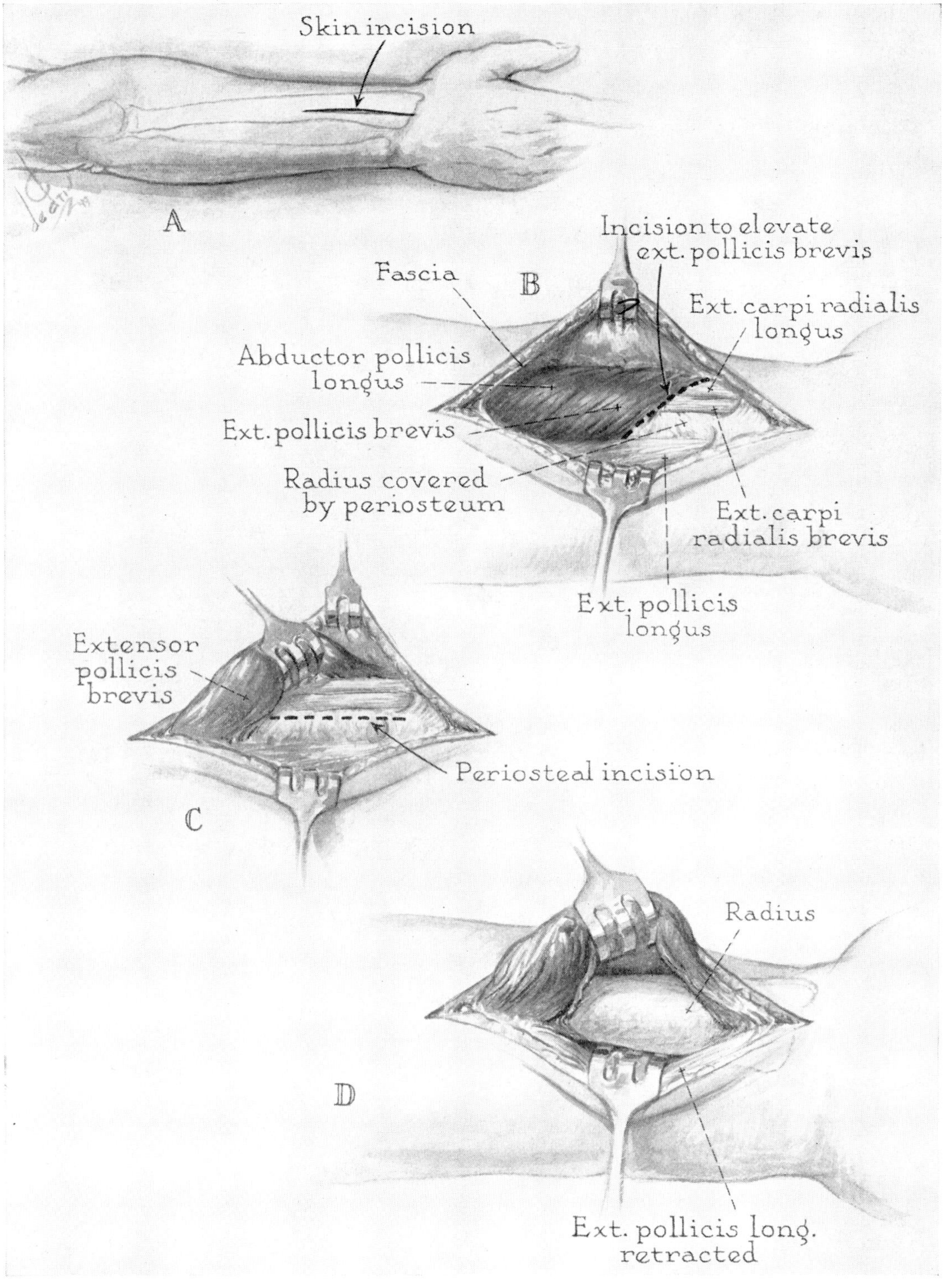

Exposure of the posterior aspect of the distal fourth of the radius through a posterior incision

EXPOSURE OF THE OLECRANON PROCESS AND THE ADJACENT PORTION OF THE ULNA THROUGH A POSTERIOR INCISION

Indications: 1. Open Reduction of Fractures of the Olecranon Process

2. Treatment of Un-united Fractures of the Olecranon Process

3. Repair of Avulsions of the Triceps Tendon

4. Partial Ostectomy for Osteomyelitis

Plate 78: Description of Procedure

A The skin incision begins at the tip of the olecranon process, and extends distally over the subcutaneous margin of the ulna for the desired distance.

B The fascia is opened, and the incision is carried down through the periosteum to the ulna.

C The olecranon process and the adjacent portion of the ulna are exposed subperiosteally. The flexor carpi ulnaris muscle is retracted medially, and the anconeus and supinator muscles are reflected radially. The posterior capsule of the elbow may be exposed in the wound. The ulnar nerve lies medially to the end of the olecranon process, but at a slightly lower level its location is within the flexor carpi ulnaris muscle. The nerve should be exposed and protected by being kept under direct vision during extensive surgery in this region.

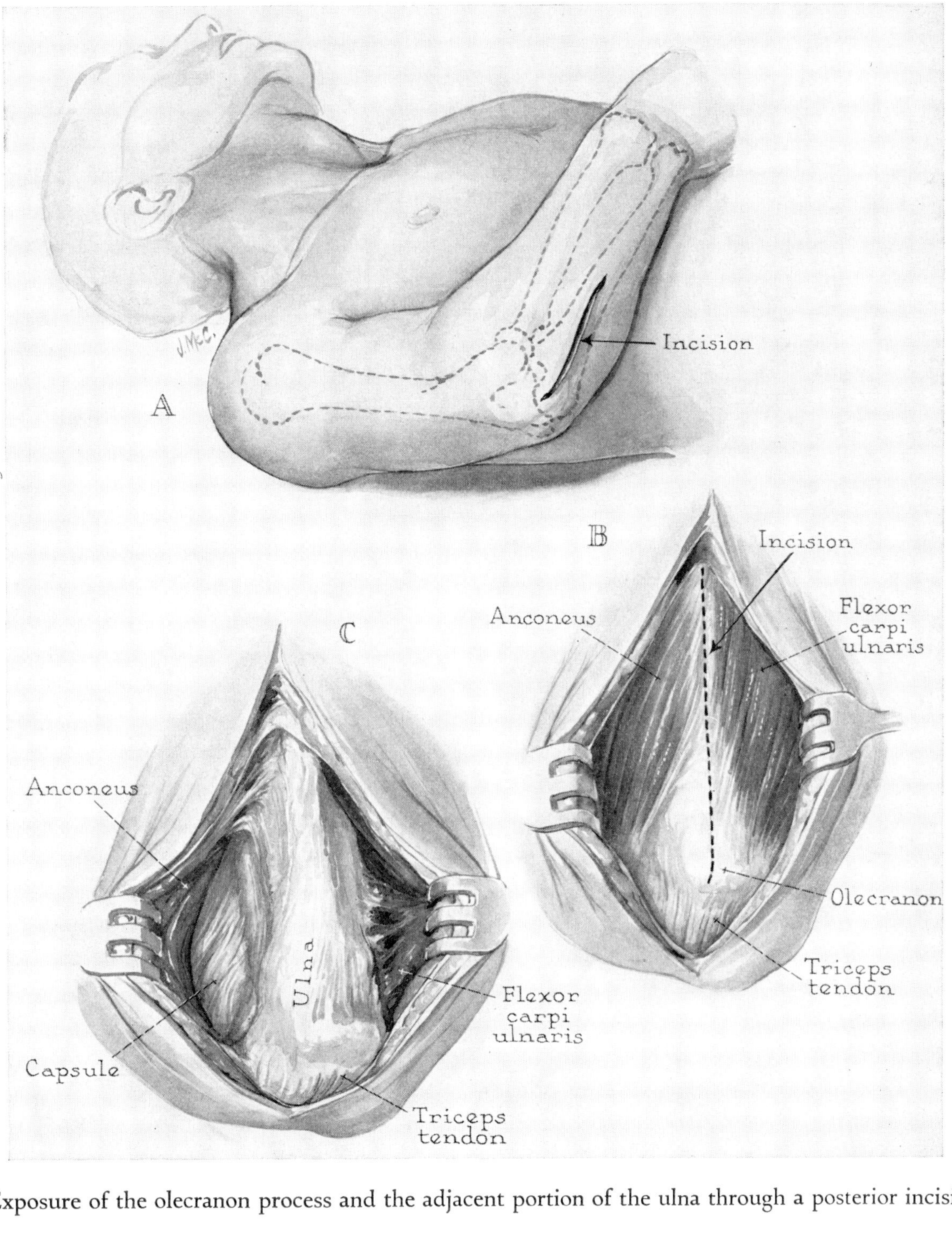

Exposure of the olecranon process and the adjacent portion of the ulna through a posterior incision

EXPOSURE OF THE PROXIMAL HALF OF THE ULNA THROUGH A POSTERIOR INCISION

Indications: 1. Open Reduction of Recent Fractures of the Ulna

2. Treatment of Un-united Fractures of the Ulna

3. Excision of Benign and Malignant Lesions

Plate 79: Description of Procedure

A An incision 6 inches long begins at the tip of the olecranon process and extends downward over the posterior margin of the ulna.

B The deep fascia is opened, undermined and retracted with the skin. The posterior margin of the ulna is now exposed between the anconeus and extensor carpi ulnaris laterally and the flexor carpi ulnaris medially.

C The periosteum is incised along the posterior margin of the ulna and elevated so as to expose the bone. Along the radial side of the wound are the anconeus and supinator muscles in the proximal half, while the extensor carpi ulnaris muscle flanks the distal half. On the opposite side of the ulna is the flexor carpi ulnaris muscle and tendon. The dissection can be extended distally or completely around the ulna.

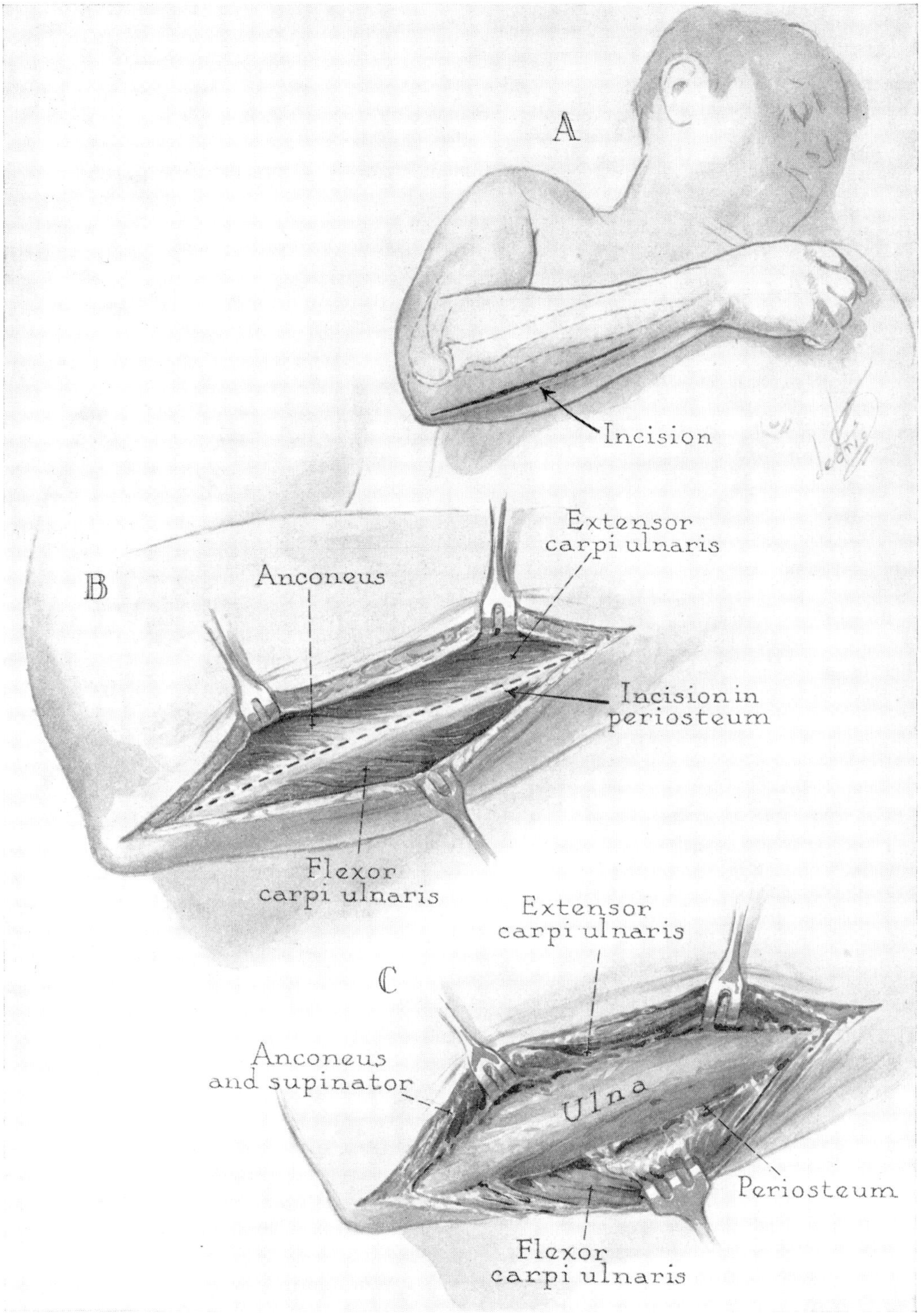

Exposure of the proximal half of the ulna through a posterior incision

EXPOSURE OF THE DISTAL HALF OF THE ULNA THROUGH A POSTERIOR INCISION

Indications: 1. Open Reduction of Recent Fractures

2. Application of Bone Grafts for Non-union and Repair of Total Bone Defects

3. Resection of Benign and Malignant Tumors

4. Correction of Deformities

Plate 80: Description of Procedure

A The skin incision begins over the posterior lateral aspect of the ulnar styloid process and extends along the subcutaneous margin of the ulna for approximately 5 inches.

B The deep fascia is incised and the margins are reflected to the sides of the wound. The subcutaneous margin of the ulnar bone is palpated and its periosteum is incised.

C The ulna is then exposed subperiosteally, and at the same time the extensor carpi ulnaris muscle and its tendon are retracted along the extensor side of the wound and the flexor carpi ulnaris muscle and tendon are retracted on the flexor side.

D The entire posterior aspect of the ulna can be exposed by a linear incision which cuts the skin, fascia and periosteum over the dorsal margin of the bone, as shown in the illustration. The anconeus, the supinator and the flexor and extensor carpi ulnaris muscles are retracted along with the periosteum to the sides of the wound.

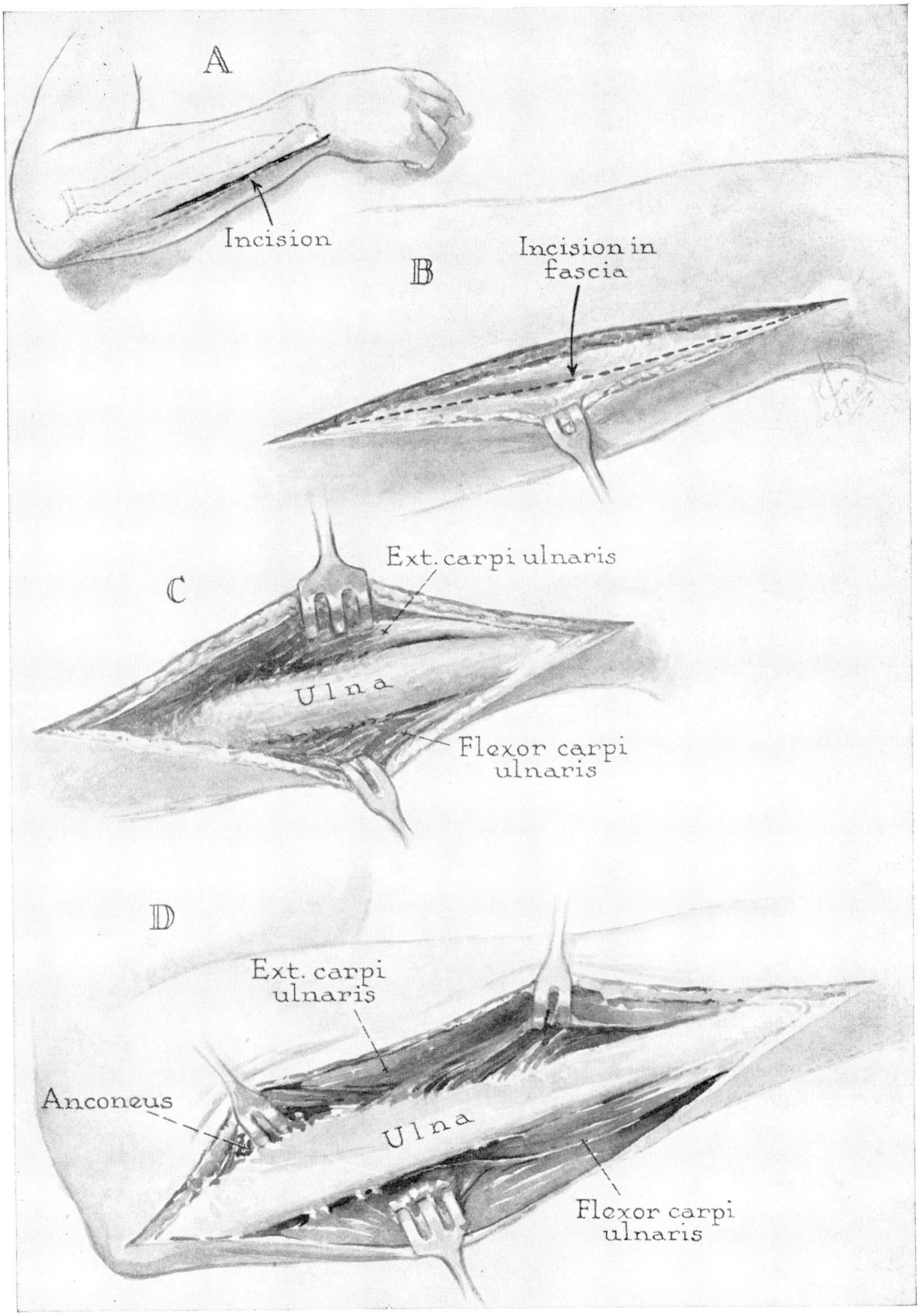

Exposure of the distal half of the ulna through a posterior incision

EXPOSURE OF THE ULNAR NERVE IN THE FOREARM THROUGH A LONGITUDINAL INCISION

Indications: 1. Neurolysis of the Ulnar Nerve

2. Suture of Lacerations of the Ulnar Nerve

Plate 81: Description of Procedure

A The skin incision, of appropriate length, follows the anterior margin of the flexor carpi ulnaris muscle, and is centered over the area of the nerve pathology.

B The skin flaps are undercut and retracted, and the deep fascia is opened in line with the incision.

C The free margin of the flexor carpi ulnaris muscle is mobilized and separated from the flexor digitorum sublimis which is lateral to it, and from the flexor digitorum profundus which is deep beneath it.

D The flexor carpi ulnaris muscle is retracted medially. The ulnar nerve is identified as it enters the forearm between the two heads of the flexor carpi ulnaris, and then is isolated the length of the wound. The ulnar artery is located on the radial side of the nerve. The sensory branch of the ulnar nerve is given off in the distal third of the forearm and then passes around the ulnar side of the arm to reach the back of the hand.

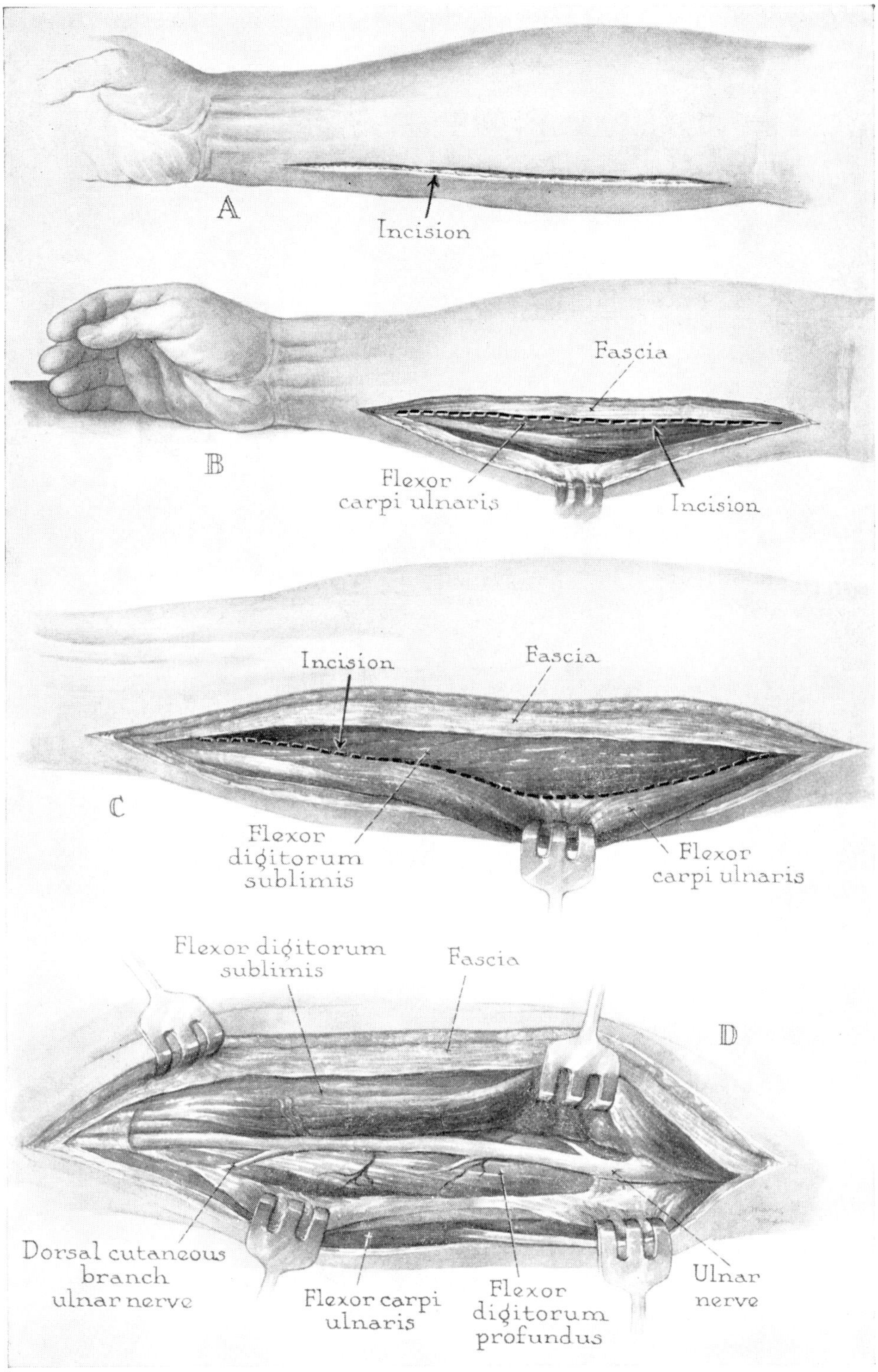

Exposure of the ulnar nerve in the forearm through a longitudinal incision

EXPOSURE OF THE DORSAL INTEROSSEOUS (RADIAL) NERVE IN THE SUPINATOR MUSCLE THROUGH A POSTERIOR INCISION BETWEEN THE EXTENSOR CARPI RADIALIS BREVIS AND THE EXTENSOR DIGITORUM COMMUNIS MUSCLES

Indications: 1. Suture of Lacerations of the Posterior Interosseous Nerve

Plate 82: Description of Procedure

A The incision begins in front of the medial epicondyle of the humerus and extends posteriorly in a gentle curve so as to find the interval between the extensor carpi radialis brevis and extensor digitorum communis muscles, where it continues distally for 3 inches. The skin is undermined widely, especially the radial flap.

B The fascia is opened between the posterior margin of the brachioradialis and the extensor carpi radialis longus muscles. The two muscles are separated to expose the supinator muscle deep to them. The supinator can be identified by the oblique downward and radial direction of its muscle fibers.

C In a similar manner the deep fascia is incised along the interval between the extensor carpi radialis brevis and the extensor digitorum communis muscles, and these are separated so as to expose the underlying supinator and abductor pollicis longus muscles. (Procedure continued on Plate 83.)

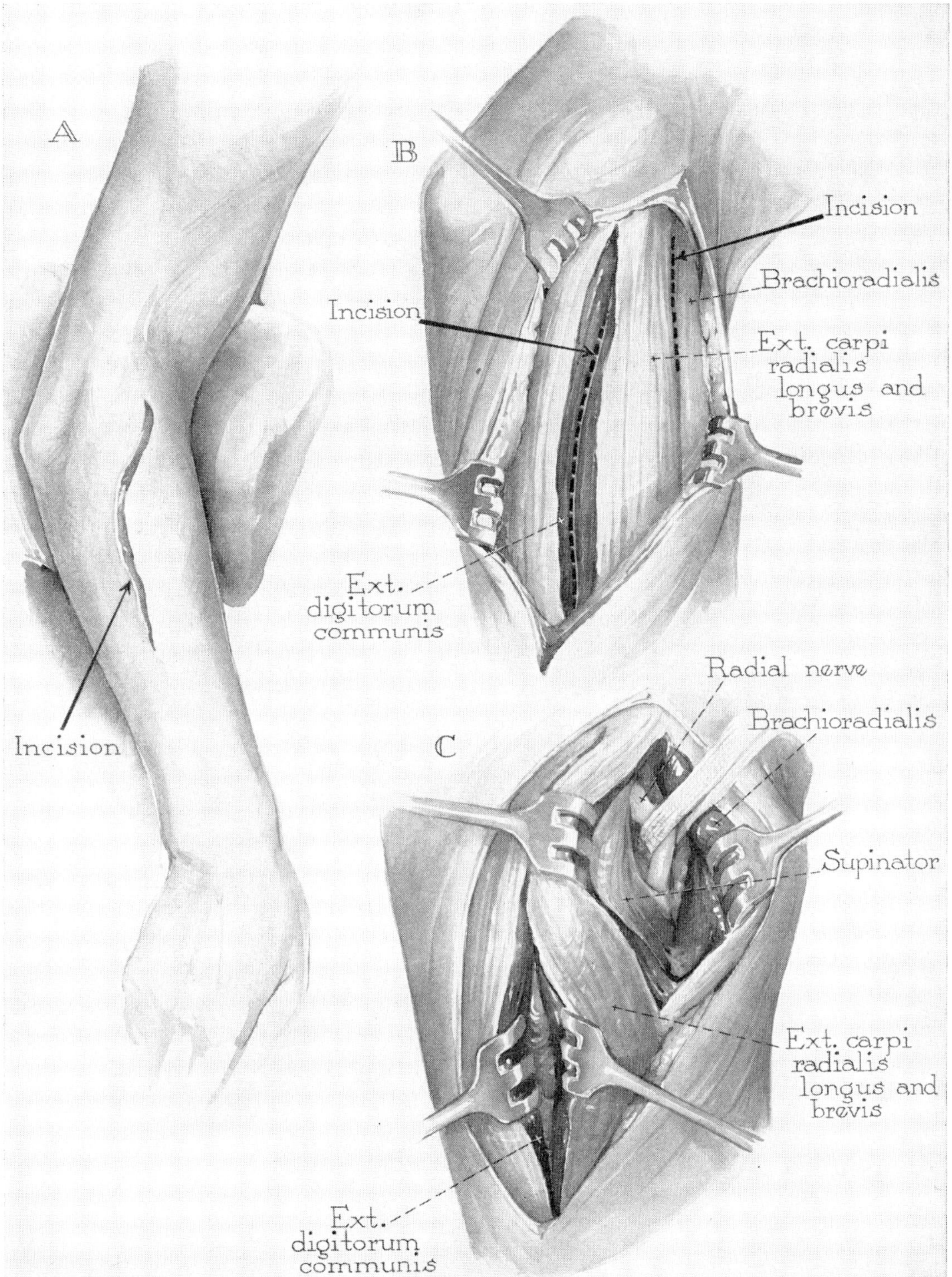

Exposure of the dorsal interosseous (radial) nerve in the supinator muscle through a posterior incision between the extensor carpi radialis brevis and the extensor digitorum communis muscles

EXPOSURE OF THE DORSAL INTEROSSEOUS (RADIAL) NERVE IN THE SUPINATOR MUSCLE THROUGH A POSTERIOR INCISION BETWEEN THE EXTENSOR CARPI RADIALIS BREVIS AND THE EXTENSOR DIGITORUM COMMUNIS MUSCLES (*Continued*)

Plate 83: Description of Procedure

D The extensor carpi radialis longus and brevis muscles are retracted maximally radialward in order to expose as much of the supinator muscle as possible. The dorsal interosseous nerve can usually be identified as it emerges from the distal margin of the supinator muscle. In some patients the severed nerve ends cannot be found because of scarring which resulted from the same injury that severed the nerve. It becomes necessary in these cases to isolate the radial nerve in the incision between the brachioradialis and the extensor carpi radialis longus, and then to trace the dorsal interosseous branch through the supinator muscle into the dorsum of the forearm.

E An incision may be made across the supinator muscle so as to connect the points of entrance and exit of the dorsal interosseous nerve when necessary for adequate exposure. The muscle wound must be opened cautiously and the nerve isolated without injury to it.

NOTE: The radial nerve is isolated beneath the brachioradialis muscle only in instances where the dorsal interosseous nerve cannot be identified at the distal margin of the supinator muscle.

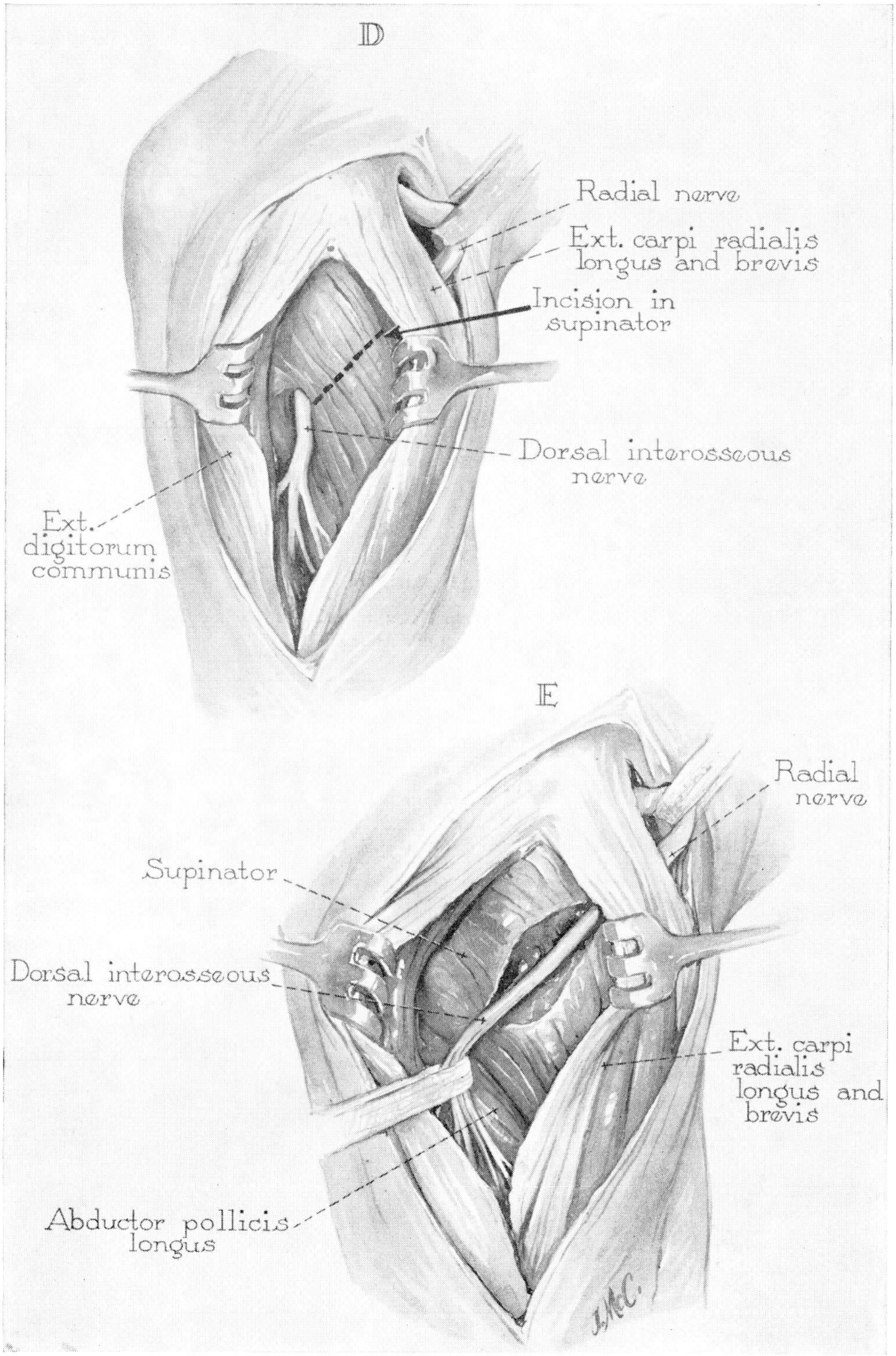

Exposure of the dorsal interosseous (radial) nerve in the supinator muscle through a posterior incision between the extensor carpi radialis brevis and the extensor digitorum communis muscles.

EXPOSURE OF THE FLEXOR POLLICIS LONGUS MUSCLE IN THE FORE-ARM THROUGH AN ANTEROLATERAL INCISION

Indications: 1. Repair of the Lacerations of the Flexor Pollicis Longus Muscle or Tendon

Plate 84: Description of Procedure

A The tendon of the flexor carpi radialis muscle must first be identified by palpation, for the incision, which starts at the flexion crease of the wrist, extends upward and directly lateral to this muscle for a distance of approximately 4 1/2 inches.

B The skin margins are retracted, and the tendon of the flexor carpi radialis and the brachio-radialis muscles can then be identified beneath the deep fascia. The radial artery courses between the two tendons and must not be injured when the deep fascia over it is being opened with the aid of a groove director for the length of the wound.

C The radial artery and the tendon of the brachioradialis muscle are now gently retracted radial-ward. The tendon of the flexor carpi radialis is pulled ulnaward to expose the lateral margin of the flexor digitorum sublimis beneath it, which muscle also must be retracted medially. The flexor pollicis longus muscle is exposed in the floor of the wound; it should be noted that its long tendon begins at a level corresponding to about the middle third of the radius. Distal to and beneath the flexor pollicis longus tendon is the quadrangular pronator muscle, which extends between the ulna and the radius. The incision can be extended so as to expose the tendon of the flexor pollicis longus muscle in the palm, as illustrated in Plate 93.

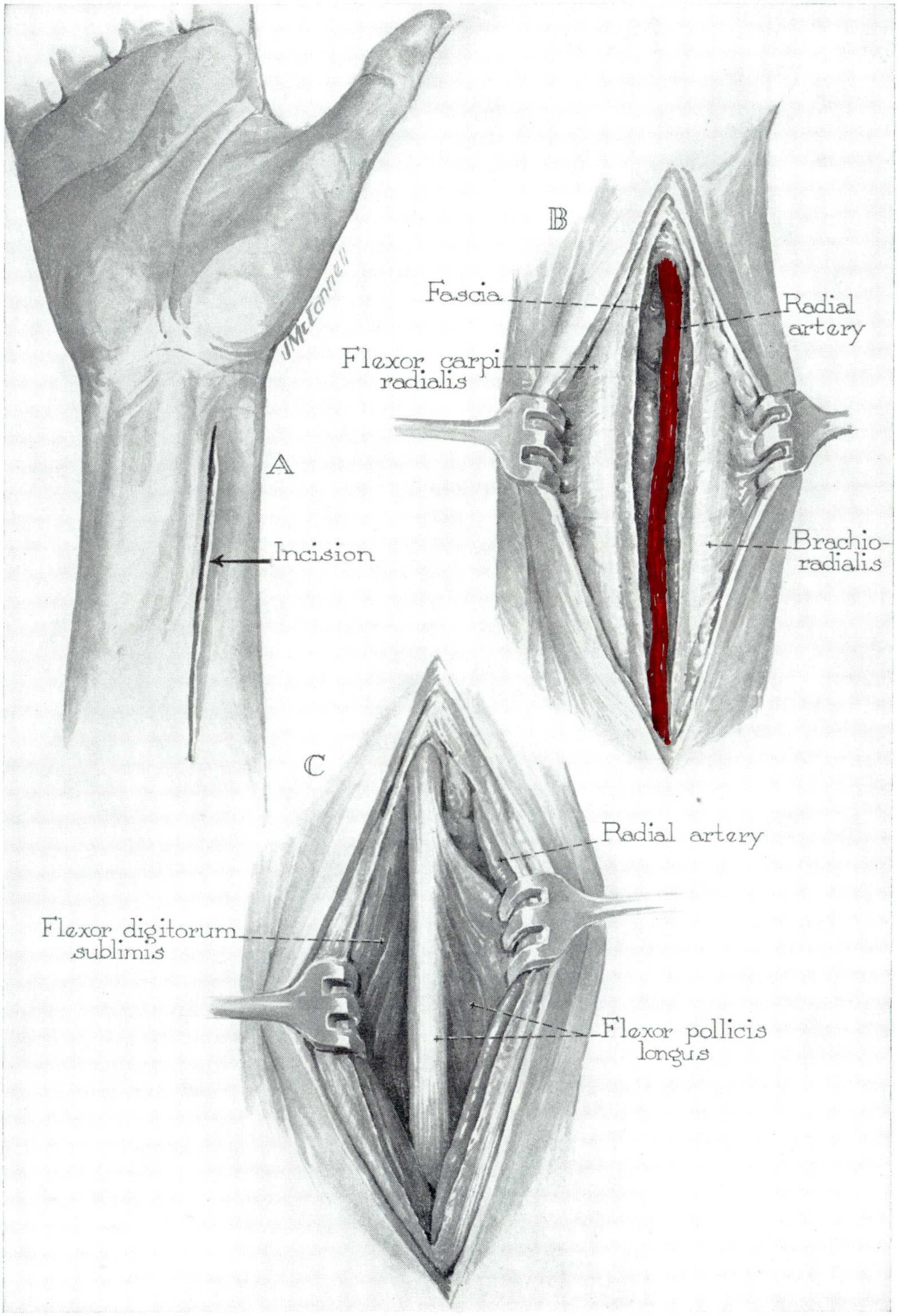

Exposure of the flexor pollicis longus muscle in the forearm through an anterolateral incision

Section VI

Region of the Wrist Joint and Hand

EXPOSURE OF THE WRIST JOINT THROUGH A DORSAL LONGITUDINAL INCISION

Indications: 1. Arthrodesis of the Wrist Joint

2. Correction of Defects of the Distal End of Radius by Bone Transplant and Arthrodesis of the Wrist Joint

3. Removal of Benign Tumors

4. Resection of the Lower End of the Radius Because of Malignant Tumors

Plate 85: Description of Procedure

A The incision begins at the proximal end of the second or third metacarpal bone and extends upward in a lazy S manner, centering on the radius and terminating some 3 inches above the wrist joint. A straight-line incision is occasionally followed by contracture, and therefore is not recommended.

B The skin flaps are undermined and the veins crossing the field are ligated or retracted to one side. The incision in the second layer cuts through the deep fascia proximally, the dorsal carpal ligament in the midportion of the wound and, distally, through the fascia over the back of the hand. The dorsal carpal ligament is opened between the extensor pollicis longus and the extensor digitorum communis tendon of the index finger.

C The extensor pollicis longus muscle is identified and lifted toward the thumb side of the wound. The ulnar half of the radius can be seen. The periosteum is incised here and the entire dorsal surface of the radius is exposed subperiosteally. The fascial canal for the extensor pollicis longus muscle is raised from the radius and retracted radially together with the tendons of the extensor carpi radialis longus and brevis muscles.

D The capsule of the wrist joint is opened in line with the radius incision and reflected from the margin of the radius and from the adjacent carpal bones. The distal row of carpal bones is best exposed by raising an osteo-periosteal flap from their dorsal surfaces.

NOTE: Care must be exercised not to injure the distal radio-ulnar articulation. The radial artery runs along the lateral aspect of the wrist joint, and cannot be injured if the operation is kept within the confines of the periosteum and capsule. The sensory branch of the radial nerve emerges at a level just proximal to the wrist joint from beneath the tendon of the brachioradialis muscle; it must not be severed.

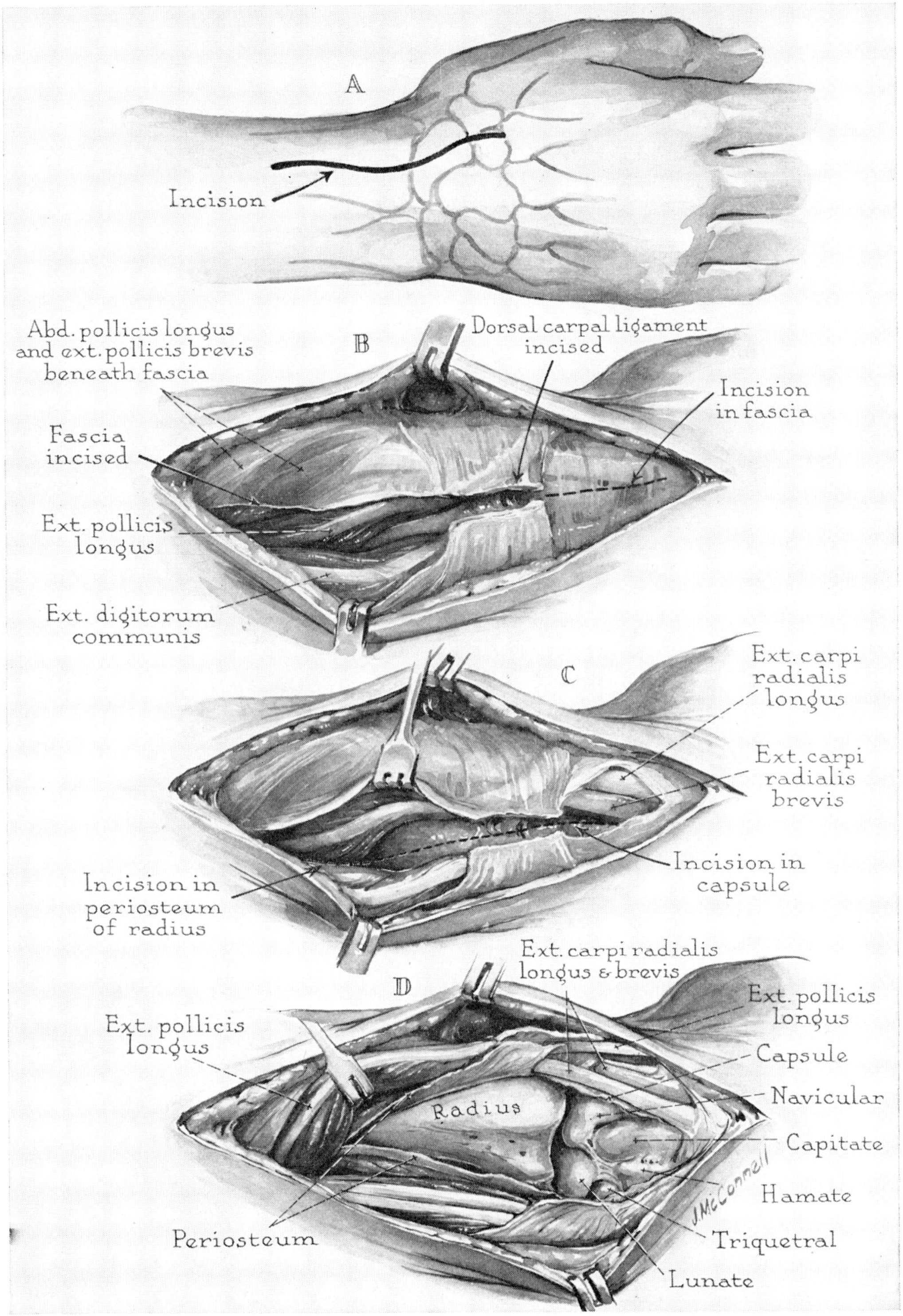

Exposure of the wrist joint through a dorsal longitudinal incision

EXPOSURE OF THE WRIST JOINT THROUGH A DORSAL TRANSVERSE INCISION

Indications: 1. Excision of a Portion of the Navicular Bone, the Lunate Bone, or Both

2. Biopsy of the Wrist Joint

Plate 86: Description of Procedure

A The skin incision, approximately 1 3/4 inches in length, is made along a prominent skin crease over the dorsal aspect of the wrist joint, at the level of the radial styloid process. The skin flaps are undermined and retracted, thus exposing the dorsal carpal ligament and the deep fascia.

B The dissection is carried longitudinally through the deep fascia over the dorsum of the hand, and thence is extended proximally across the dorsal carpal ligament and the deep fascia of the distal forearm along the interval between the tendons of the extensor pollicis longus and the extensor digitorum communis to the index finger.

C The wound is deepened between the two tendons to expose the periosteum of the subjacent portion of the radius and the capsule of the wrist joint. An incision through these structures will permit the subperiosteal exposure of a varying area of the dorsal surface of the radius and give access to the wrist joint. The dorsal surfaces of the navicular, lunate, capitate and adjacent bones can be exposed by elevating the soft tissues over them, as desired. On the other hand, it is not necessary to elevate the fascial canal of the extensor pollicis longus from the radius if only removal of the lunate and/or a portion of the navicular bone is contemplated. It is necessary, however, in arthrodesis of the wrist joint.

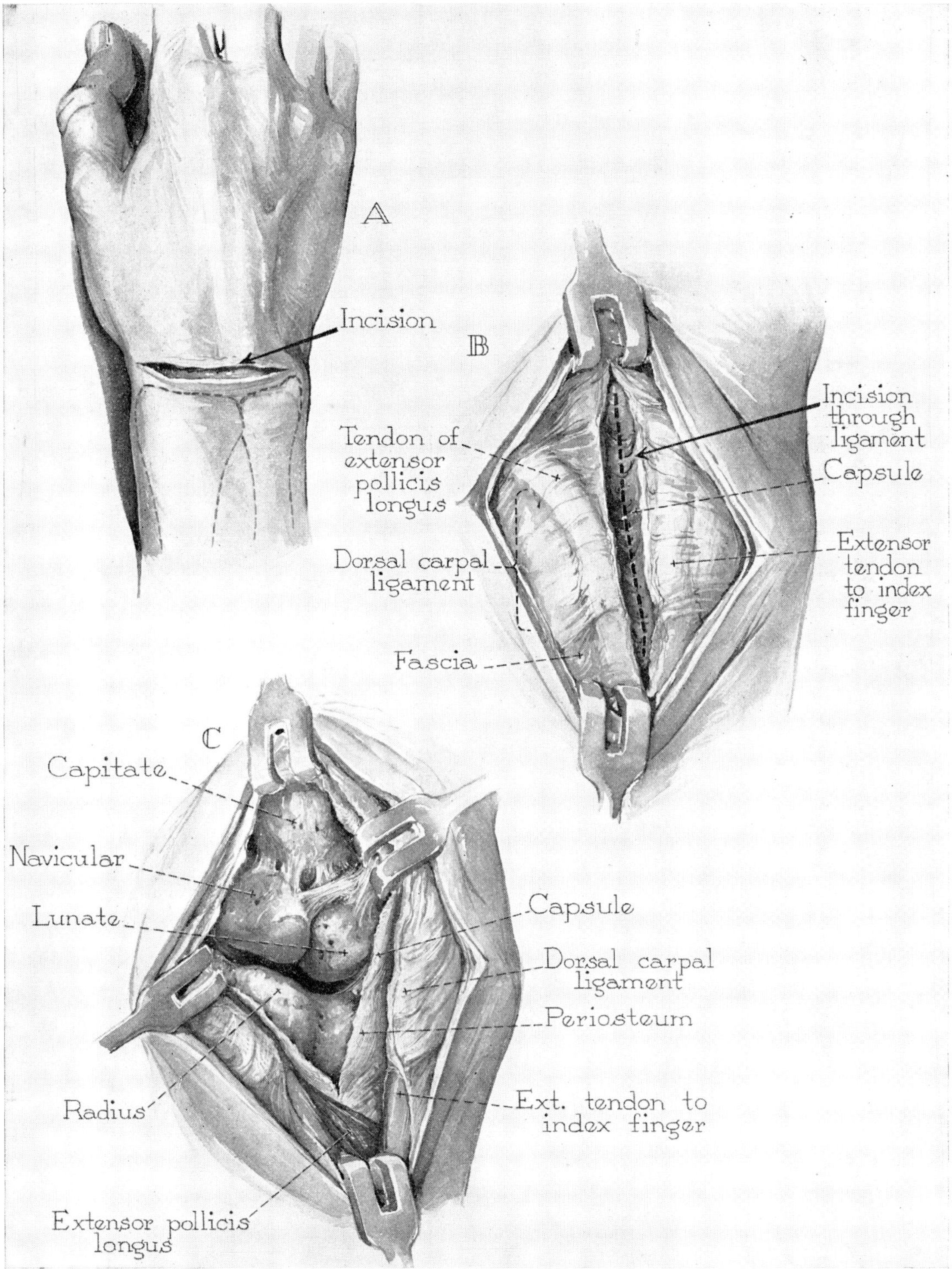

Exposure of the wrist joint through a dorsal transverse incision

EXPOSURE OF THE NAVICULAR BONE THROUGH A LATERAL WRIST INCISION

Indication: 1. Treatment of Non-union of the Navicular Bone;
Multiple Drilling, Bone Grafting, or a Combination of These

Plate 87: Description of Procedure

A The skin incision begins over the base of the first metacarpal bone and extends upward for approximately 2 1/2 inches, centering over the anatomical snuffbox.

B The fascia is opened between the extensor pollicis longus dorsally, and the extensor pollicis brevis ventrally. The sensory branch of the radial nerve, which is located beneath the tendon of the extensor pollicis longus, must not be severed during the procedure. The radial artery traverses the wound after passing beneath the extensor pollicis brevis and then disappears distally between the metacarpal bones of the thumb and index fingers; it must be identified and protected.

C The tendons of the extensor pollicis longus and of the extensor carpi radialis longus are mobilized from the underlying capsule of the wrist joint and retracted ulnaward. The dorsal carpal ligament is exposed proximally.

D The wrist joint is opened through a linear incision in the capsule. The navicular bone is seen as the wound margins are retracted. The lower end of the radius can be exposed by extending the dissection proximally. Next, an incision is made through the dorsal carpal ligament and the periosteum lateral to the extensor pollicis longus, as shown in the illustration. Access to the navicular bone may be further facilitated by stripping the capsule from the adjacent radius and by placing the wrist in ulnar deviation.

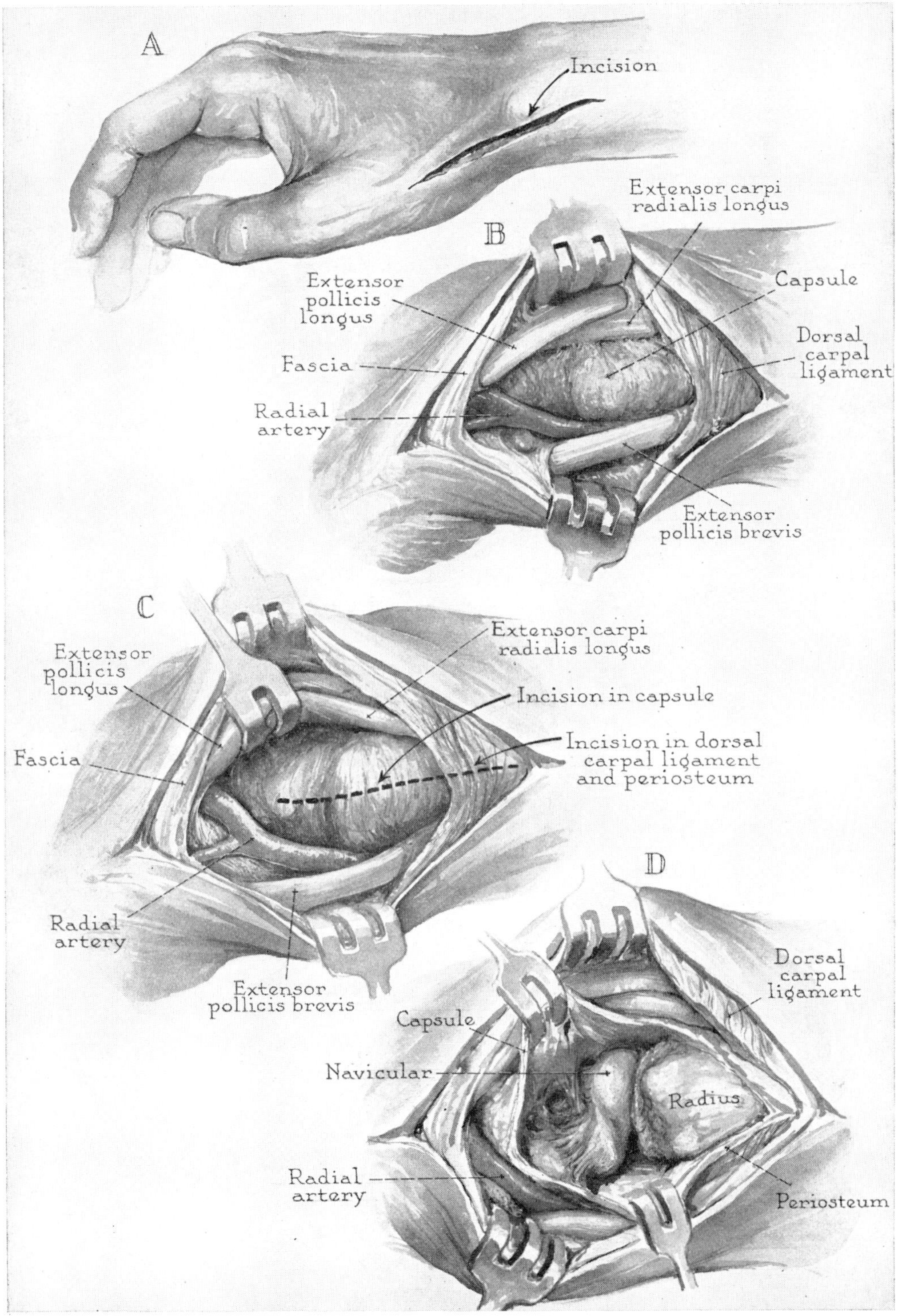

Exposure of the navicular bone through a lateral wrist incision

EXPOSURE OF THE ULNAR NERVE IN THE REGION OF THE FOREARM, THE WRIST JOINT AND THE ADJACENT PORTION OF THE HAND THROUGH A CURVED PALMAR, TRANSVERSE WRIST, MEDIAL FOREARM INCISION

Indications: 1. Repair of Laceration of the Ulnar Nerve

2. Resection of Neuromas of the Ulnar Nerve

Plate 88: Description of Procedure

A The skin incision begins at the proximal flexion crease of the palm and extends upward between the thenar and hypothenar eminences, to the flexion crease at the wrist joint. The incision curves gently medially in this flexion crease to its ulnar extremity, and then turns upward along the side of the forearm for a distance of approximately 2 1/2 inches. The skin margins are mobilized in the palm and the forearm. The palmar fascia is incised in line with the skin incision and the exposure is continued upward through the deep fascia of the forearm.

B The palmaris brevis muscle at the level of the pisiform bone and the volar carpal ligament proximal to it are cut. The tendon of the flexor carpi ulnaris muscle is identified by palpation along the ulnar side of the forearm portion of the wound, although in some patients the tendon is visible through the overlying fascia. The fascia is incised along the lateral aspect of the tendon of the flexor carpi ulnaris muscle.

C The margins of the fascia are separated and carefully retracted to expose the ulnar nerve skirting the outer border of the flexor carpi ulnaris tendon and the ulnar artery located on the radial side of this nerve. The flexor digitorum sublimis lies along the outer aspect of the ulnar artery. It need not be disturbed.

Distally, the ulnar nerve divides into a deep branch and a superficial branch. The deep branch disappears between the flexor and abductor digiti muscles to reach the deeper layer of the palm. The superficial branch gives off a branch to supply the palmaris brevis muscle and an anastomosing branch to the median nerve. It then terminates by dividing into digital branches which supply the skin over the hypothenar eminence, the fifth digit and half of the fourth digit.

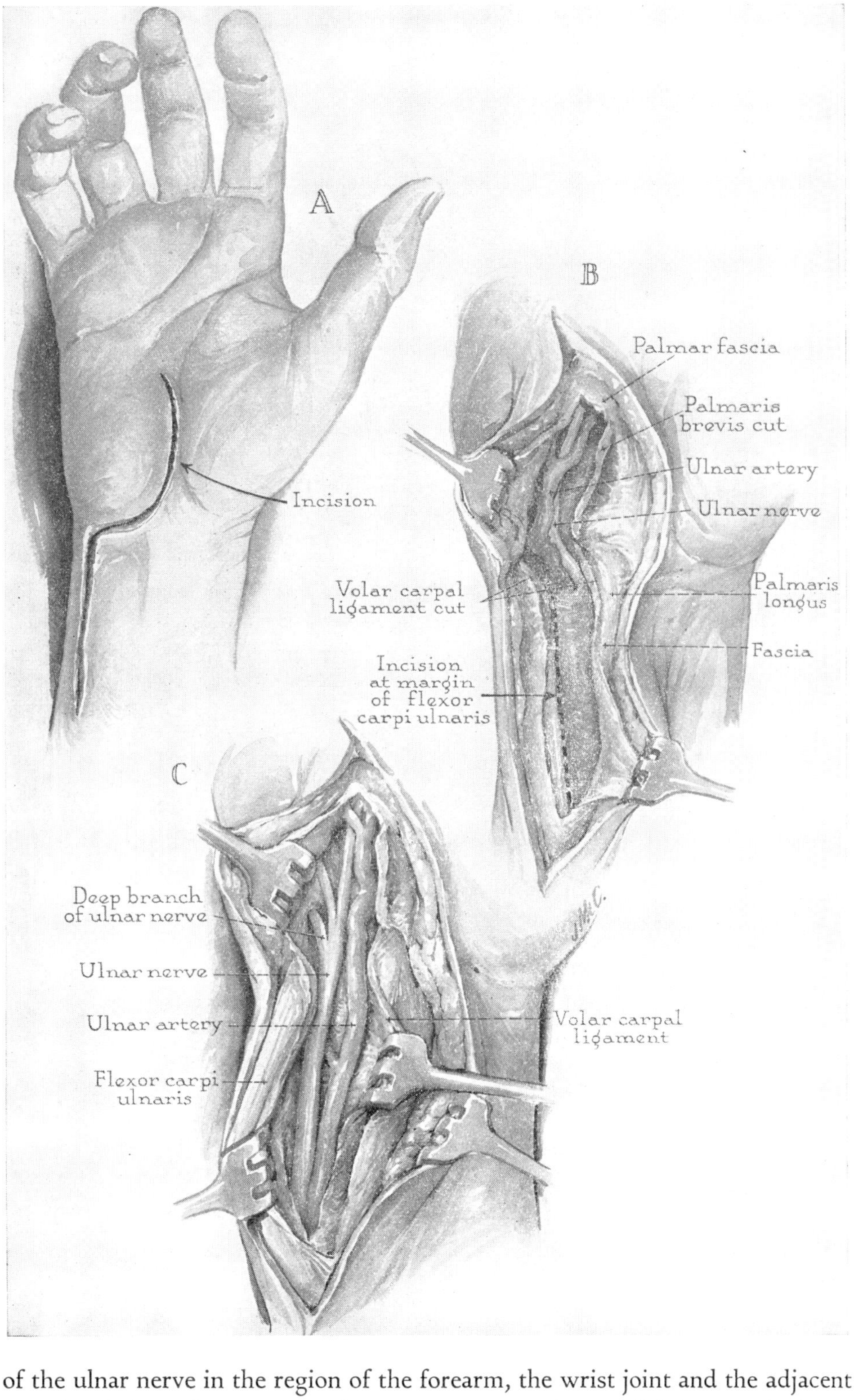

Exposure of the ulnar nerve in the region of the forearm, the wrist joint and the adjacent portion of the hand through a curved palmar, transverse wrist, medial forearm incision

EXPOSURE OF THE MEDIAN NERVE IN THE DISTAL PORTION OF THE FOREARM, AT THE WRIST JOINT, AND IN THE PALM, THROUGH A CURVED PALMAR, LATERAL WRIST JOINT AND FOREARM INCISION

Indication: 1. Repair of Lacerations of the Median Nerve

Plate 89: Description of Procedure

A The incision is made in both the palmar region of the hand and the forearm, as shown in the illustration. The incision in the hand begins at the proximal flexion crease in line with the index finger and then follows along the base of the thenar eminence to end at the wrist. A still wider exposure of the palm can be obtained by placing the incision closer to the hypothenar eminence. The incision in the forearm starts at a point one inch above the flexion crease of the wrist and then extends upward for 4 inches in an S-shaped curve just to the ulnar side of the tendon of the flexor carpi radialis muscle.

B The skin flaps of the two wounds are mobilized and retracted. A curved incision is then made in the palmar fascia and the branches of the median nerve are isolated in the hand.

C Next, a linear cut is made in the fascia of the forearm between the palmaris longus and the flexor carpi radialis tendons. The flexor digitorum sublimis muscle is identified as the wound is retracted and the tendon of the flexor carpi radialis is pulled radially. The lateral margin of the flexor digitorum sublimis is raised and the muscle is retracted medially, after it is carefully separated from the underlying structures. The median nerve and its accompanying artery at the bottom of the wound are next exposed. (Procedure continued on Plate 90.)

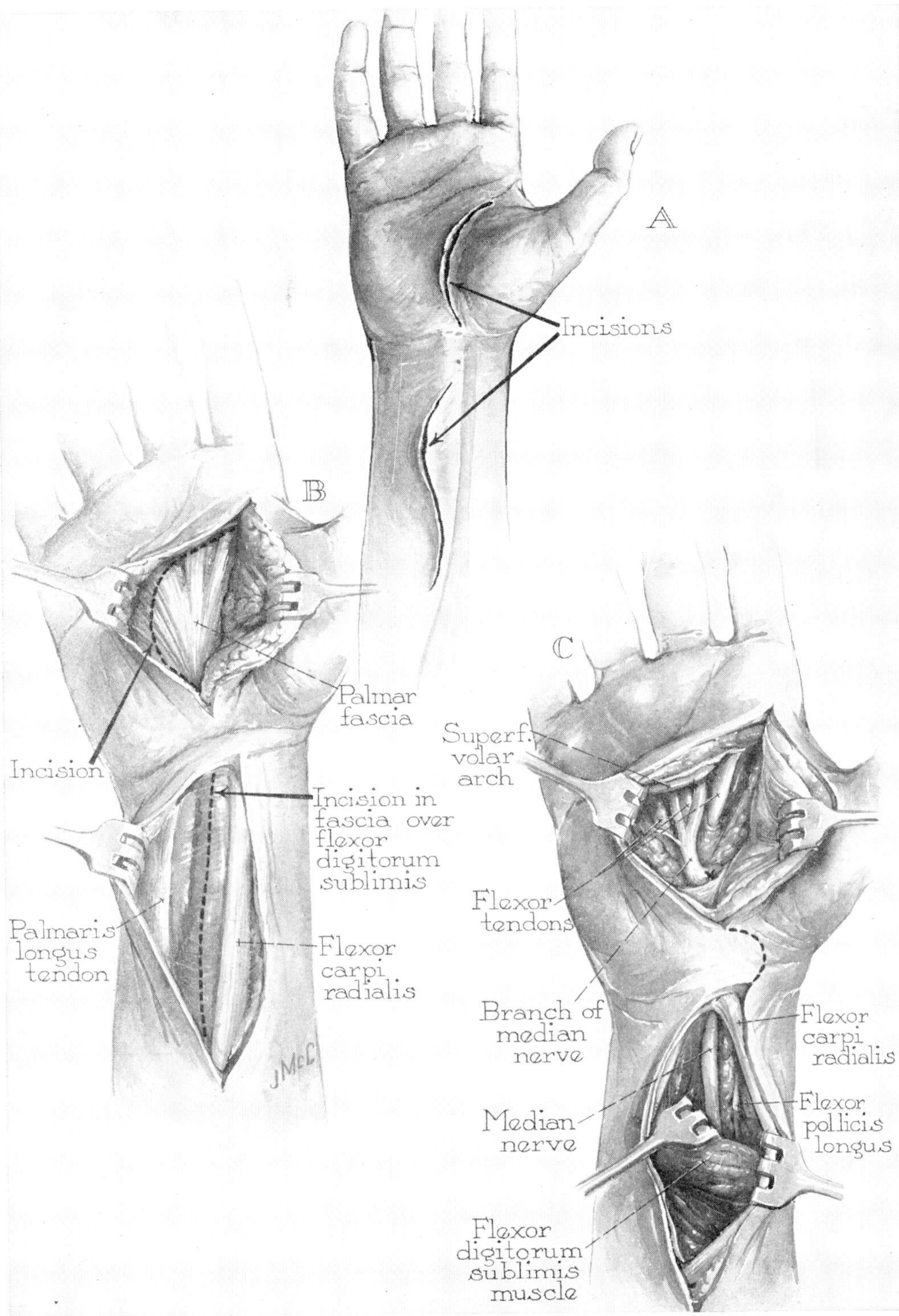

Exposure of the median nerve in the distal portion of the forearm, at the wrist joint, and in the palm through a curved palmar, lateral wrist joint and forearm incision

EXPOSURE OF THE MEDIAN NERVE IN THE DISTAL PORTION OF THE FOREARM, AT THE WRIST JOINT, AND IN THE PALM, THROUGH A CURVED PALMAR, LATERAL WRIST JOINT AND FOREARM INCISION *(Continued)*

Plate 90: Description of Procedure

D The exposure of the median nerve just effected in the distal third of the forearm and in the palm will ordinarily suffice for the repair of most lacerations. In some instances, however, it will also be necessary to isolate the median nerve beneath the transverse carpal ligament. This can be done by joining the dissections in the forearm and palm by a curved incision at the radial side of the wrist, as outlined in Illustration C. A straight-line skin incision is contraindicated because it produces a keloid and a resulting flexion contracture of the wrist. The curved incision having been made, the skin is mobilized and retracted. A vertical cut then is made in the transverse carpal ligament, which affords access to the median nerve at the radial side of the carpal canal.

E The nerve is easily identified and separated from the adjacent tendons at the wrist, but there may be considerable difficulty in dissecting out the several terminal branches of the nerve in the palm.

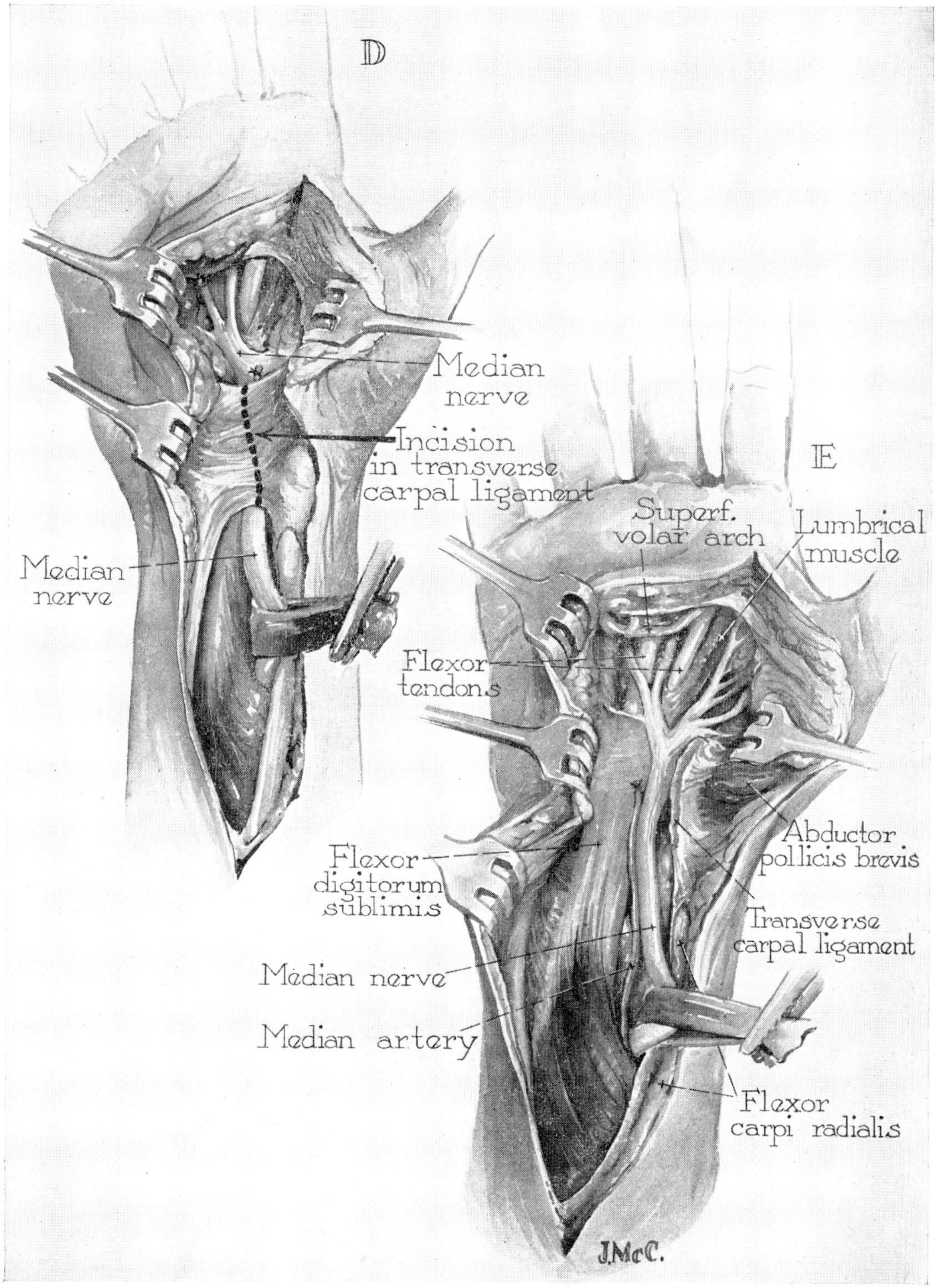

Exposure of the median nerve in the distal portion of the forearm, at the wrist joint, and in the palm through a curved palmar, lateral wrist joint and forearm incision

EXPOSURE OF THE CONTENTS OF THE DISTAL FOREARM, WRIST AND PALM THROUGH A CURVED HAND, TRANSVERSE WRIST AND ULNAR FOREARM INCISION

Indications: 1. Suture of Multiple Lacerations of Tendons and Nerves

2. Reconstruction of Disabled Hands Following Infections and Trauma

Plate 91: Description of Procedure

A The skin incision, as shown, begins at the medial margin of the palm; it proceeds in a curved manner to the wrist joint by following along the skin creases as much as possible and then turns ulnaward to the pisiform bone, where it continues halfway up the forearm in the S-shaped form illustrated. Abrupt turns in direction are to be avoided.

B The palmar fascia is opened along the line of incision and the skin and fascial flaps are retracted to their respective sides. The transverse carpal ligament and the fascia of the forearm are sectioned by a midline incision, as indicated. It is to be noted that the ulnar nerve and artery are located beneath the volar carpal ligament and above the transverse carpal ligament. The ulnar nerve divides into two branches: a deep and a superficial one. The profunda branch passes into the deep portion of the palm between the flexor and abductor digiti quinti muscles; it supplies the muscles of the little finger, the interossei, lumbrical 4, and occasionally 3, the adductor pollicis and the deep head of the flexor pollicis brevis. The superficial branch of the ulnar nerve divides into digital branches which supply the skin over the hypothenar eminence, the little finger and the ulnar half of the ring finger.

The ulnar artery ends in the volar carpal arch after it gives off a profunda branch, which accompanies the deep portion of the ulnar nerve; it also provides branches to the adjacent muscles and skin. The volar carpal arch lies just beneath the palmar fascia and provides three common digital arteries which terminate in digital branches that supply the contacting surfaces of the index, long, ring and small fingers.

C The ulnar nerve and artery are located between the flexor digitorum sublimis and the flexor carpi ulnaris muscles in the forearm. These structures are exposed as the fascial flap, including the palmaris longus, is retracted medially and the flexor carpi radialis is mobilized laterally. The median nerve and its accompanying artery can now be isolated along the outer margin of the flexor digitorum sublimis muscle, and also, more proximally, beneath this muscle. (Procedure continued on Plate 92.)

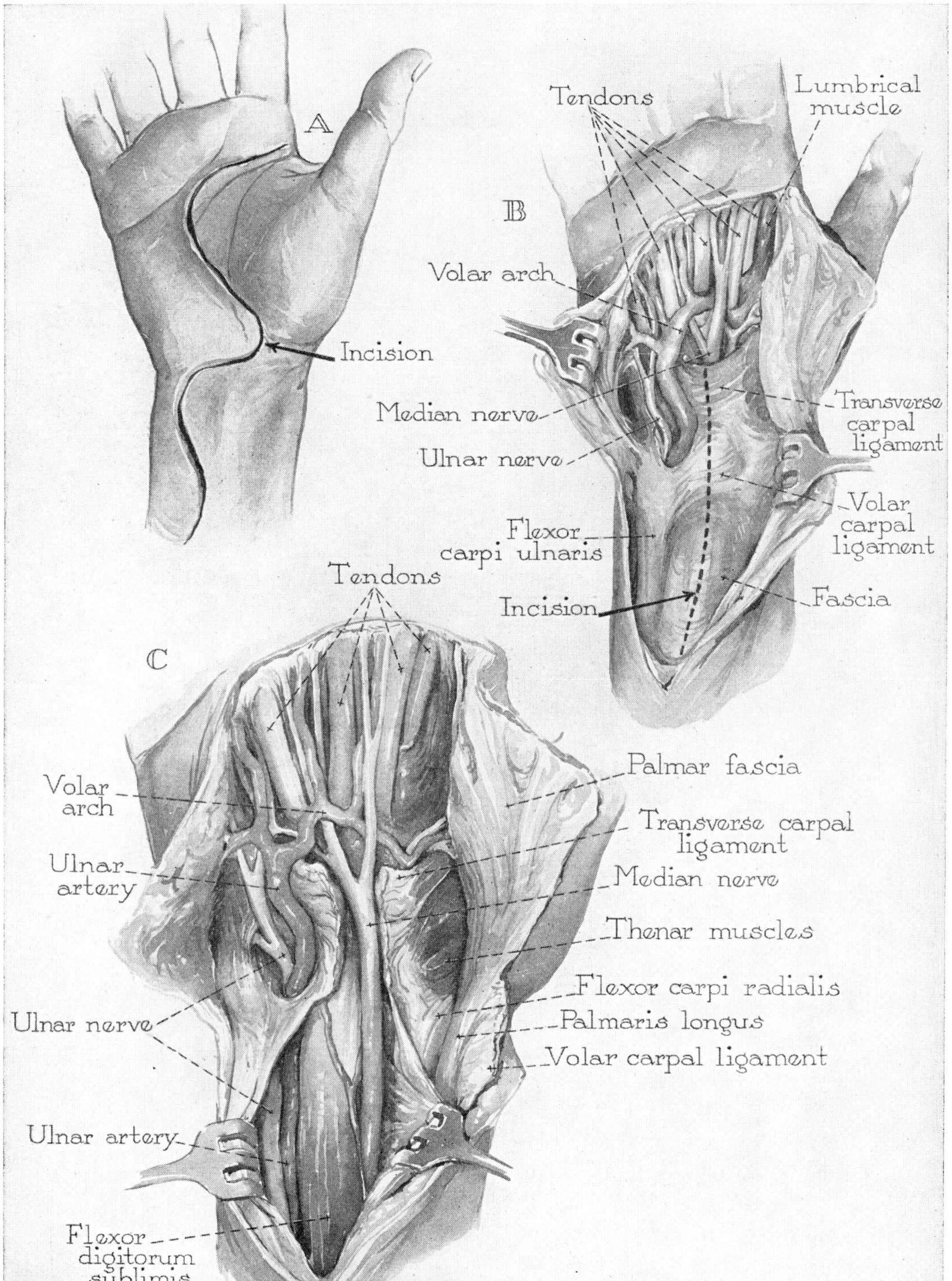

Exposure of the contents of the distal forearm, wrist and palm through a curved hand, transverse wrist and ulnar forarem incision

EXPOSURE OF THE CONTENTS OF THE DISTAL FOREARM, WRIST AND PALM THROUGH A CURVED HAND, TRANSVERSE WRIST AND ULNAR FOREARM INCISION *(Continued)*

Plate 92: Description of Procedure

D The median nerve may be traced into the hand. It passes distally at the radial side of the carpal canal beneath the transverse carpal ligament into the palm. The nerve then divides into the following branches: (1) the thenar branch to the abductor pollicis brevis, opponens pollicis and flexor pollicis brevis muscles; (2) two sensory branches to the thumb; (3) one sensory branch to the radial side of the index finger, and (4) two digital branches which, after supplying the first two or three lumbrical muscles, divide at the clefts between the index and long, and the long and ring fingers to reach the skin of the adjacent portions of these digits.

The flexor digitorum sublimis muscle gives rise to four tendons, each of which inserts at the two sides of the second phalanx of the index to small fingers, respectively. In the carpal tunnel the tendons are arranged in pairs, so that those for the middle and ring fingers are in front, while those for the index and small fingers are behind. All of the tendons, including those of the flexor digitorum profundus, are surrounded by a synovial sheath which facilitates their movement beneath the ligament and over the underlying carpal bones.

E The flexor digitorum profundus is brought into view as the flexor digitorum sublimis is retracted medially out of the way. The muscle arises primarily from the front of the ulna and the adjacent interosseous membrane. The muscle gives off four tendons which traverse the distal forearm and carpal canal to enter the palm and are concealed from view by the overlying tendons of the flexor digitorum sublimis. At the digital canals, the tendons enter the fingers along with, but deep to, those of the sublimis and finally insert at the proximal margin of the distal phalanx of the fingers.

The flexor pollicis longus muscle covers the front of the radius and adjacent portion of the interosseous membrane, and may be exposed by strong radial retraction of the tendon of the flexor carpi radialis, and by lifting the median nerve gently out of the way. The tendon of the flexor pollicis longus sweeps around the base of the thenar eminence after emerging from beneath the transverse carpal ligament, and inserts at the base of the volar aspect of the terminal phalanx of the thumb.

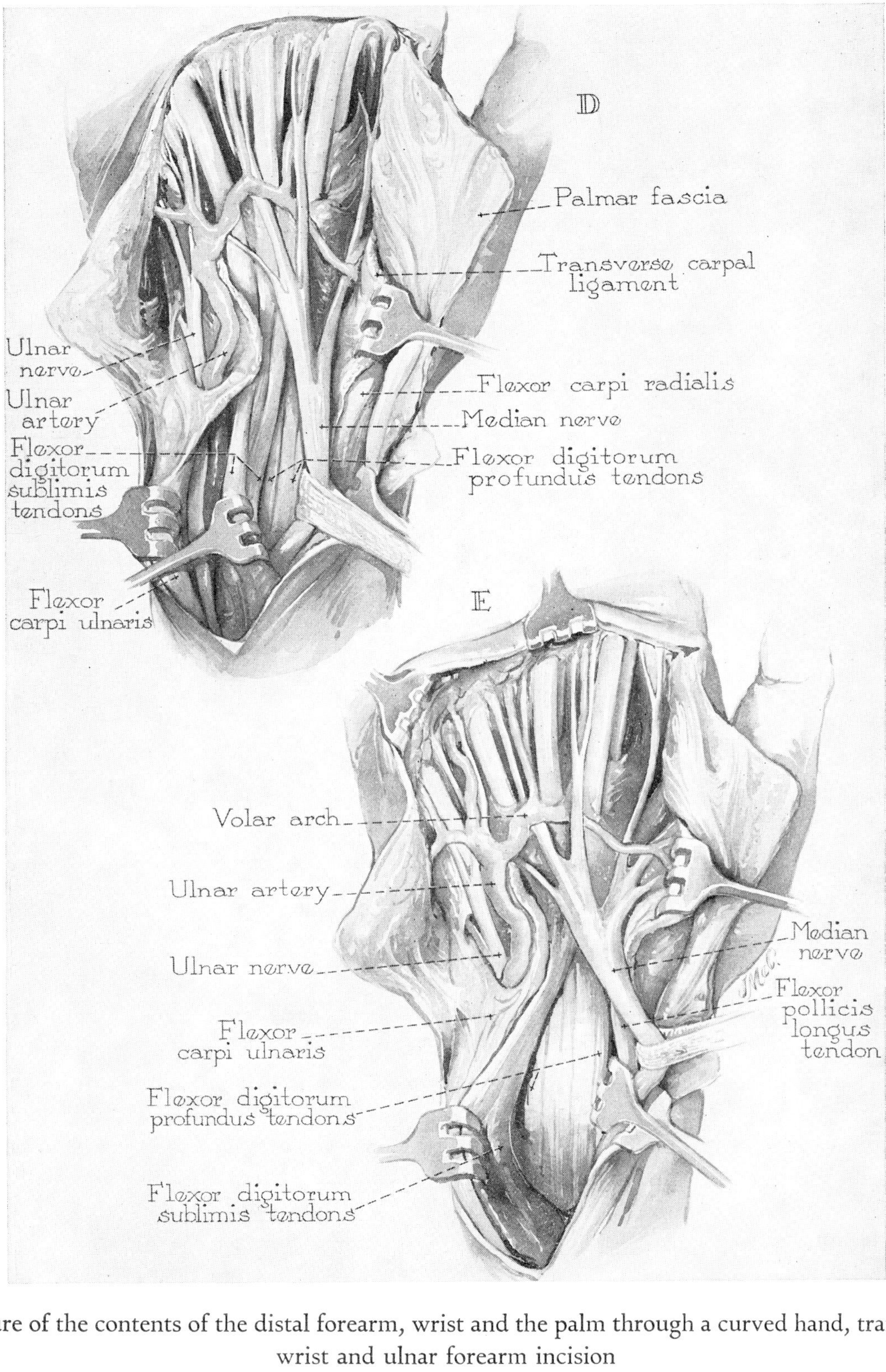

Exposure of the contents of the distal forearm, wrist and the palm through a curved hand, transverse wrist and ulnar forearm incision

EXPOSURE OF THE FLEXOR POLLICIS LONGUS MUSCLE IN THE FORE-ARM AND HAND THROUGH A CURVED PALMAR AND LATERAL FOREARM INCISION

Indications: 1. Repair of Lacerations of the Flexor Pollicis Longus Tendon

2. Restoration of Function of the Flexor Pollicis Longus by Tendon Graft

Plate 93: Description of Procedure

A A palmar and a lateral forearm incision are made. The palmar incision starts at the radial side of the hand in the flexion crease at the base of the thenar eminence, and extends along this crease to within one inch of the distal flexion crease of the wrist. The forearm incision is made along the distal third of the arm; it is centered over the interval between the tendons of the brachioradialis laterally, and the flexor carpi radialis medially, both of which can be located by palpation. The distal end of this incision may curve into the flexion crease of the wrist, as illustrated, or stop short of it.

B The skin flaps are developed and retracted. The palmar fascia is opened in line with the incision, and the radial flap is mobilized to expose the underlying structures. The thenar branch of the median nerve, as well as the two sensory branches to the thumb, must be isolated and protected.

Next, the deep fascia of the forearm is opened through a linear incision. This is best done with the aid of a groove director, to avoid cutting the radial artery which lies just beneath the fascia.

C The flexor carpi radialis tendon is pulled ulnaward to expose the flexor digitorum sublimis, which then is mobilized medially. Note must be made of the location of the median nerve at a deeper level beneath these two structures. Next, the radial artery is identified and protected, and the brachioradialis is pulled outward. The flexor digitorum profundus is exposed at the bottom of the dissection; it has a prominent tendon which extends for a considerable distance up the forearm along the medial margin of the muscle. The pronator quadratus muscle is crossed by the tendon just above the wrist as the latter enters the carpal canal. The location of the tendon at the base of the thenar muscles is determined by means of palpation as the muscle is being pulled in the forearm. It is rarely necessary to uncover the tendon beneath the transverse ligament. A lateral thumb incision permits adequate exposure for passage of the tendon or tendon graft along the digital canal, or for access to the distal phalanx so that the end of the tendon can be anchored to bone.

Page 196

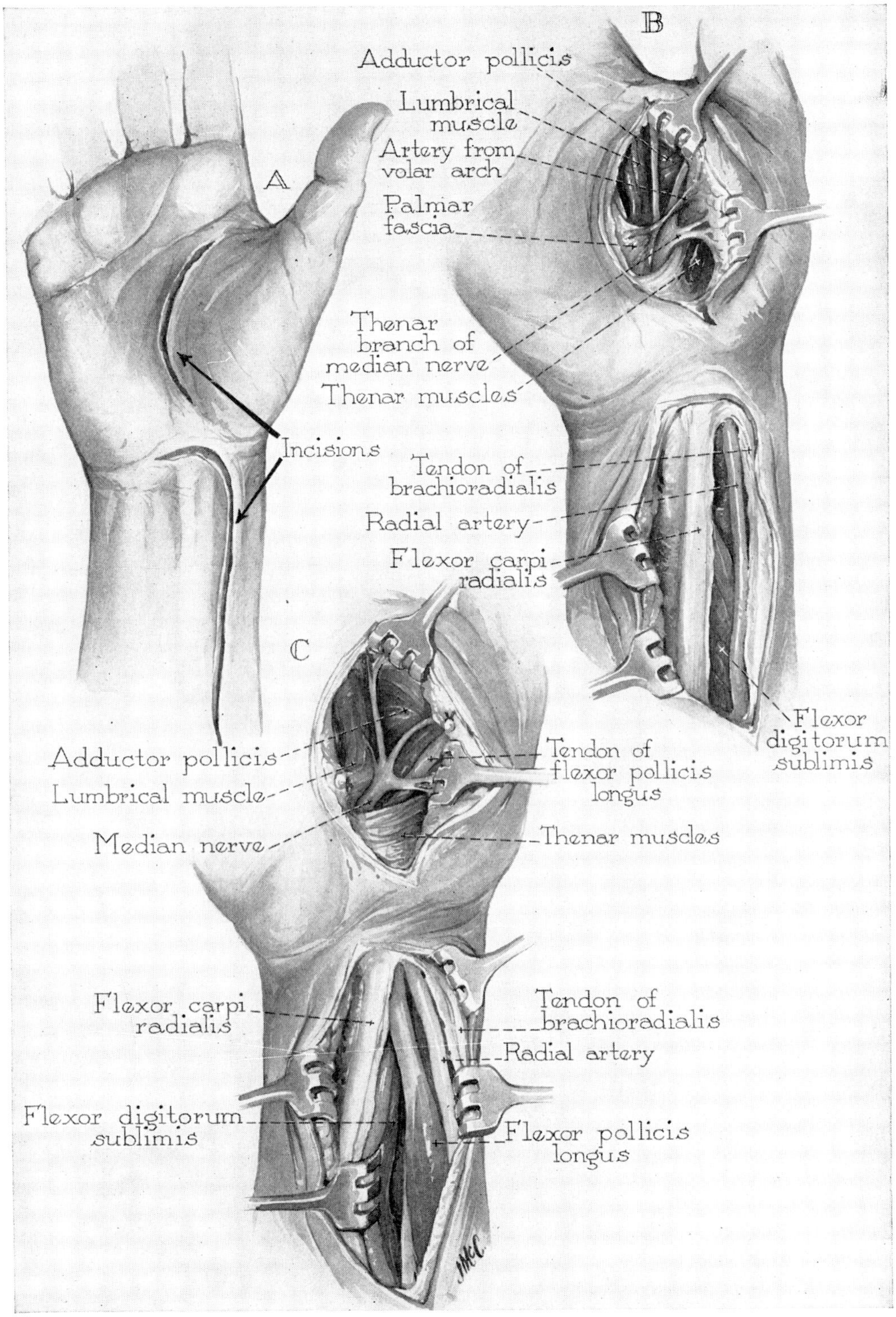

Exposure of the flexor pollicis longus muscle in the forearm and hand through a curved palmar **and** lateral forearm incision

EXPOSURE OF THE MEDIAN NERVE IN THE RADIAL HALF OF THE PALM THROUGH A CURVED VOLAR INCISION

Indications: 1. Repair of Lacerations of the Median Nerve

Plate 94: Description of Procedure

A The incision is made along the flexion crease at the base of the thenar eminence; it starts directly distal to the wrist and ends at the medial margin of the palm.

B The palmar fascia is cut the length of the skin incision. The radial flap is undermined carefully as far as the first metacarpal bone. The medial flap is mobilized for a short distance and retracted. The superficial volar arch is cut between ligatures. The digital branch of the median nerve to the radial side of the index finger is easily identified at the distal end of the wound. This nerve can be traced proximally so as to locate the main portion of the median nerve from which it arises. The median nerve enters the palm beneath the transverse carpal ligament, and the latter may be cut if it should be necessary for obtaining additional exposure of the nerve.

C The remaining branches of the median nerve in the radial half of the palm can now be isolated. Several of them enter and innervate the muscles of the thenar eminence. Two branches pass toward the base of the proximal phalanx of the thumb, from whence they proceed separately along the sides of this digit to supply the skin.

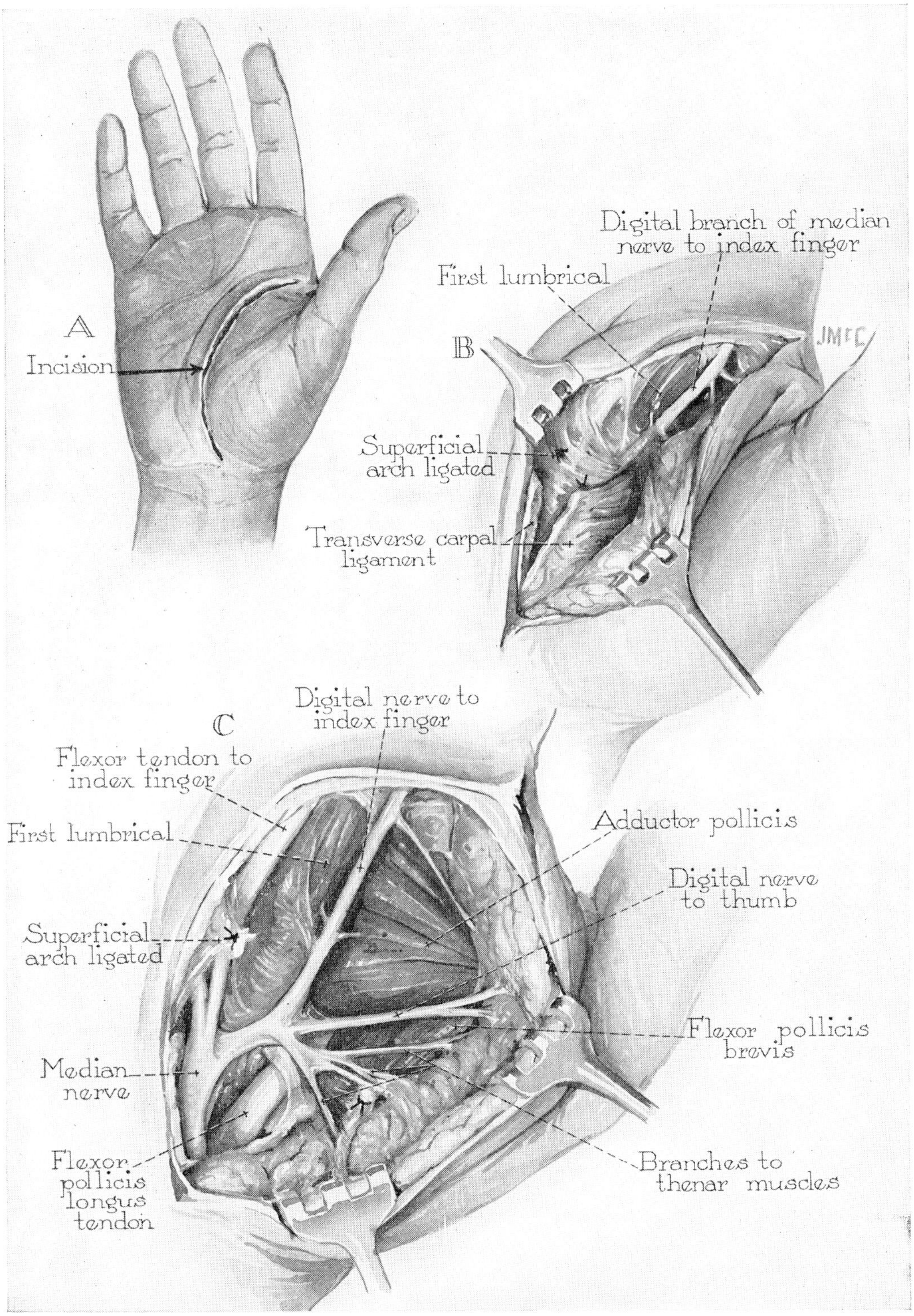

Exposure of the median nerve in the radial half of the palm through a curved volar incision

EXPOSURE OF THE CONTENTS OF THE PALM THROUGH A CURVED HAND INCISION

Indications: 1. Resection of the Palmar Fascia

2. Repair of the Median Nerve in the Palm

3. Repair of Lacerations of the Flexor Tendons

Plate 95: Description of Procedure

A The incision begins at the lateral margin of the palm and extends to the midline in the proximal flexion crease before it curves gently to the wrist between the thenar and hypothenar eminences. The incision should be directed along the skin creases wherever possible.

B The radial skin flap is undercut as far as the thumb. The palmar fascia is opened as shown in the illustration or may be mobilized with the skin.

C The flexor tendons to the index and long fingers are isolated together with their corresponding digital nerves, which are branches of the median nerve. The superficial volar arch crosses the field proximally and may be ligated if necessary to facilitate the exposure. (Procedure continued on Plate 96.)

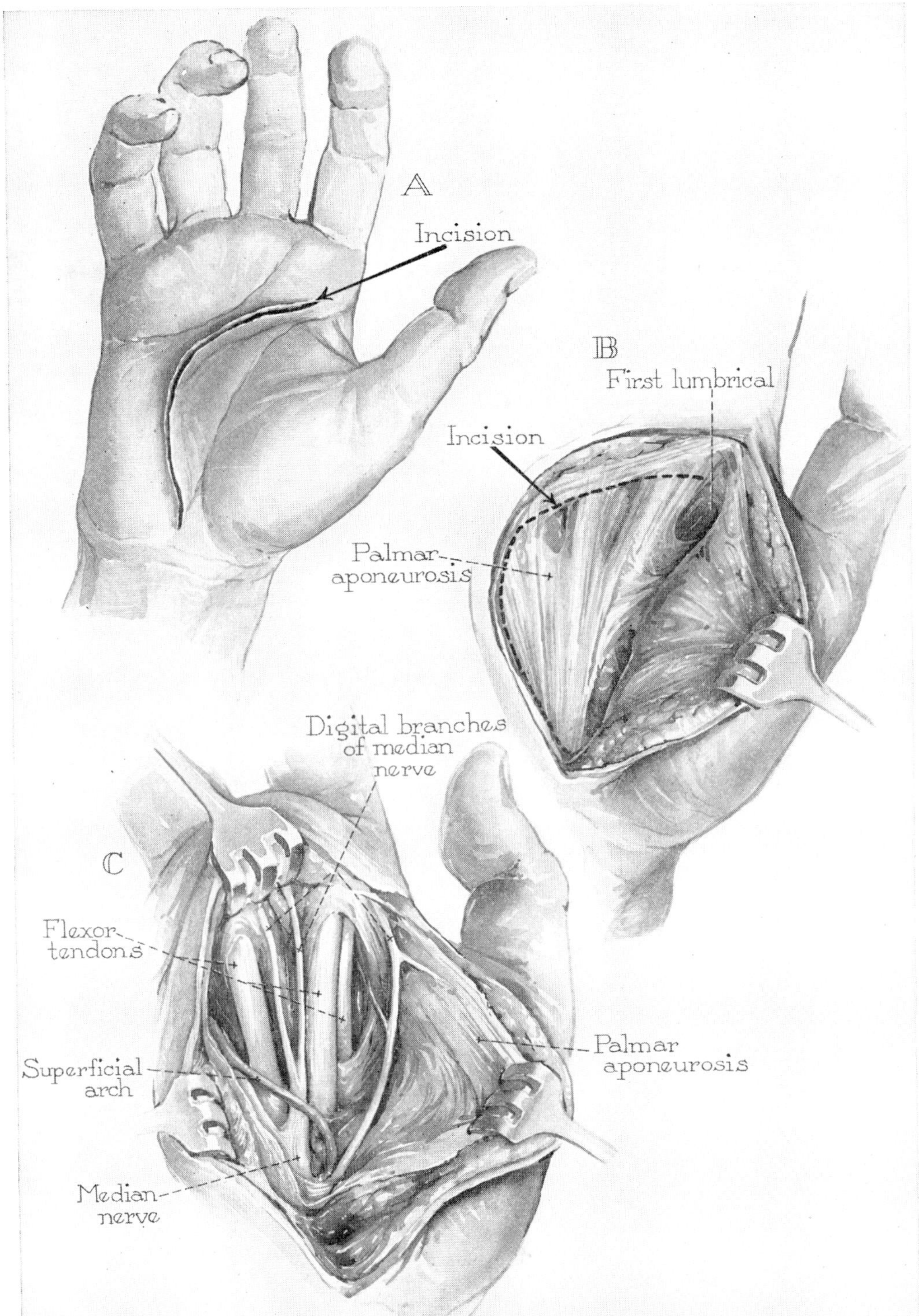

Exposure of the contents of the palm through a curved hand incision

EXPOSURE OF THE CONTENTS OF THE PALM THROUGH A CURVED HAND INCISION *(Continued)*

Plate 96: Description of Procedure

D The ulnar skin flap and palmar fascia are now mobilized from the underlying structures and retracted so as to extend the exposure to the medial margin of the palm. The ulnar artery and nerve enter the hand from beneath the volar carpal ligament and superficial to the transverse carpal ligament. The artery gives off a profunda branch which, together with the deep branch of the ulnar nerve, passes between the abductor and the flexor digiti quinti muscles to enter the deep portion of the palm and complete the deep palmar arch. The main portion of the ulnar artery provides branches to the hypothenar muscles before it passes radialward to form the superficial volar arch. Four common digital arteries arise from this arch; they accompany the digital branches of the ulnar and median nerves to the index, long, ring and small fingers.

The tendons of the flexor digitorum sublimis and profundus muscles are now exposed; they can be traced from beneath the transverse carpal ligament to the proximal ends of the digital canals. Each of the four lumbrical muscles is found on the radial side of the corresponding flexor digitorum sublimis tendon.

The adductor pollicis brevis and the muscles of the thenar eminence, together with their nerve supply, are now uncovered radially.

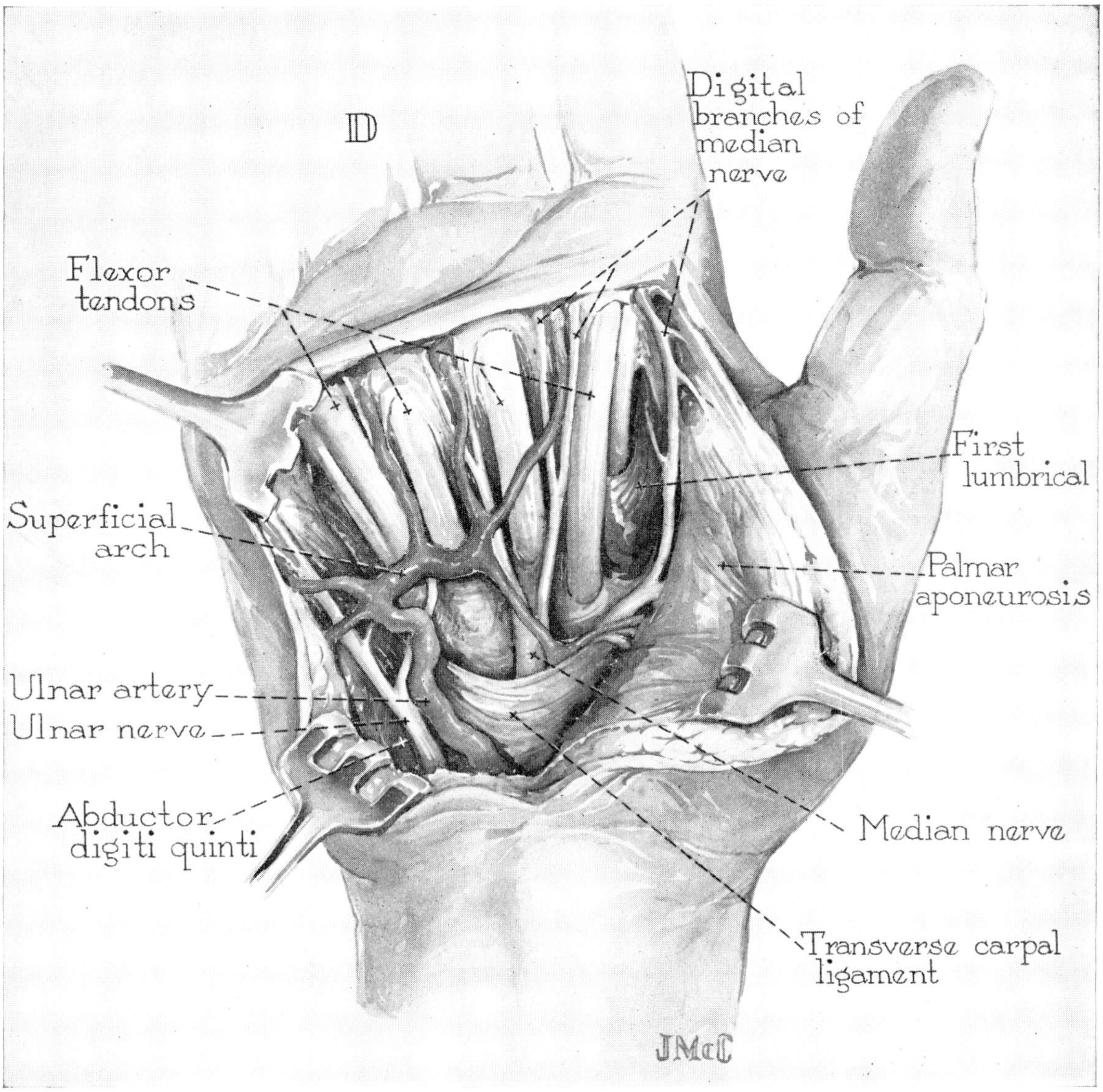

Exposure of the contents of the palm through a curved hand incision

EXPOSURE OF THE THENAR SPACE OF THE PALM THROUGH A LINEAR INCISION OVER THE FIRST DORSAL INTEROSSEOUS MUSCLE

Indications: 1. Drainage of Abscess

2. Removal of Benign Growths Which Cannot Be Resected Satisfactorily through a Volar Incision

Plate 97: Description of Procedure

A The anatomical landmark for placing the incision is the free margin of the first dorsal interosseous muscle. The length of the incision depends on the particular surgical objective. Thus, if the objective is the drainage of an abscess, the incision, made over its summit, may be a short one.

B The skin and the deep fascia are retracted, and the radial margin of the first dorsal interosseous is freed and pulled toward the second metacarpal bone. The adductor pollicis muscle now is seen in the floor of the wound. It is fan-shaped, and its muscle fibers run in the direction of their attachment onto the first metacarpal bone.

C The distal or free margin of the adductor pollicis muscle is separated from the tendons anterior to it, and the muscle is pulled dorsally to expose the intermediate thenar space.

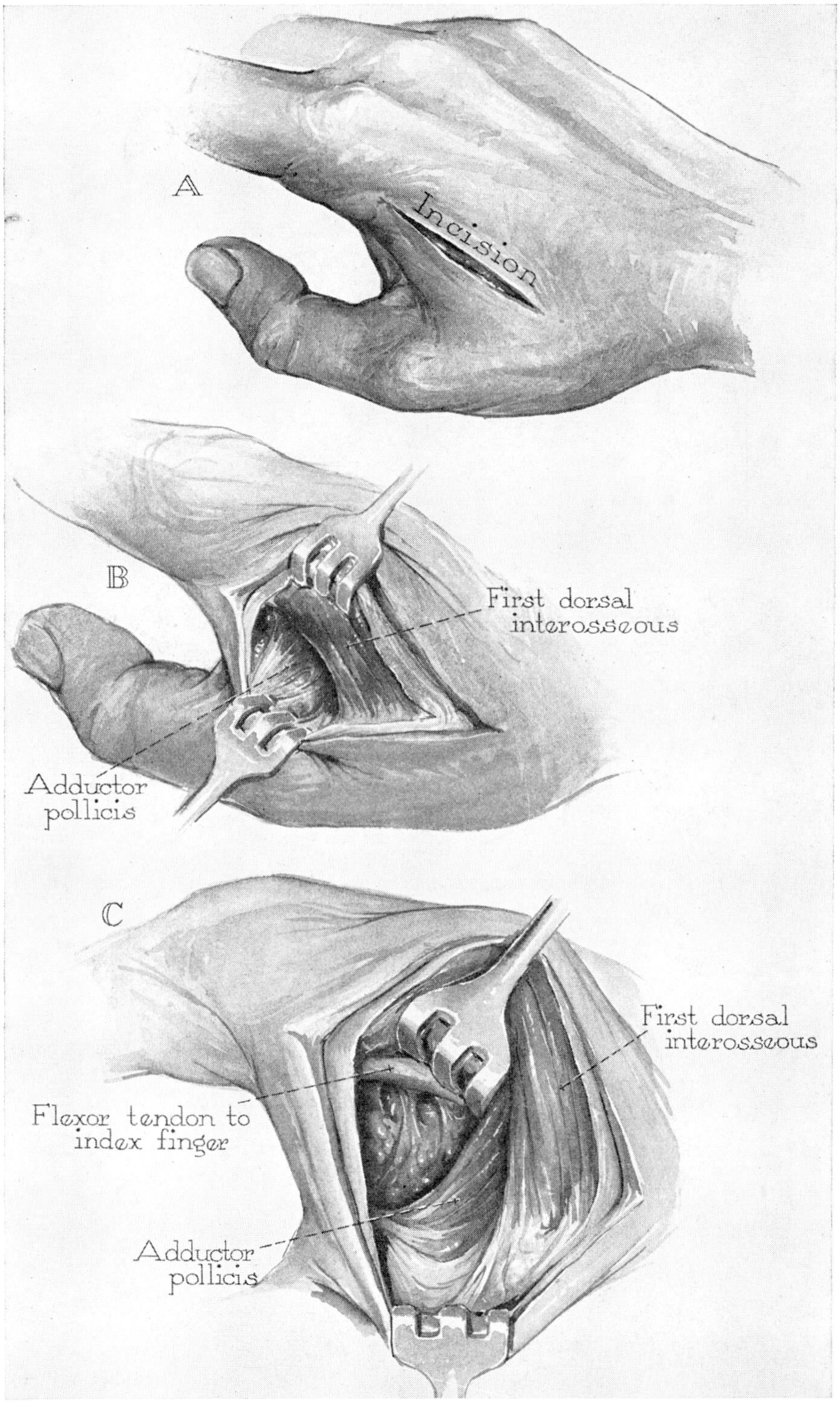

Exposure of the thenar space of the palm through a linear incision over the first dorsal interosseous muscle

EXPOSURE OF THE FIRST METACARPAL BONE AND THE METACARPAL MULTANGULAR MAJOR JOINT THROUGH A CURVED INCISION

Indications: 1. Partial Ostectomy for Osteomyelitis

2. Resection of Benign Tumors

3. Open Reduction of Bennett Fractures Which Cannot Be Reduced by Skeletal Traction

Plate 98: Description of Procedure

A The incision begins at the midpoint of the flexion crease over the metacarpal phalangeal joint of the thumb, and extends posteriorly in this crease to the dorsum of the first metacarpal bone; it then curves upward, while centering over this structure, and ends at the anatomical snuffbox. The deep fascia is incised in line with the skin incision.

B The abductor pollicis brevis muscle is located along the radial side of the incision, and the tendon of the extensor pollicis longus is identified along the opposite side. The periosteum is opened over the dorsum of the first metacarpal bone between the abductor pollicis brevis and the dorsal first interosseous muscles. The bone is exposed subperiosteally for the desired distance.

C The capsule of the first metacarpal multangular joint is located in the proximal end of the wound; the capsule is incised and its edges retracted to expose the interior of this joint.

NOTE: The incision may be shortened proximally if exposure of the metacarpal multangular major joint is not desired; on the other hand, the joint and the adjacent portion of the first metacarpal bone can be adequately exposed without extending the incision beyond the middle third of this bone.

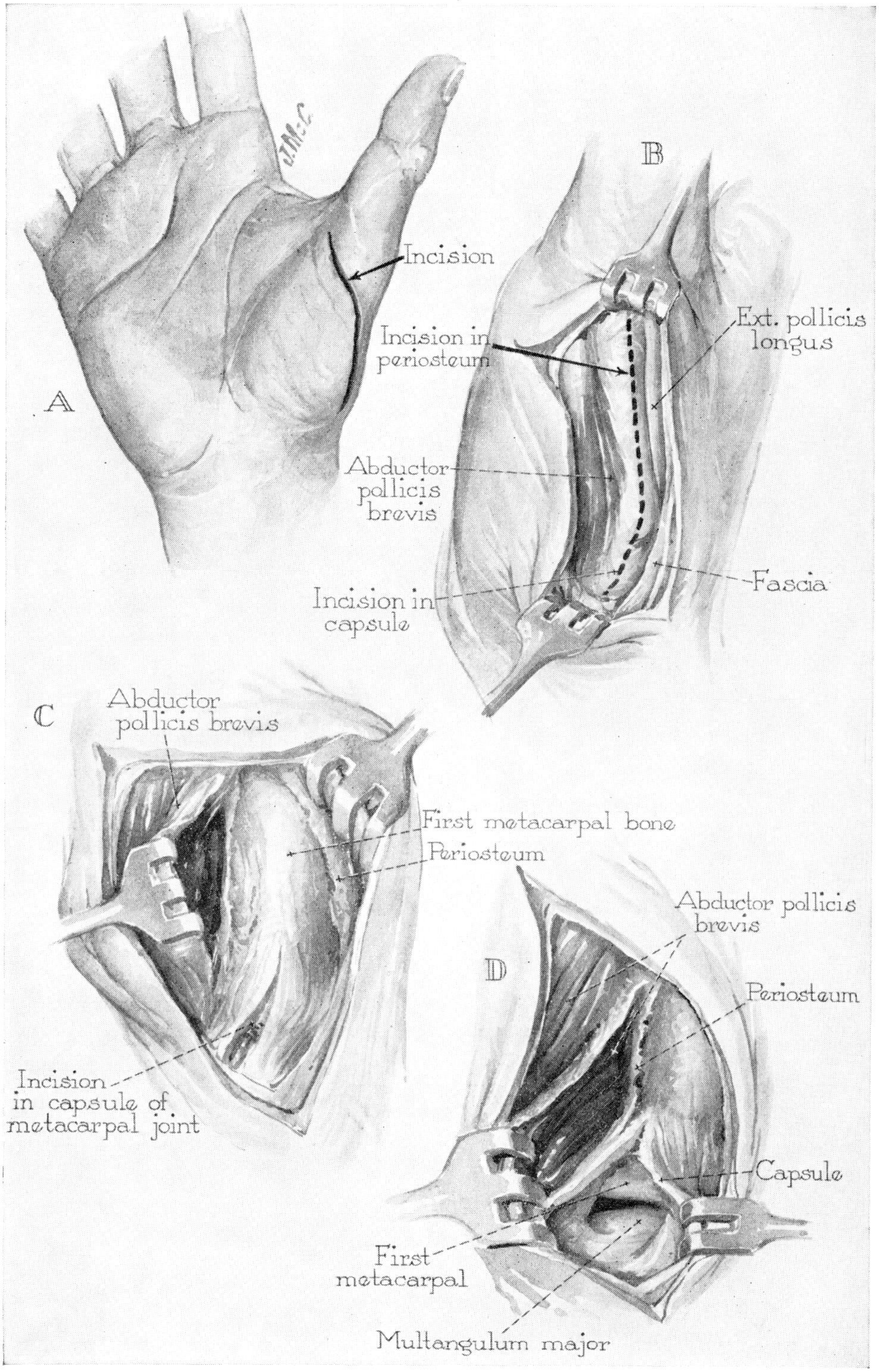

Exposure of the first metacarpal bone and the metacarpal multangular major joint through a curved incision

EXPOSURE OF THE SECOND METACARPAL BONE THROUGH A DORSAL LINEAR INCISION

Indications: 1. Open Reduction of Acute Fractures

2. Treatment of Mal-united and Un-united Fractures

3. Removal of Benign Tumors

4. Partial Ostectomy for Osteomyelitis

Plate 99: Description of Procedure

A An incision, about 2 1/4 inches in length, is made over the dorsal surface of the second metacarpal bone. The incision is placed slightly to the radial side of the midline of the bone in order to avoid the extensor tendons.

B The deep fascia is cut and the wound edges are retracted. The extensor tendons to the index finger are located along the ulnar side of the incision. Beneath them can be seen the second dorsal interosseous muscle, the first dorsal interosseous muscle being visible on the other side of the wound.

C The second metacarpal bone and periosteum is located dorsally between the first and second dorsal interosseous muscles. This bone is exposed subperiosteally after incising the periosteum along the line shown in the illustration. This dissection can be carried completely around the bone without endangering the surrounding tissues, because of the protection afforded by the periosteum.

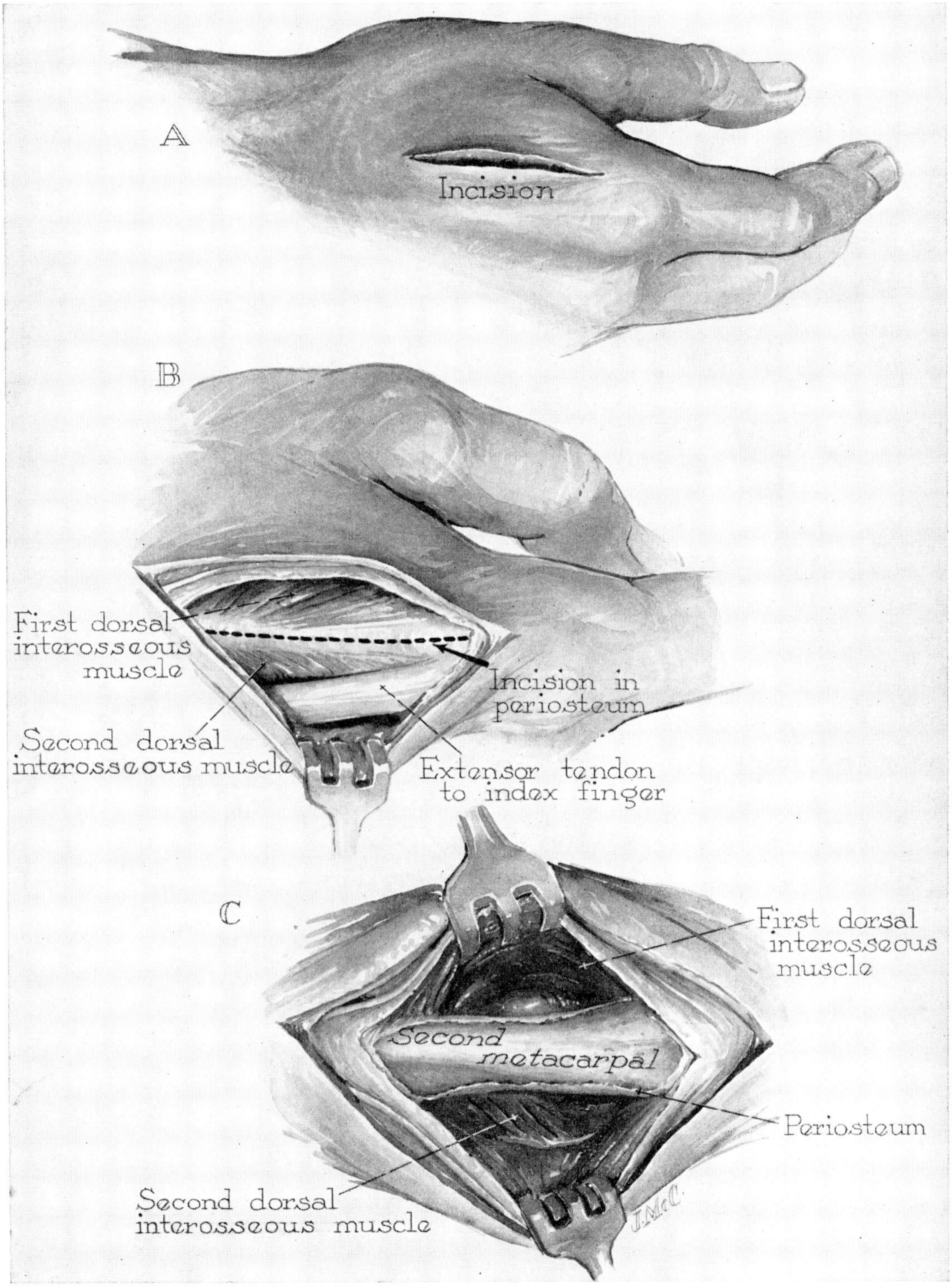

Exposure of the second metacarpal bone through a dorsal linear incision

EXPOSURE OF THE FIFTH METACARPAL BONE THROUGH A DORSAL LATERAL INCISION

Indications: 1. Open Reduction of Acute Fractures

2. Treatment of Mal-united and Un-united Fractures

3. Removal of Benign Tumors

4. Partial Ostectomy for Osteomyelitis

Plate 100: Description of Procedure

A The skin incision is placed over the dorsal lateral surface of the fifth metacarpal bone, which can be identified by palpation. The length of the incision is determined by the desired bone exposure.

B The deep fascia is incised and its margins and the skin are retracted. The abductor digiti quinti muscle is located along the ulnar side of the wound. Radially to the bone are the fourth dorsal interosseous muscle and the extensor tendons to the small finger.

C Flanked by the soft tissues just described is the fifth metacarpal bone, covered dorsally only by the periosteum. The periosteum is incised and reflected from the bone for the desired distance. Firm downward retraction of the abductor digiti quinti will expose the opponens digiti quinti muscle.

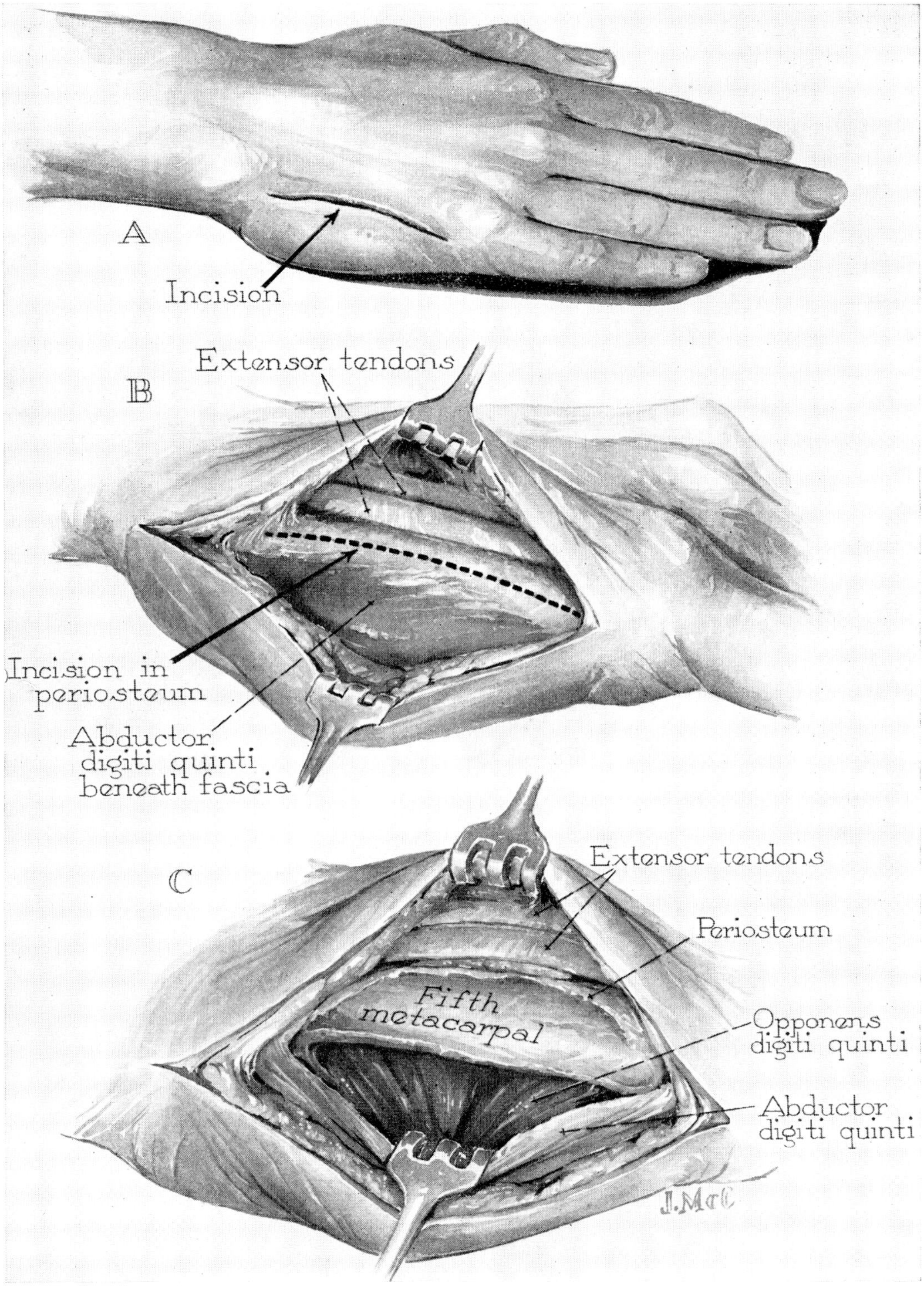

Exposure of the fifth metacarpal bone through a dorsal lateral incision

Section VII

Region of the Hip Joint

EXPOSURE OF THE HIP JOINT THROUGH AN ANTERIOR FEMORAL INCISION

Indications: 1. Biopsy of the Hip Joint

2. Removal of the Loose Bodies from the Hip Joint

3. Open Reduction of Congenital Dislocation of the Hip

4. Arthroplasty of the Hip in Certain Cases

Plate 101: Description of Procedure

A The skin incision extends along the interval between the tensor fasciae latae laterally and the sartorius medially; it begins at the anterior superior iliac spine and is directed distally for approximately 5 inches.

B The skin margins are undercut and retracted, and the fascia lata is opened in line with the skin incision. The anterior margin of the tensor fasciae latae muscle is separated from the sartorius muscle and retracted laterally; the wound then is deepened by cutting through the loose areolar tissue which separates these structures. The ascending branch of the lateral circumflex artery and accompanying vein which cross the field must be carefully clamped, severed and ligated.

C The wound is deepened down to the anterior capsule of the hip joint, which will bring into view the rectus femoris muscle lying beneath the sartorius along the inner wall of the incision and the gluteus medius muscle laterally beneath the tensor fasciae latae.

D The fatty layer is removed from the front of the capsule and, if necessary, the reflected head of the rectus femoris muscle is retracted out of the way. This portion of the rectus muscle may be transected to enlarge the wound, while the tendon of the iliopsoas is pulled medially. The hip joint is exposed through a T incision made into the capsule.

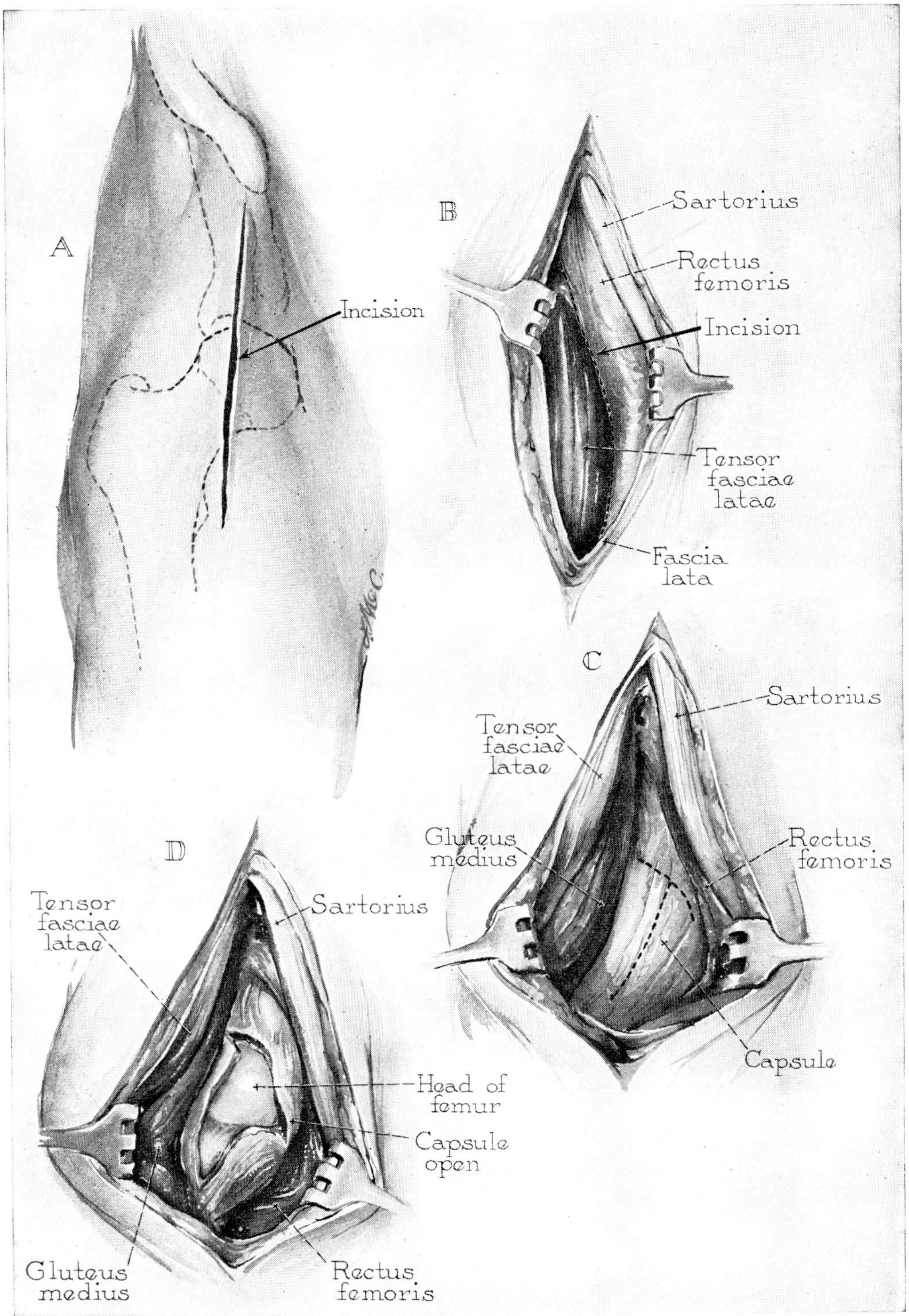

Exposure of the hip joint through an anterior femoral incision

EXPOSURE OF THE HIP JOINT AND SUBTROCHANTERIC REGION OF THE FEMUR THROUGH AN ANTERIOR FEMORAL INCISION WHICH TRANSECTS THE TENSOR FASCIAE LATAE MUSCLE

Indications: 1. Open Reduction and Internal Fixation of Fractures of the Neck of the Femur

2. Osteotomy and Internal Fixation of the Neck of the Femur for Correction of Slipped Femoral Epiphysis

Plate 102: Description of Procedure

A The incision starts downward from the anterior superior iliac spine, in the interval between the tensor fasciae latae and the sartorius muscle, and, in its lower end, gradually curves posteriorly to terminate over the side of the femur, some 2 1/2 inches below the greater trochanter.

B The skin margins are undermined adequately, and the fascia lata is opened in line with the skin incision.

C The dissection is then developed through the loose areolar tissue between the tensor fasciae latae laterally, and the sartorius and rectus femoris medially. The ascending branch of the lateral circumflex artery is ligated. In the lower portion of the wound, the incision crosses the tensor fasciae latae muscle and sections it. This dissection will likewise expose the vastus lateralis muscle which lies below the tensor fasciae latae. (Procedure continued on Plate 103.)

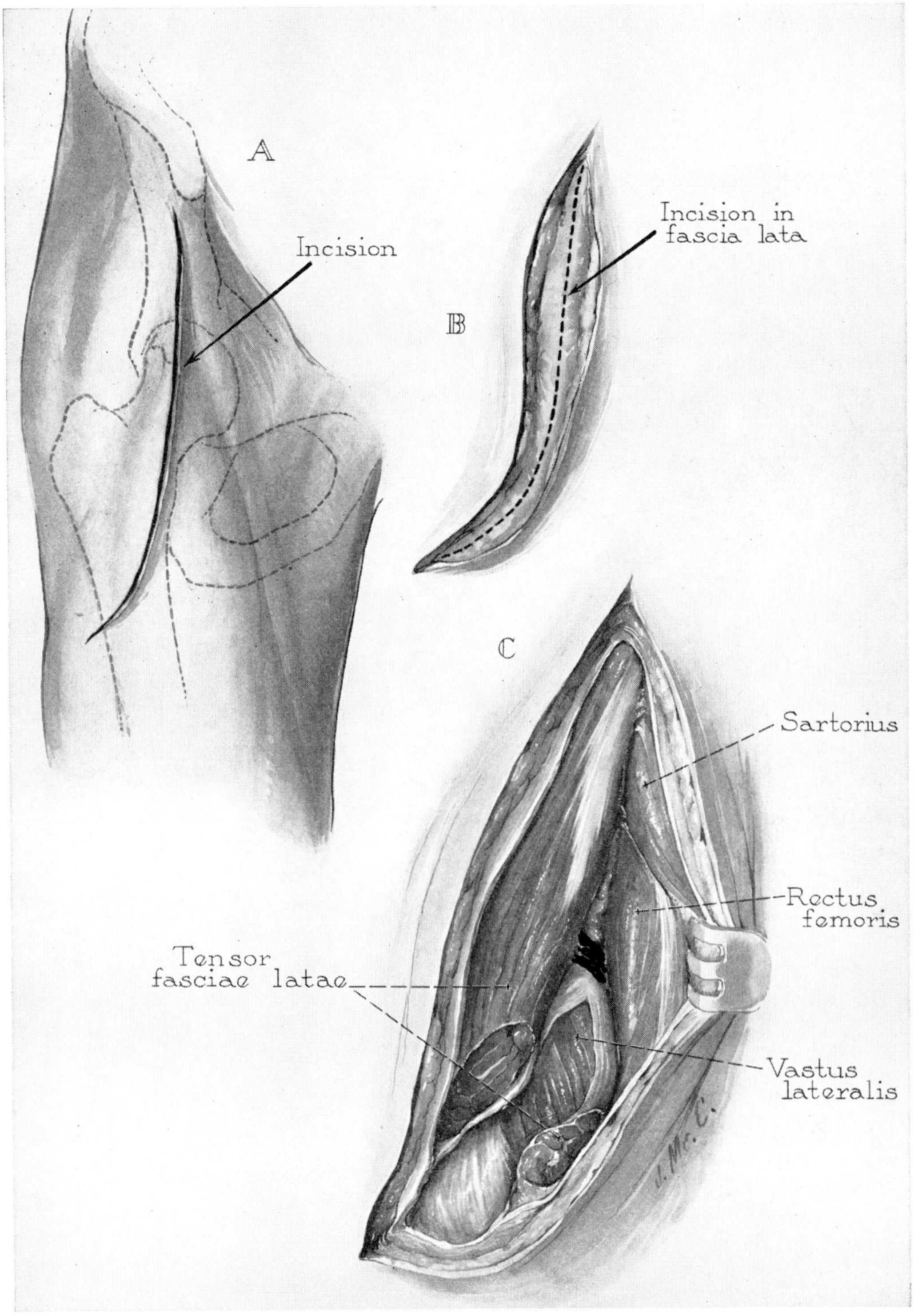

Exposure of the hip joint and subtrochanteric region of the femur through an anterior femoral incision which transects the tensor fasciae latae muscle

EXPOSURE OF THE HIP JOINT AND SUBTROCHANTERIC REGION OF THE FEMUR THROUGH AN ANTERIOR FEMORAL INCISION WHICH TRANSECTS THE TENSOR FASCIAE LATAE MUSCLE *(Continued)*

Plate 103: Description of Procedure

D The tensor fasciae latae then is retracted firmly toward the lateral side, thereby exposing the gluteus medius muscle. The capsule of the hip joint is cleared of the overlying fatty tissue and the iliopsoas tendon is pulled medially. The proximal end of the vastus lateralis is identified below the greater trochanter.

E The hip joint is opened by a T incision, and the subtrochanteric region of the shaft of the femur is exposed by reflecting the vastus lateralis subperiosteally in a downward direction away from the bone.

NOTE: The only nerve which may be encountered in this incision is the lateral femoral cutaneous, which enters the thigh at the level of and just medial to the anterior superior iliac spine. It is located usually along the medial skin flap and easily escapes attention. The exposure can be enlarged by extending the wound along the iliac crest and by denuding the surface of the ilium subperiosteally.

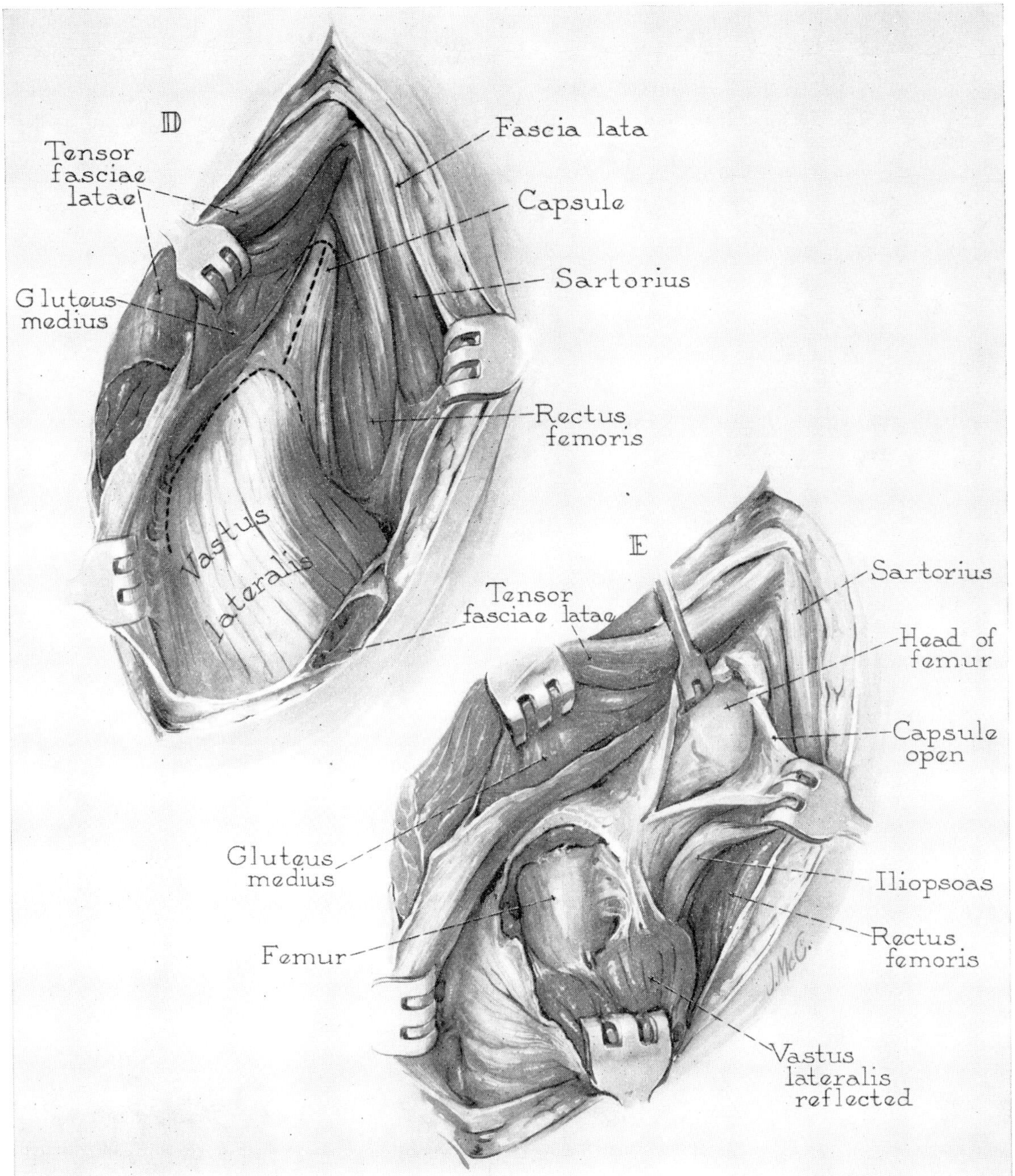

Exposure of the hip joint and subtrochanteric region of the femur through an anterior femoral incision which transects the tensor fasciae latae muscle

EXPOSURE OF THE HIP JOINT THROUGH AN ANTERIOR ILIOFEMORAL INCISION

Indications: 1. Arthroplasty of the Hip Joint

2. Reconstruction Operations for Un-united Fractures of the Neck of the Femur

3. Arthrodesis of the Hip Joint

4. Open Reduction of Some Cases of Traumatic Dislocation of the Hip

Plate 104: Description of Procedure

A The skin incision, approximately 9 inches in length, begins over the iliac crest 3 inches posteriorly to the anterior superior iliac spine. The cut extends forward along the iliac crest to the spine and downward into the leg between the tensor fasciae latae and the rectus femoris muscles for the required distance.

B The deep fascia is opened and the flaps are retracted.

C The incision is deepened along the iliac crest down to the bone, and the fascia lata, gluteus medius and gluteus minimus muscles are separated subperiosteally from the ilium. A gauze pack is inserted to control bleeding. The dissection in the leg separates the tensor fasciae latae muscle from the sartorius muscle medially. The ascending branch of the lateral femoral circumflex artery crosses the operative field, and must be ligated. (Procedure continued on Plate 105.)

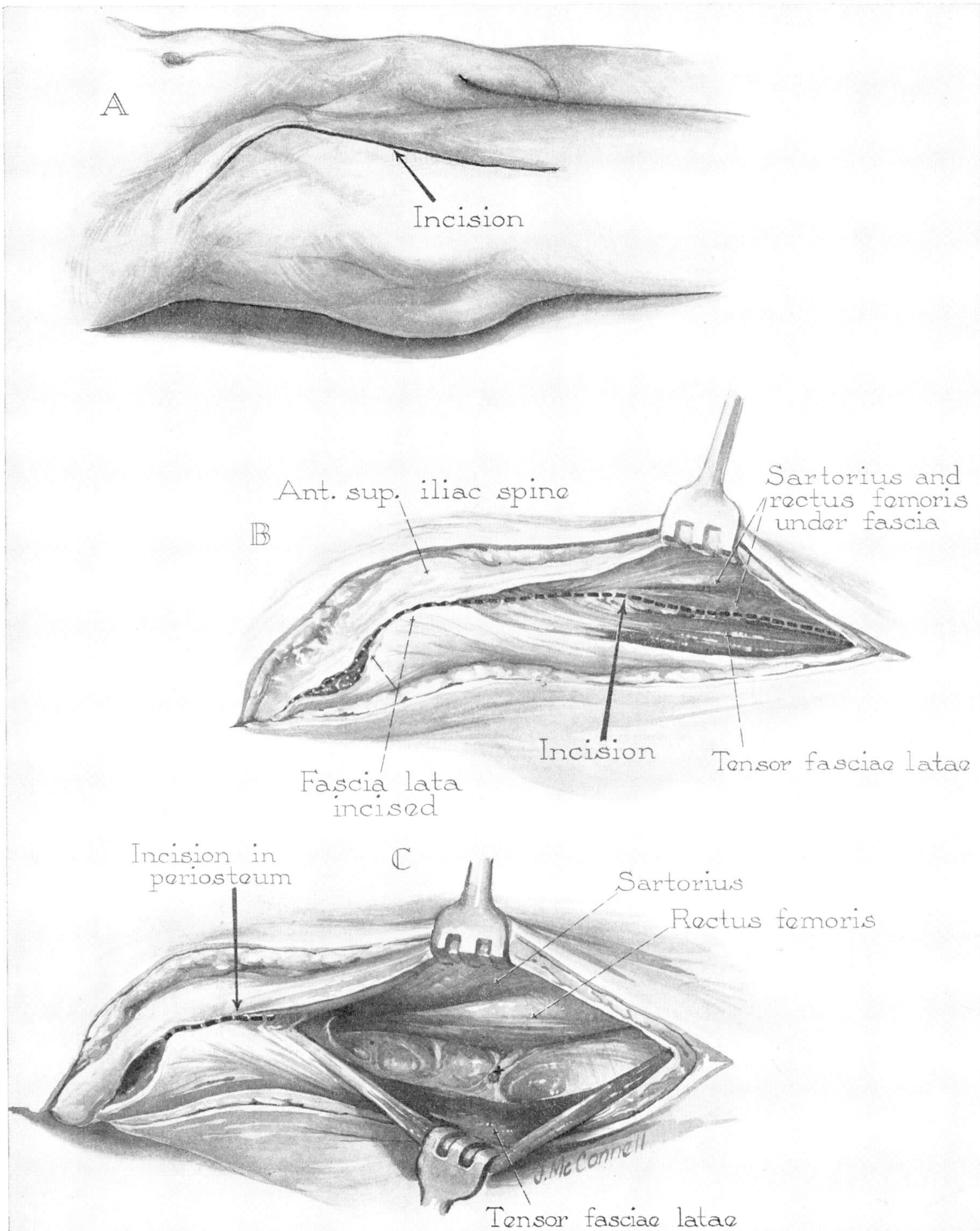

Exposure of the hip joint through an anterior iliofemoral incision

EXPOSURE OF THE HIP JOINT THROUGH AN ANTERIOR ILIOFEMORAL INCISION *(Continued)*

Plate 105: Description of Procedure

D The outer flap of tissue, consisting of the tensor fasciae latae and the gluteus medius and minimus muscles, is pulled as far laterally as possible. The inner aspect of the wound is lined by the sartorius and rectus femoris muscles. The vastus lateralis muscle covers the femur distal to the capsule of the hip joint, at the bottom of the incision.

E The exposure then is continued down to the hip joint capsule, which is isolated beneath the pad of fat that covers it. The reflected tendon of origin of the rectus femoris muscle can be cut if it interferes with the exposure. The tendon of the iliopsoas muscle usually must be pulled medially out of the way with a rake retractor. The capsule is opened to expose the interior of the joint.

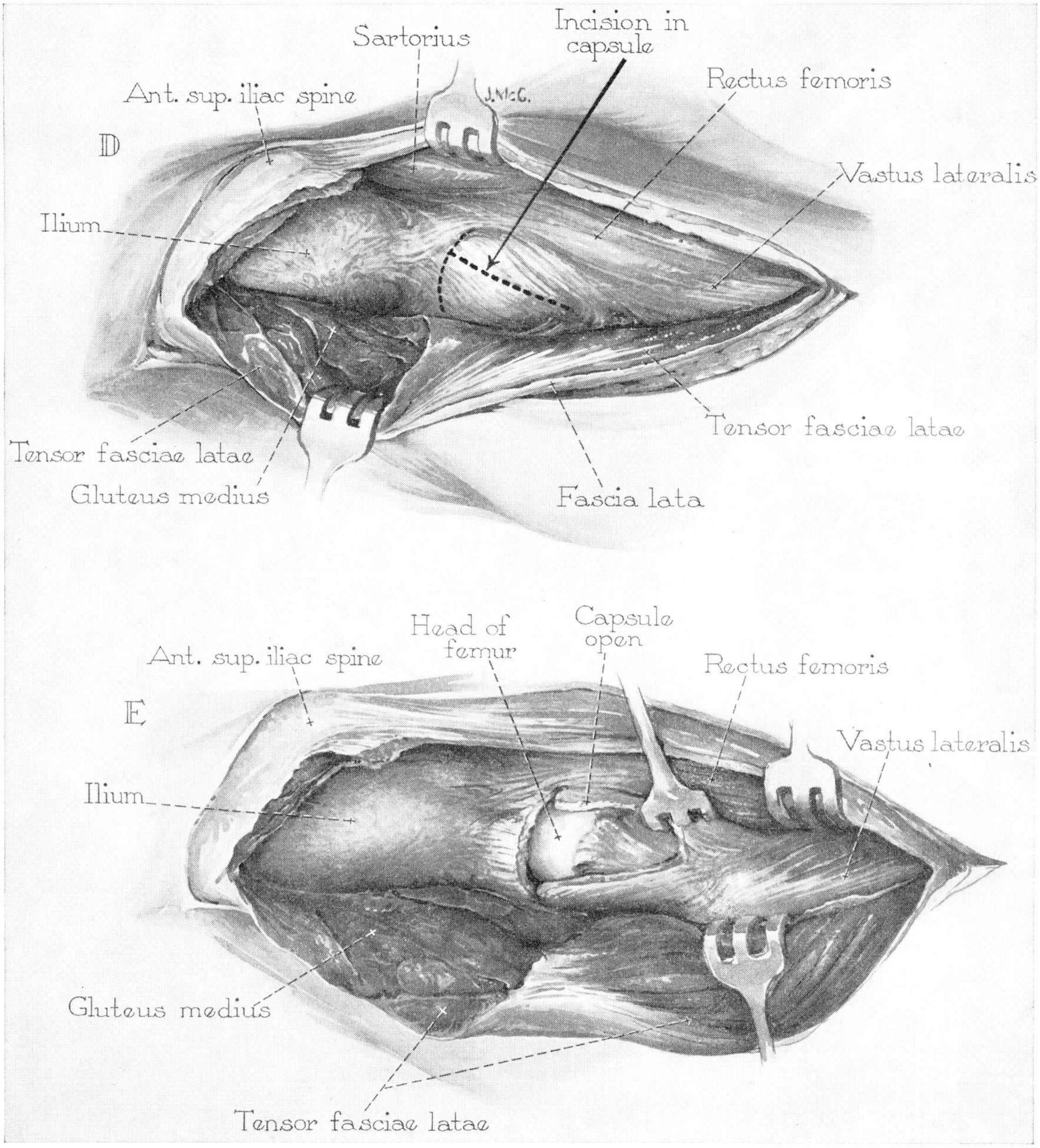

Exposure of the hip joint through an anterior iliofemoral incision

EXPOSURE OF THE HIP JOINT AND SUBTROCHANTERIC REGION OF THE FEMUR THROUGH AN ANTERIOR ILIOFEMORAL INCISION TRANSECTING THE TENSOR FASCIAE LATAE MUSCLE

Indications: 1. Arthrodesis of the Hip Joint

2. Arthroplasty of the Hip Joint

3. Open Reduction and Internal Fixation of an Intracapsular Fracture of the Hip

Plate 106: Description of Procedure

A The incision extends forward from the middle third of the iliac crest to the anterior superior iliac spine, and then turns distally into the thigh, following for 5 inches along the groove between the tensor fasciae latae and the sartorius muscle before it curves gently posteriorly to end over the lateral aspect of the femur.

B The deep fascia is incised throughout the course of the skin incision.

C The dissection is extended to the crest of the ilium above, and across the tensor fasciae latae muscle distally. By incising the fascia lata connecting the two, the groove between the tensor fasciae latae laterally and the sartorius and rectus femoris muscles medially is opened. The dissection is continued down to the fatty layer which covers the front of the hip joint. The ascending branch of the lateral femoral circumflex artery crosses the midportion of the wound and must be isolated, cut between forceps and then ligated. (Procedure continued on Plate 107.)

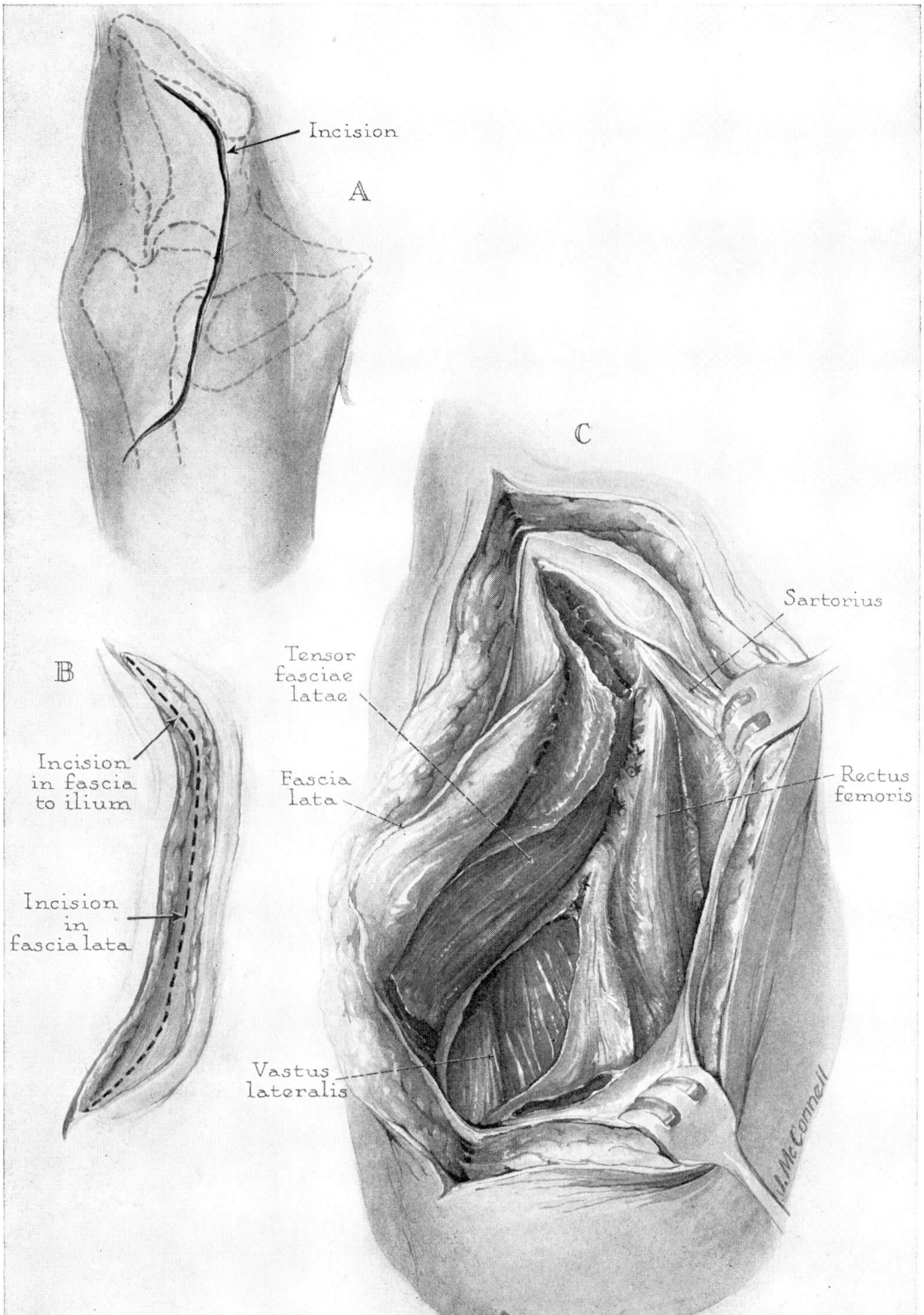

Exposure of the hip joint and subtrochanteric region of the femur through an anterior iliofemoral incision transecting the tensor fasciae latae muscle

EXPOSURE OF THE HIP JOINT AND SUBTROCHANTERIC REGION OF THE FEMUR THROUGH AN ANTERIOR ILIOFEMORAL INCISION TRANSECTING THE TENSOR FASCIAE LATAE MUSCLE *(Continued)*

Plate 107: Description of Procedure

D The tensor fasciae latae and the gluteus medius and gluteus minimus muscles are stripped subperiosteally from the outer surface of the wing of the ilium. The muscular flap consisting of these muscles can be retracted far laterally to expose the greater trochanter and the adjacent portion of the thigh.

E The capsule is opened after excision of its overlying fatty layer, and the iliopsoas tendon and the medial muscles are pulled toward the midline. The reflected head of the rectus femoris muscle is cut if it obscures the upper aspect of the capsule.

The subtrochanteric portion of the femur then is exposed by lifting the vastus lateralis muscle subperiosteally from the bone and retracting it downward and medially.

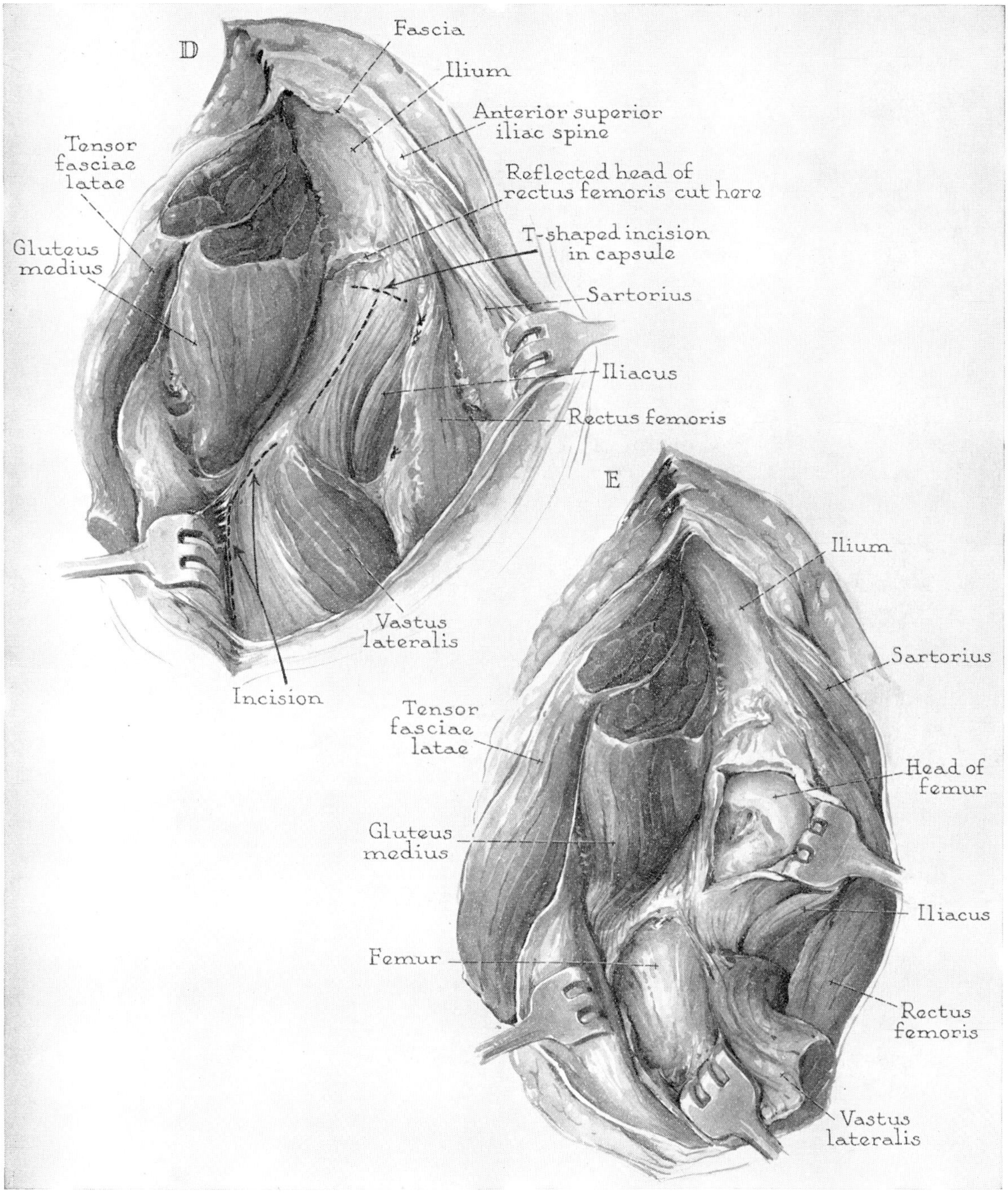

Exposure of the hip joint and subtrochanteric region of the femur through an anterior iliofemoral incision transecting the tensor fasciae latae muscle

EXPOSURE OF THE HIP JOINT AND THE SUPRA-ACETABULAR PORTION OF THE PELVIS THROUGH AN ANTERIOR ILIOFEMORAL INCISION WITH REFLECTION DOWNWARD OF THE RECTUS FEMORIS MUSCLE

Indication: 1. Arthroplasty of the Hip Joint

Plate 108: Description of Procedure

A The incision begins over the iliac crest from a point about 3 inches back of the anterior superior iliac spine, and then continues straight downward from the spine for approximately 6 inches or more over the thigh.

B The skin margins are mobilized and retracted widely. The deep fascia is incised over the iliac crest and the interval between the tensor fasciae latae and sartorius muscles.

C The wound is deepened to the iliac crest by an incision through the periosteum. The tensor fasciae latae and the gluteus medius and gluteus minimus muscles are reflected subperiosteally from the lateral surface of the wing of the ilium. The dissection then is continued into the thigh. The tensor fasciae latae is separated from the sartorius and the rectus femoris muscle. The ascending branch of the lateral circumflex artery which traverses this portion of the wound is ligated. (Procedure continued on Plate 109.)

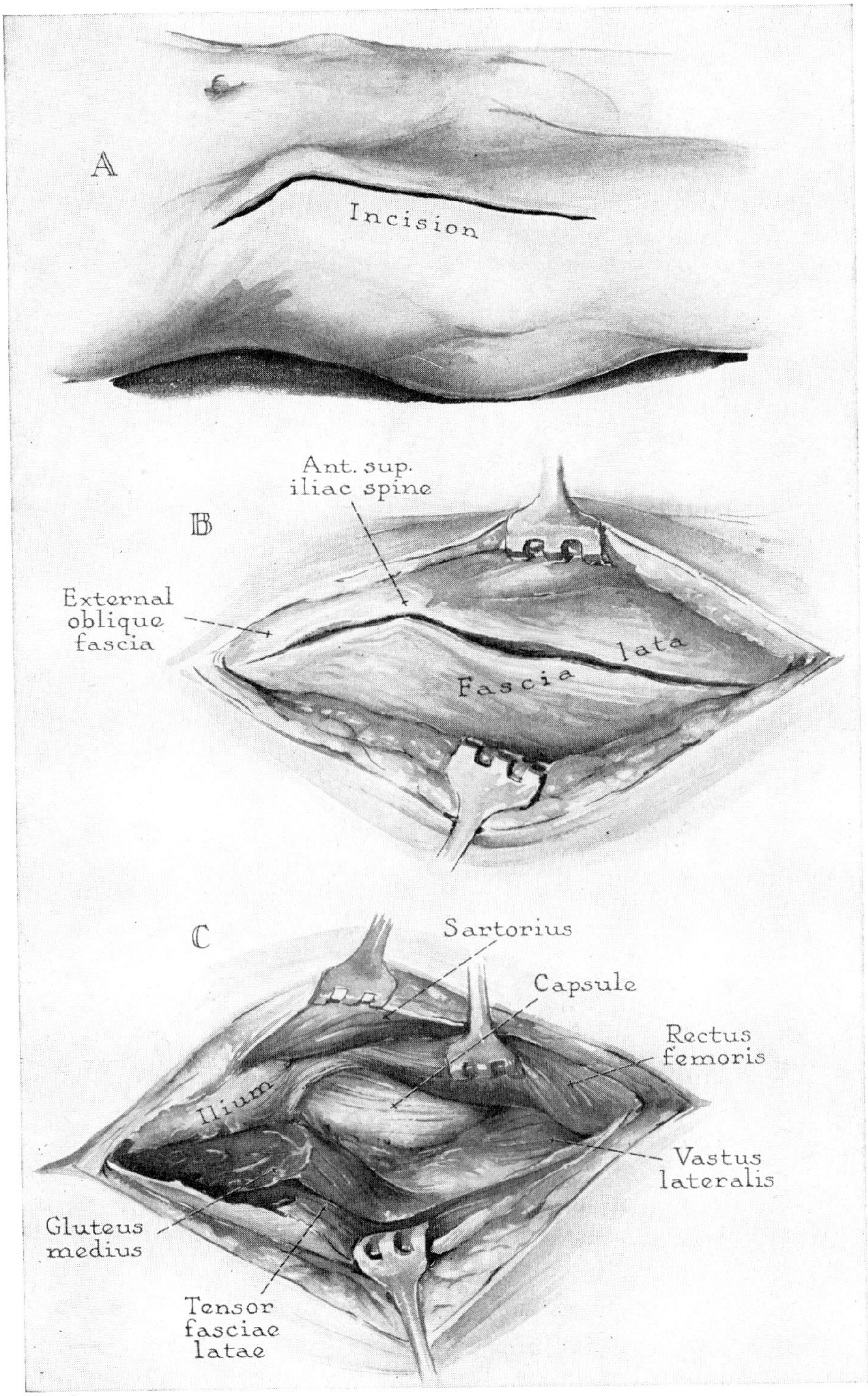

Exposure of the hip joint and the supra-acetabular portion of the pelvis through an anterior ilio-femoral incision, with reflection downward of the rectus femoris muscle

EXPOSURE OF THE HIP JOINT AND THE SUPRA-ACETABULAR PORTION OF THE PELVIS THROUGH AN ANTERIOR ILIOFEMORAL INCISION WITH REFLECTION DOWNWARD OF THE RECTUS FEMORIS MUSCLE *(Continued)*

Plate 109: Description of Procedure

D The two heads of origin of the rectus femoris muscle, the direct head from the anterior inferior iliac spine and the reflected head from above the acetabulum, are exposed by cleaning the fatty tissue in front of the hip joint and by firmly retracting the sartorius muscle medially.

E The rectus femoris muscle is reflected downward, as illustrated, after severance of its origins from the ilium.

F The dissection is carried subperiosteally into the pelvis by separating, respectively, the abdominal muscles from the crest of the ilium, and the iliac muscle from the inner aspect of the wing of the ilium. At the same time, the sartorius muscle is separated from the anterior superior iliac spine and reflected medially with the abdominal and iliopsoas muscles. The hip joint is opened through an appropriate incision into the capsule.

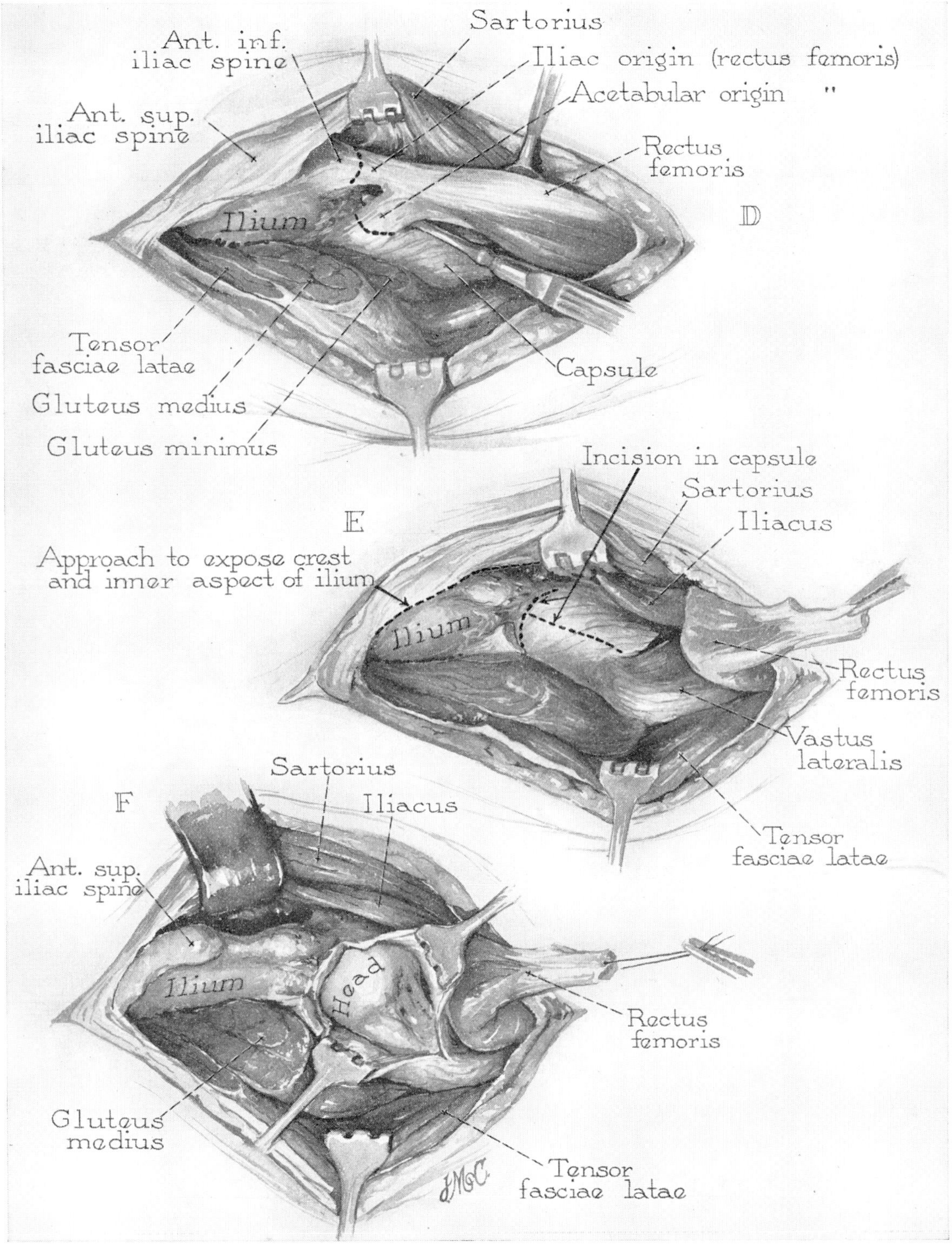

Exposure of the hip joint and the supra-acetabular portion of the pelvis through an anterior ilio-femoral incision with reflection downward of the rectus femoris muscle

EXPOSURE OF THE HIP JOINT AND THE SUBTROCHANTERIC REGION OF THE FEMUR THROUGH A LATERAL HIP AND THIGH INCISION

Indications: 1. Open Reduction and Internal Fixation of Fractures of the Neck of the Femur

2. Treatment of Un-united Fractures of the Femur

Plate 110: Description of Procedure

A The skin incision, approximately 8 inches long, begins at the iliac crest and extends vertically downward along the anterior margin of the gluteus medius muscle to end 3 inches distally to the greater trochanter.

B The skin margins are retracted, and the fascia lata is opened the length of the wound. The tensor fasciae latae is identified, its lateral margin is freed, and the muscle is separated from the underlying structures so that it can be retracted medially. It then becomes necessary to cut the reflection of the fascia lata beneath the tensor fasciae latae and to pull it medially with the muscle. Several small arteries will be severed during this part of the operation, and the bleeding must be controlled.

C The gluteus medius lies partly uncovered in the proximal half of the wound, and is separated by blunt dissection from the anterolateral aspect of the capsule of the hip joint, which will permit its retraction posteriorly.

D The capsule is cleared of the overlying fat, and the interior of the joint is exposed by an adequate incision. Attention is now directed to the presence of the vastus lateralis muscle in the lower half of the wound. The fascia lata and the lateral intermuscular septum are retracted posteriorly as the vastus lateralis is separated subperiosteally from the subtrochanteric portion of the femur. Note should be made of the tendon of the gluteus maximus as it approaches its place of insertion onto the femur.

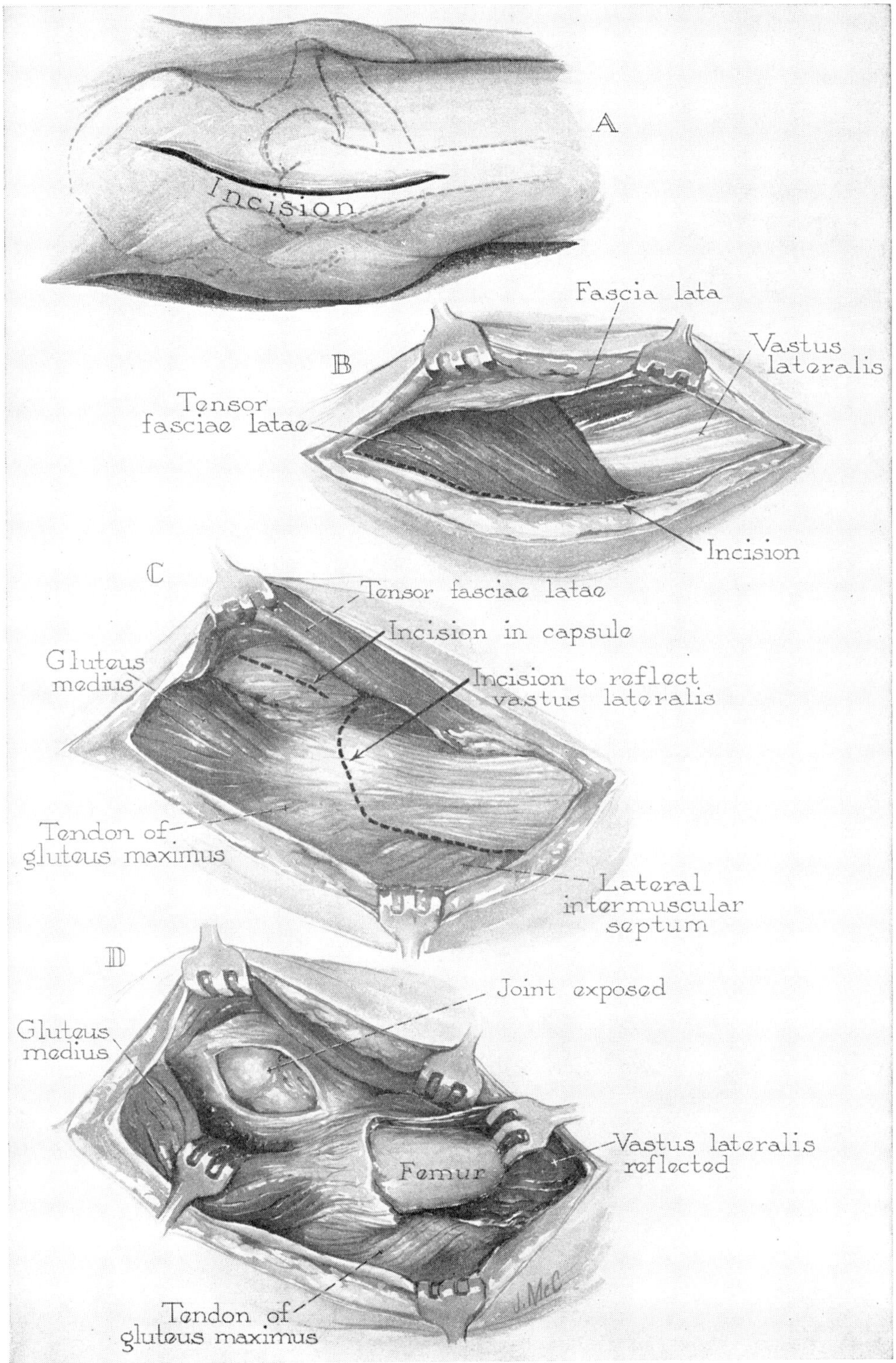

Exposure of the hip joint and subtrochanteric region of the femur through a lateral hip and thigh incision

EXPOSURE OF THE HIP JOINT THROUGH A LATERAL INCISION WITH UPWARD REFLECTION OF THE GREATER TROCHANTER

Indications: 1. Reconstruction of the Hip for Un-united Fracture of the Neck of the Femur

2. Arthrodesis of the Hip Joint

3. Arthroplasties of the Hip

Plate 111: Description of Procedure

A The incision begins at the iliac crest approximately 2 inches behind the anterior superior iliac spine and extends downward for a distance of 8 inches, while centered over the greater trochanter.

B The skin flaps are retracted, and the fascia over the gluteus medius muscle is opened along the line of the incision, and reflected. This fascial layer is continuous with the one which covers the greater trochanter and the vastus lateralis muscle; the latter will be seen in the distal third of the wound when the fascia has been opened.

C The interval between the anterior margin of the gluteus medius muscle and the posterior edge of the tensor fasciae latae muscle is located, and the two muscles are separated by blunt dissection. The operational field can be enlarged by cutting the anterior layer of the fascia near the iliac crest. Care must be taken, however, not to sever the nerve supplying the tensor fasciae latae muscle which enters near by. The wound is deepened in the interval between the inner surfaces of the gluteus medius and minimus muscles, and the lateral aspect of the capsule of the hip joint. (Procedure continued on Plate 112.)

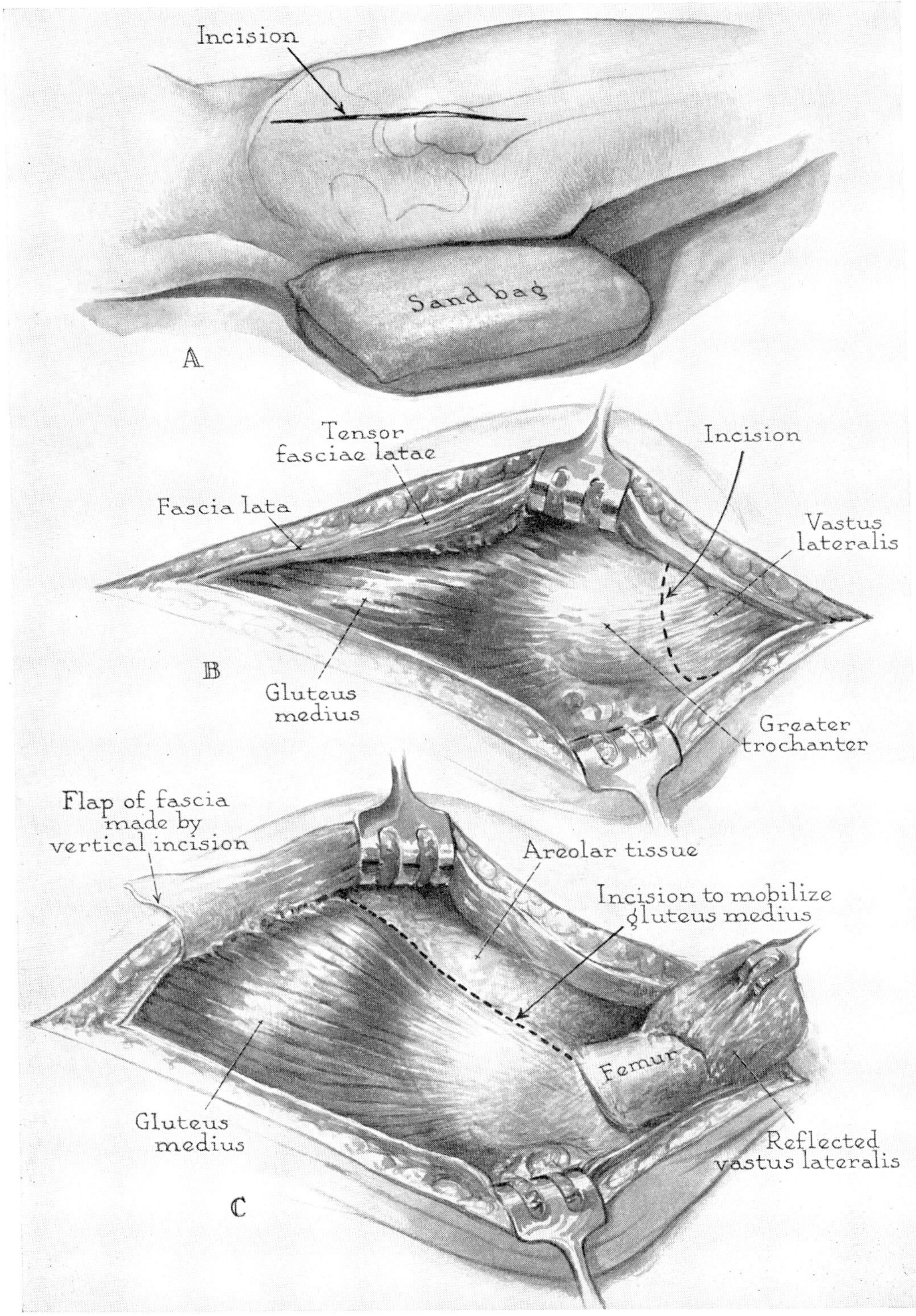

Exposure of the hip joint through a lateral incision with upward reflection of the greater trochanter

EXPOSURE OF THE HIP JOINT THROUGH A LATERAL INCISION WITH UPWARD REFLECTION OF THE GREATER TROCHANTER

(Continued)

Plate 112: Description of Procedure

D The vastus lateralis muscle is reflected downward subperiosteally from its origin on the anterior and lateral aspects of the subtrochanteric region of the femur, to expose the base of the greater trochanter and the adjacent 2 inches of the lateral surface of the shaft of the femur.

E The greater trochanter is separated from the shaft of the femur by means of an osteotome, and then is reflected upward with the attached tendons of the gluteus medius and gluteus minimus muscles. Reflection of this fragment from its site will make it necessary to separate the posterior margin of the gluteus medius from the anterior fibers of the gluteus maximus muscle.

F The lateral aspect of the capsule of the hip joint and the superior and lateral dortions of the acetabulum can be clearly seen. The anterior capsule is exposed by retracting the rectus femoris muscle and the iliopsoas tendon medially, and then is incised to afford access to the hip joint and the head of the femur.

NOTE: Relatively little bleeding occurs in this incision. Several small arteries must be ligated when the gluteus medius muscle is being separated from the tensor fasciae latae. The dissection between the gluteus medius and gluteus maximus muscles must not be extended too far proximally, or else the nerve supply to the gluteus medius and tensor fasciae latae muscles will be severed. In closing the wound, the greater trochanter is replaced accurately on the shaft of the femur or transplanted distally as indicated, and fixed with metal screws.

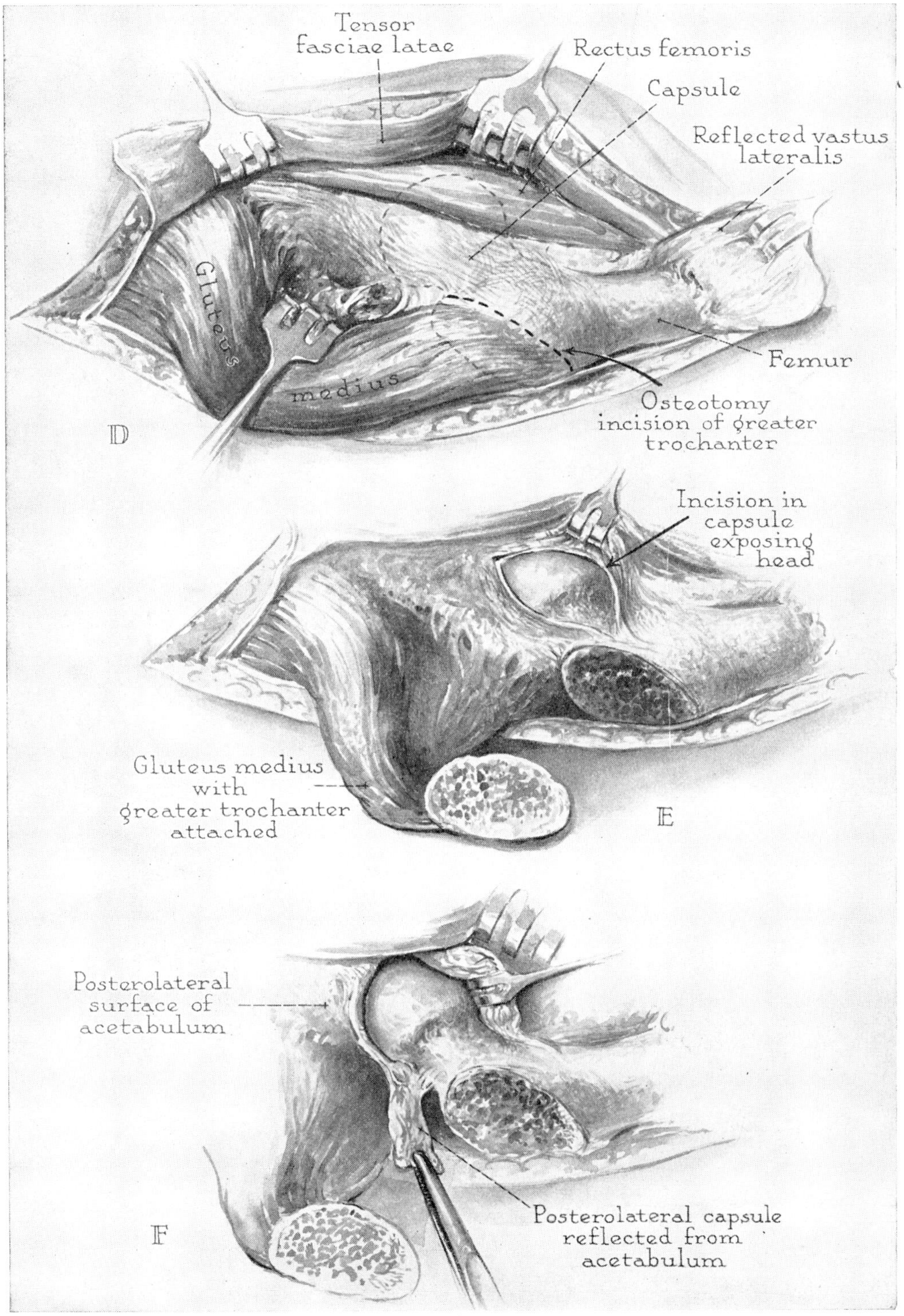

Exposure of the hip joint through a lateral incision with upward reflection of the greater trochanter

EXPOSURE OF THE HIP JOINT THROUGH A POSTERIOR CURVED GLUTEAL INCISION REFLECTING THE GLUTEUS MAXIMUS, WITH TENOTOMY OF THE PIRIFORMIS, OBTURATOR INTERNUS AND THE GEMELLI MUSCLES

Indications: 1. Open Reduction of Posterior Dislocations and Fracture Dislocations of the Hip Joint

2 Removal of Regional Benign and Malignant Lesions

3. Removal of Loose Bodies from the Posterior Portion of the Hip Joint

Plate 113: Description of Procedure

A The skin incision, about 10 inches long, begins some 5 inches distal to the greater trochanter, over the lateral aspect of the thigh. It extends upward in a straight line to the top of the greater trochanter, and then curves posteriorly to parallel the anterior margin of the gluteus maximus muscle.

B The skin flaps are undermined and the deep fascia is opened in line with the incision.

C The anterior margin of the gluteus maximus muscle is mobilized from the fascia lata laterally, and as far distally as the insertion of the muscle onto the shaft of the femur. The lower portion of the gluteus medius muscle with its insertion onto the greater trochanter, and also the quadratus femoris muscle, are seen as the gluteus maximus muscle is retracted toward the midline. (Procedure continued on Plate 114.)

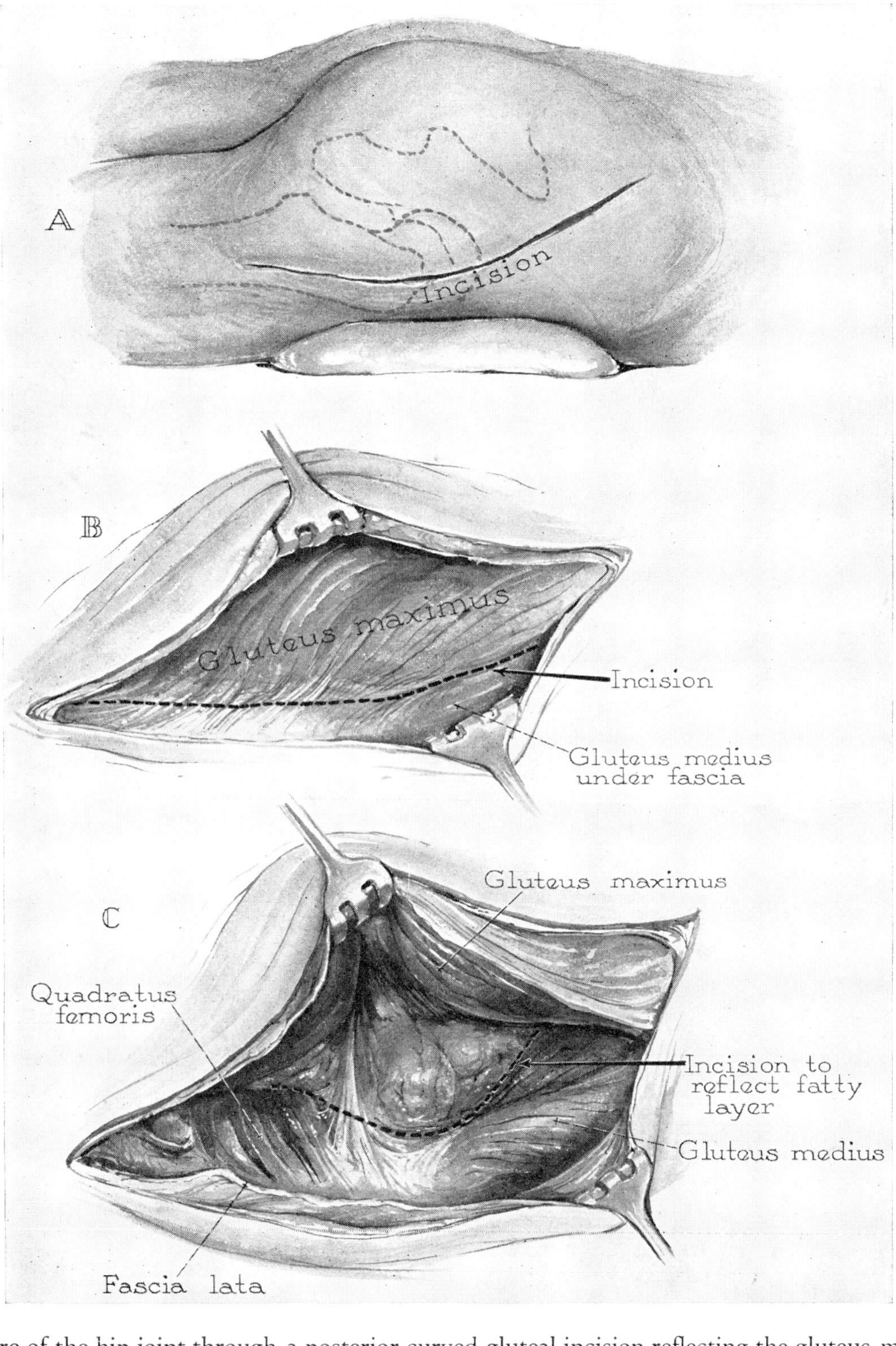

Exposure of the hip joint through a posterior curved gluteal incision reflecting the gluteus maximus. with tenotomy of the piriformis, obturator internus and the gemelli muscles

EXPOSURE OF THE HIP JOINT THROUGH A POSTERIOR CURVED GLUTEAL INCISION REFLECTING THE GLUTEUS MAXIMUS, WITH TENOTOMY OF THE PIRIFORMIS, OBTURATOR INTERNUS AND THE GEMELLI MUSCLES *(Continued)*

Plate 114: Description of Procedure

D The sciatic nerve is located beneath the gluteus maximus muscle, and must be identified and protected. The layer of fat covering the floor of the wound is raised (as illustrated), in order to uncover the piriformis, superior gemellus, obturator internus and inferior gemellus muscles and tendons, as they pass laterally to gain attachment to the femur in the region of the greater trochanter.

E The posterior aspect of the capsule of the hip joint is brought into view by transecting these tendons over an instrument placed beneath them and then retracting the muscles and tendons toward the midline.

F A T incision made in the capsule then permits access to the posterior aspect of the head and neck of the femur. The supra-acetabular portion of the pelvis can be exposed by stripping forward the oblique head of the rectus femoris muscle and raising the adjacent soft tissues subperiosteally, superiorly and posteriorly.

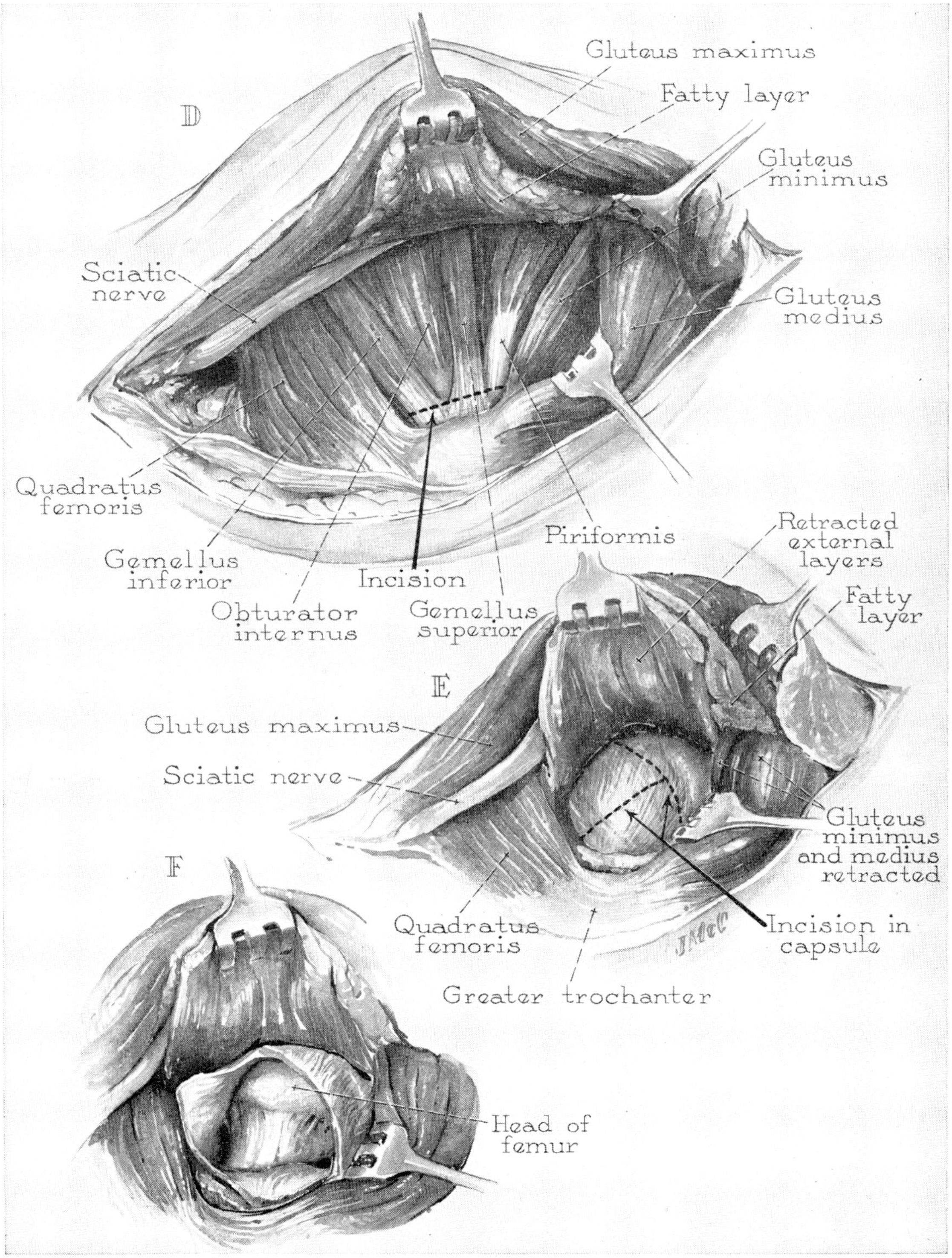

Exposure of the hip joint through a posterior curved gluteal incision reflecting the gluteus maximus, with tenotomy of the piriformis, obturator internus and the gemelli muscles

EXPOSURE OF THE HIP JOINT THROUGH A POSTERIOR CURVED GLUTEAL INCISION WITH REFLECTION OF THE GLUTEUS MAXIMUS AND DETACHMENT OF THE TENDONS OF THE GLUTEUS MEDIUS AND MINIMUS AND PIRIFORMIS MUSCLES

Indications: 1. Arthroplasty of the Hip Joint

2. Osteotomy of the Neck of the Femur for Slipped Femoral Epiphysis

3. Open Reduction of Traumatic Dislocation of the Hip

Plate 115: Description of Procedure

A The patient is placed on the operating table in either a prone or lateral recumbent position. The incision first follows the lateral margins of the gluteus maximus muscle from a point near the iliac crest to the greater trochanter, before it turns vertically downward over the thigh for approximately 4 inches. The skin margins are adequately mobilized and retracted.

B The junction of the gluteus maximus and medius is located by palpation, and the overlying fascia is opened by sharp dissection. The incision then is continued distally through the fascia lata along the line where the gluteus maximus muscle attaches to it.

C The gluteus maximus is pulled medially. The fascia lata is retracted laterally to expose the gluteus medius muscle, as well as the lateral surface of the greater trochanter and the proximal portion of the vastus lateralis distal to it. A pad of fat deep in the wound separates the gluteus maximus and medius muscles. The sciatic nerve lies deep and medially to the gluteus maximus and need not be exposed if the dissection is to be confined to the immediate area of the hip joint. (Procedure continued on Plate 116.)

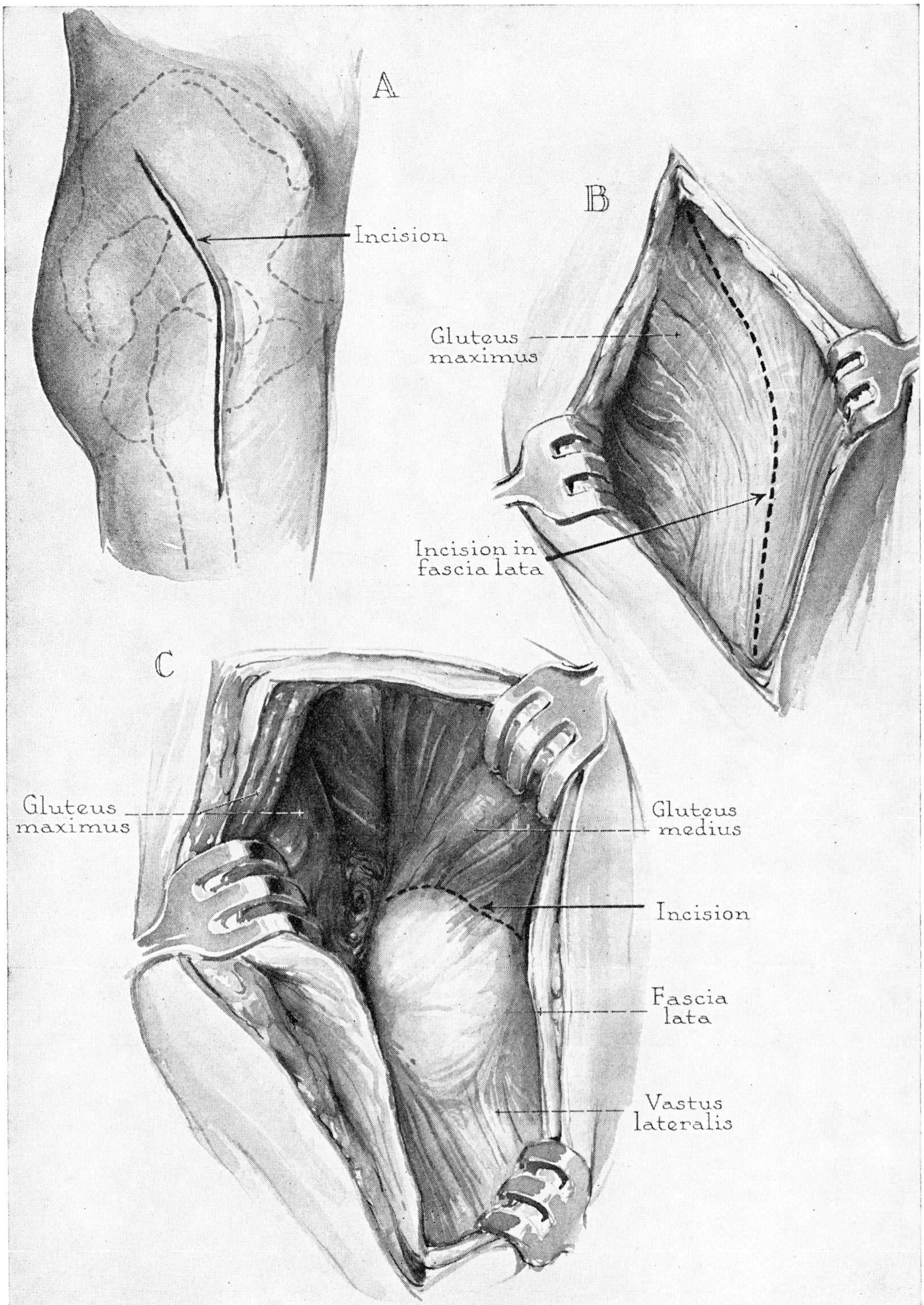

Exposure of the hip joint through a posterior curved gluteal incision with reflection of the gluteus maximus and detachment of the tendons of the gluteus medius and minimus and piriformis muscles

EXPOSURE OF THE HIP JOINT THROUGH A POSTERIOR CURVED GLUTEAL INCISION WITH REFLECTION OF THE GLUTEUS MAXIMUS AND DETACHMENT OF THE TENDONS OF THE GLUTEUS MEDIUS AND MINIMUS AND PIRIFORMIS MUSCLES *(Continued)*

Plate 116: Description of Procedure

D The tendons of the gluteus medius and minimus muscles are cut at their attachment to the greater trochanter and are retracted proximally, as shown. The lateral and anterior surfaces of the capsule of the hip joint are now in the wound. The head of the femur can be exposed by an adequate incision through the capsule.

E Additional room can be obtained by tenotomy of the piriformis at its point of attachment to the greater trochanter. When maximum exposure is required, the obturator internus and the superior and inferior gemellus muscles may be separated from the greater trochanter with the scalpel.

NOTE: This incision is becoming increasingly popular because it provides a wide exposure of the hip joint, with encounter of few vessels and no major nerves. The tendons are reattached as the wound is closed.

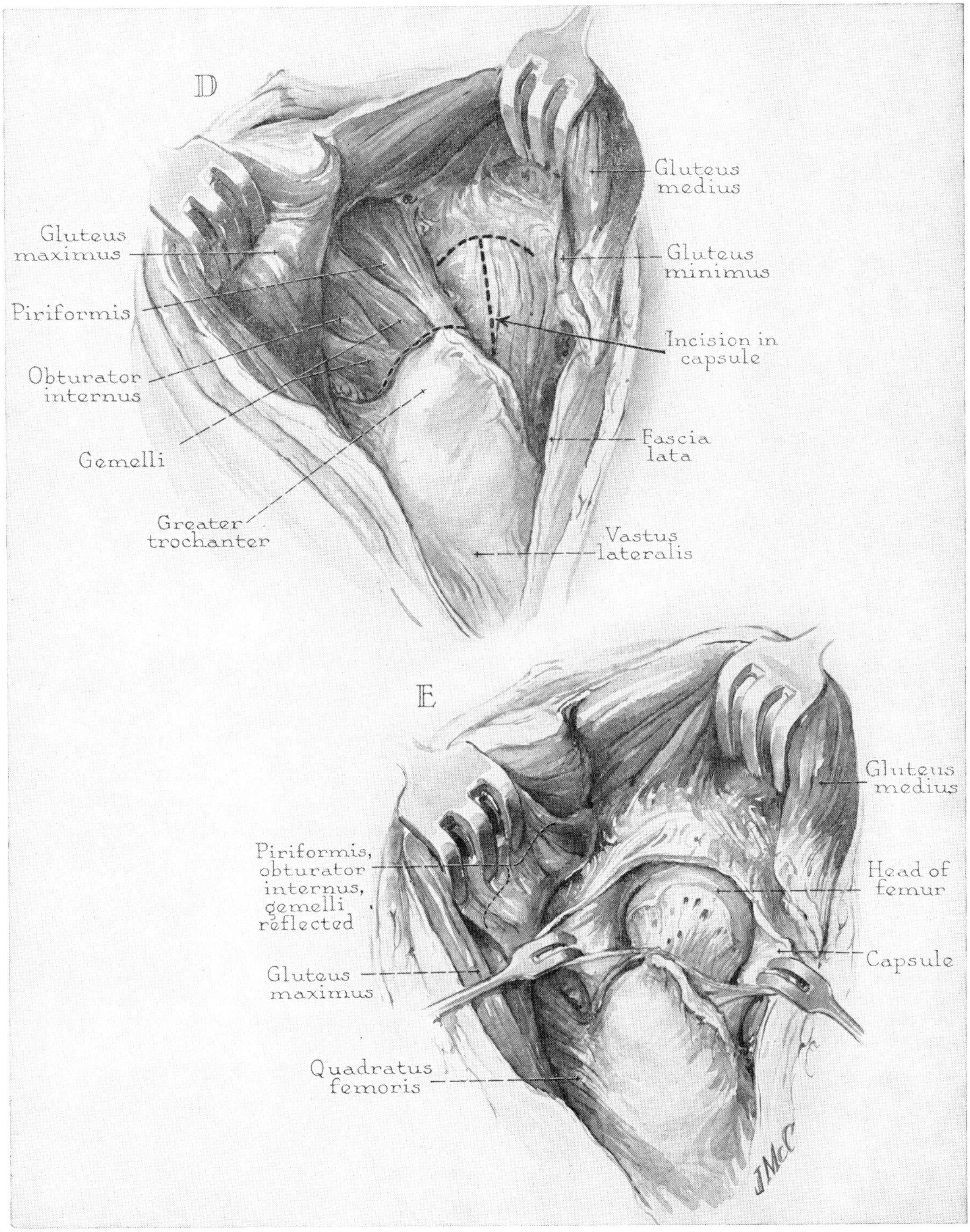

Exposure of the hip joint through a posterior curved gluteal incision with reflection of the gluteus maximus and detachment of the tendons of the gluteus medius and minimus and piriformis muscles

EXPOSURE OF THE ISCHIAL TUBEROSITY AND THE SUBTROCHANTERIC REGION OF THE FEMUR THROUGH A POSTERIOR CURVED GLUTEAL INCISION

Indications: 1. Arthrodesis of the Hip by Ischial-Femoral Bone Graft

Plate 117: Description of Procedure

A The operation is performed with the patient in the prone position. A two-step skin incision is made by using the superior margin of the gluteus maximus muscle and the greater trochanter of the femur as positional reference points. One section of the incision starts at the greater trochanter and extends distally for approximately 5 inches; the other section begins at the tip of the greater trochanter and then runs upward and backward along the groove between the gluteus maximus and gluteus medius muscles for about 4 inches.

B The next cut, at the upper end of the incision, opens the fascia between gluteus maximus and gluteus medius. Then it extends distally through the fascia lata at the attachment of the gluteus maximus muscle to it and, beyond this, over the vastus lateralis.

C The gluteus maximus muscle is mobilized from the gluteus medius and the greater trochanter and retracted towards the midline. The attachment of the gluteus medius muscle to the greater trochanter is then identified. The sciatic nerve is isolated and kept protected under cover of the gluteus maximus muscle. The quadratus femoris muscle can easily be recognized as it extends transversely across the field, from the ischial tuberosity (identified by palpation) to its insertion on the intertrochanteric crest of the femur. (Procedure continued on Plate 118.)

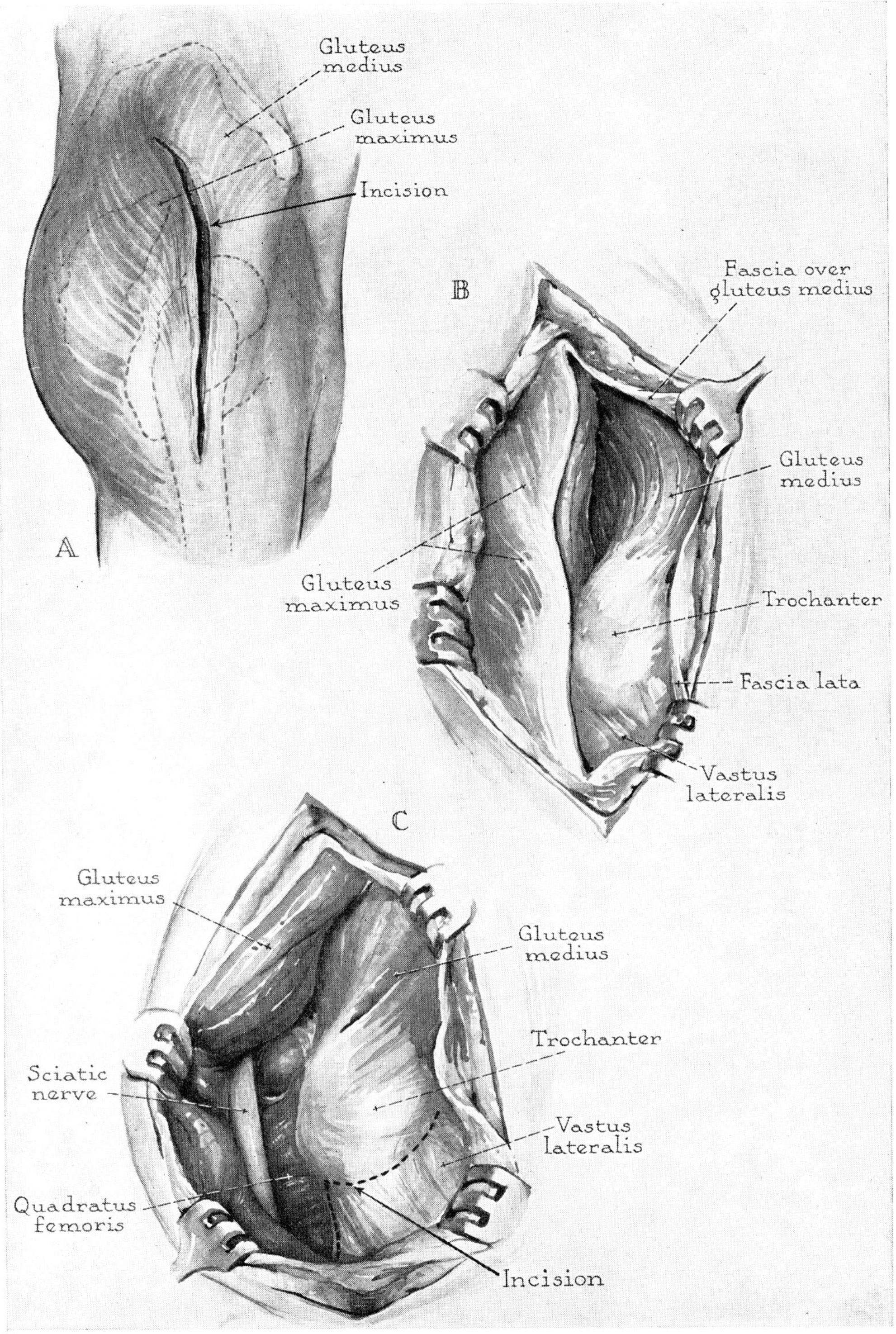

Exposure of the ischial tuberosity and the subtrochanteric region of the femur through a posterior curved gluteal incision

EXPOSURE OF THE ISCHIAL TUBEROSITY AND THE SUBTROCHANTERIC REGION OF THE FEMUR THROUGH A POSTERIOR CURVED GLUTEAL INCISION *(Continued)*

Plate 118: Description of Procedure

D The quadratus femoris muscle is detached subperiosteally from the ischial tuberosity and the intertrochanteric portion of the femur, and retracted proximally. No injury is done to this muscle, for the nerve which supplies it enters at its upper margin as an offshoot of the nerve which innervates the inferior gemellus muscle. The quadratus femoris muscle, on closure of the wound, is resutured into its original position.

E Exposure of the subtrochanteric region of the femur is brought about by pulling the proximal portion of the vastus lateralis muscle off the bone and then retracting it distally. In a similar manner the ischial tuberosity is exposed subperiosteally.

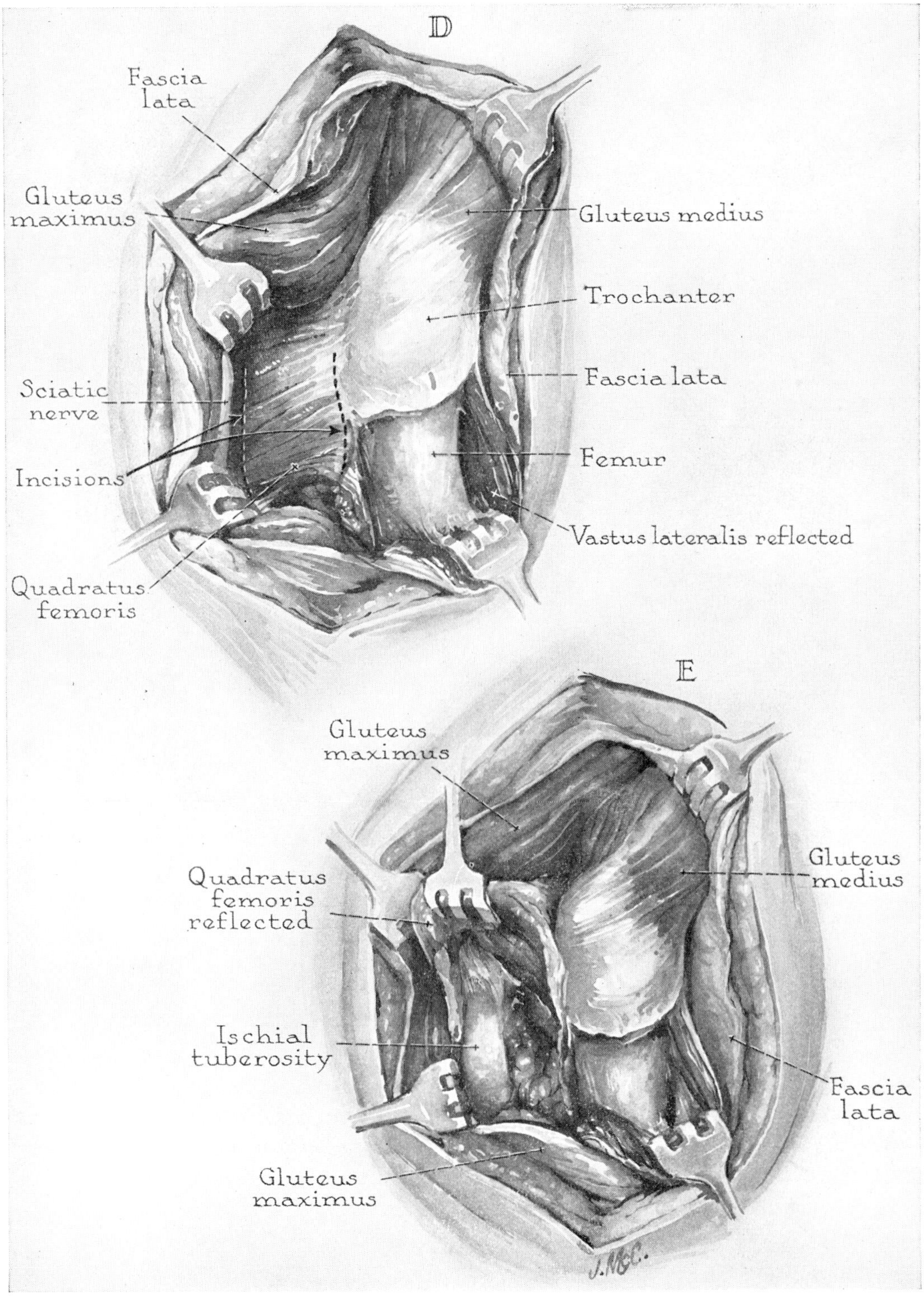

Exposure of the ischial tuberosity and the subtrochanteric region of the femur through a posterior curved gluteal incision

Section VIII

Region of the Femur

EXPOSURE OF THE BASE OF THE NECK AND OF THE SUBTROCHANTERIC REGION OF THE FEMUR THROUGH A LATERAL THIGH INCISION

Indications: 1. Treatment of Recent Fractures of the Neck and Intertrochanteric Region of the Femur

2. Subtrochanteric Osteotomy

3. Extra-articular Arthrodesis of the Hip Joint, Utilizing a Femoral-Ischial Bone Graft

4. Partial Ostectomy for Osteomyelitis and Benign New Growths

5. Femoral Shortening

Plate 119: Description of Procedure

A The skin incision begins over the midportion of the greater trochanter and extends distally over the side of the femur for approximately 5 1/2 inches or more, depending on the surgical objective.

B With this incision the tensor fasciae latae muscle will be encountered as the deep fascia is opened in the proximal half of the wound. The lateral margin of the tensor fasciae latae is mobilized by sharp dissection from the deep fascia, and the muscle and fascia layer beneath it are retracted medially. If, on the other hand, the incision is made posteriorly to the greater trochanter, the muscle can be retracted together with its intact fascial covering.

C Next, a retractor is placed on the margin of the fascia lata, and the vastus lateralis muscle is lifted forward by means of rake retractors as it is separated from the lateral intramuscular septum by blunt dissection down to the posterior lateral aspect of the femur. The oblique fibers of the tendon of the gluteus maximus pass medially downward to their insertion onto the femur, as shown in the illustration. A linear incision is made through the vastus lateralis and the periosteum at the point of attachment of the muscle and the lateral intramuscular septum. (Procedure continued on Plate 120.)

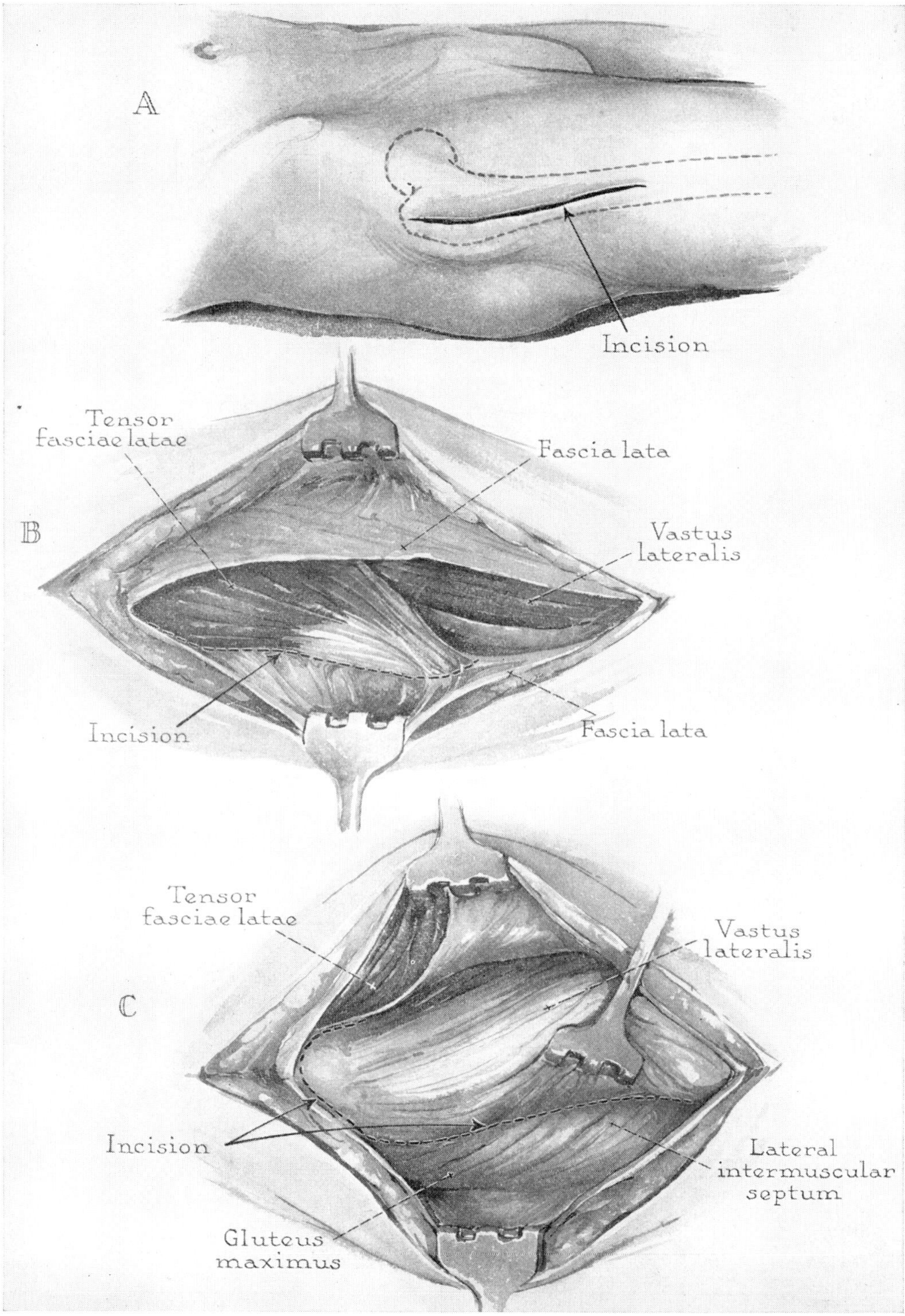

Exposure of the base of the neck and of the subtrochanteric region of the femur through a lateral thigh incision

EXPOSURE OF THE BASE OF THE NECK AND OF THE SUBTROCHANTERIC REGION OF THE FEMUR THROUGH A LATERAL THIGH INCISION *(Continued)*

Plate 120: Description of Procedure

D The muscle then is elevated subperiosteally from the underlying bone and retracted medially to expose the subtrochanteric region of the femur. Exposure of the base of the neck and the intertrochanteric region of the femur can be obtained by transecting the chevron-shaped proximal attachment of the vastus lateralis muscle to the anterior surface of the femur, and retracting the muscle medially and downward.

E The anterior capsule of the hip joint is made accessible by strongly retracting the proximal medial angle of the wound. This incision affords, however, only a limited exposure of the head of the femur.

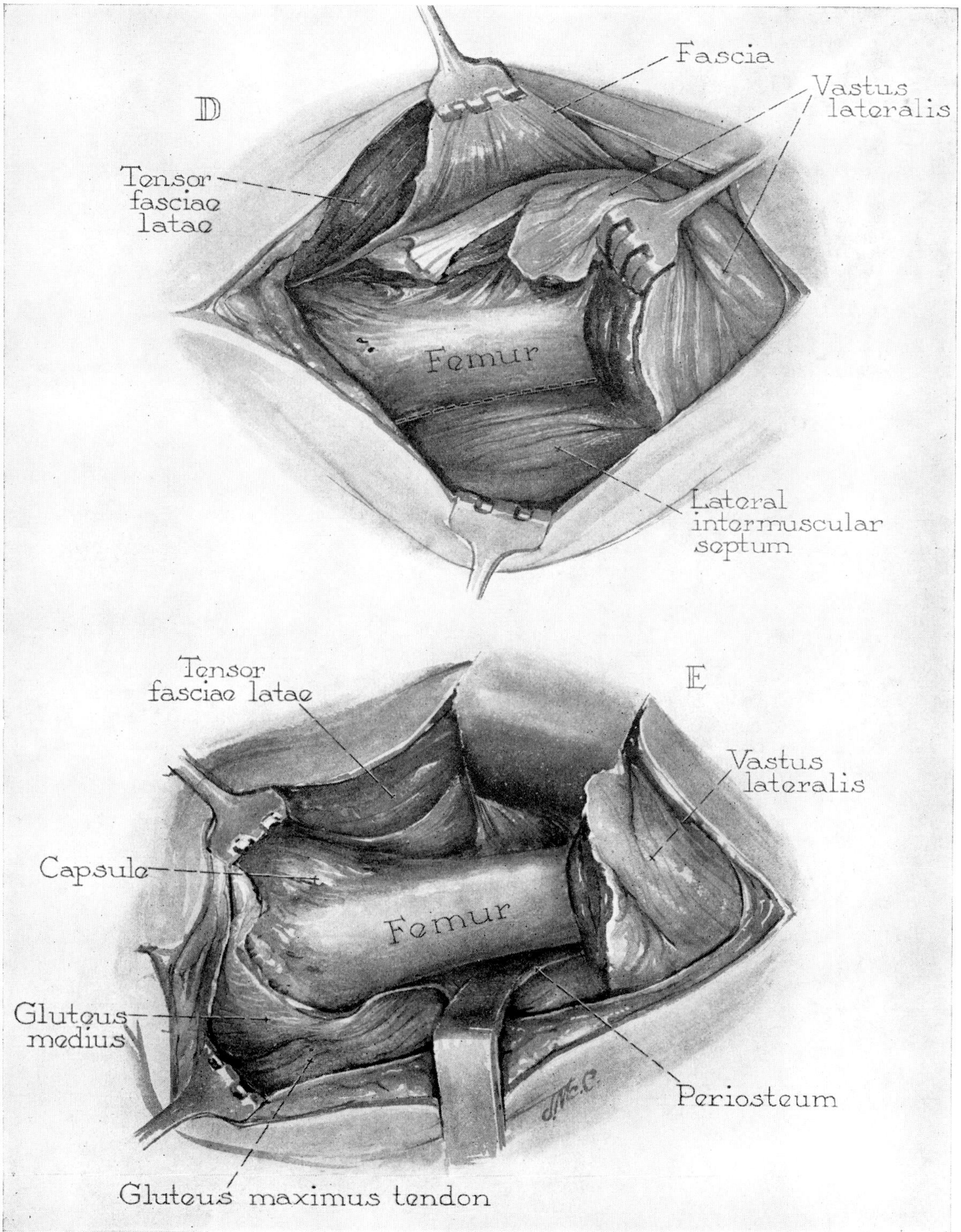

Exposure of the base of the neck and of the subtrochanteric region of the femur through a lateral thigh incision

EXPOSURE OF THE PROXIMAL THIRD OF THE SHAFT OF THE FEMUR THROUGH A POSTERIOR LATERAL INCISION

Indications: 1. Partial Ostectomy for Acute and Chronic Infections

2. Removal of Benign Tumors

3. Open Reduction of Recent Fractures

4. Treatment of Un-united Fractures

Plate 121: Description of Procedure

A The incision begins at the posterior margin of the base of the greater trochanter and extends distally for 7 inches, in line with the femur. The skin margins are mobilized and retracted.

B The fascia lata is incised in line with the skin incision. The posterior margin is retracted backward, and rake retractors are placed on the posterolateral aspect of the vastus lateralis muscle, which, in turn, is lifted forward and medially to permit its blunt dissection (through loose areolar tissue) from the lateral intramuscular septum. The exposure is then carried down to the femur along the line of attachment thereto of the lateral intramuscular septum. If branches of the perforating arteries are encountered, they must be spared, if possible, by keeping the dissection on the forward side with respect to them. The tendon of the gluteus maximus muscle is exposed as shown in the illustration.

C The periosteum is incised in the interval formed by the vastus lateralis muscle and the attachment of the lateral intermuscular septum.

D The femur is exposed by elevating the vastus lateralis muscle and retracting it toward the midline. The danger of injuring the femoral artery, vein or nerve is largely circumvented by keeping the dissection subperiosteally to the vastus medialis muscle.

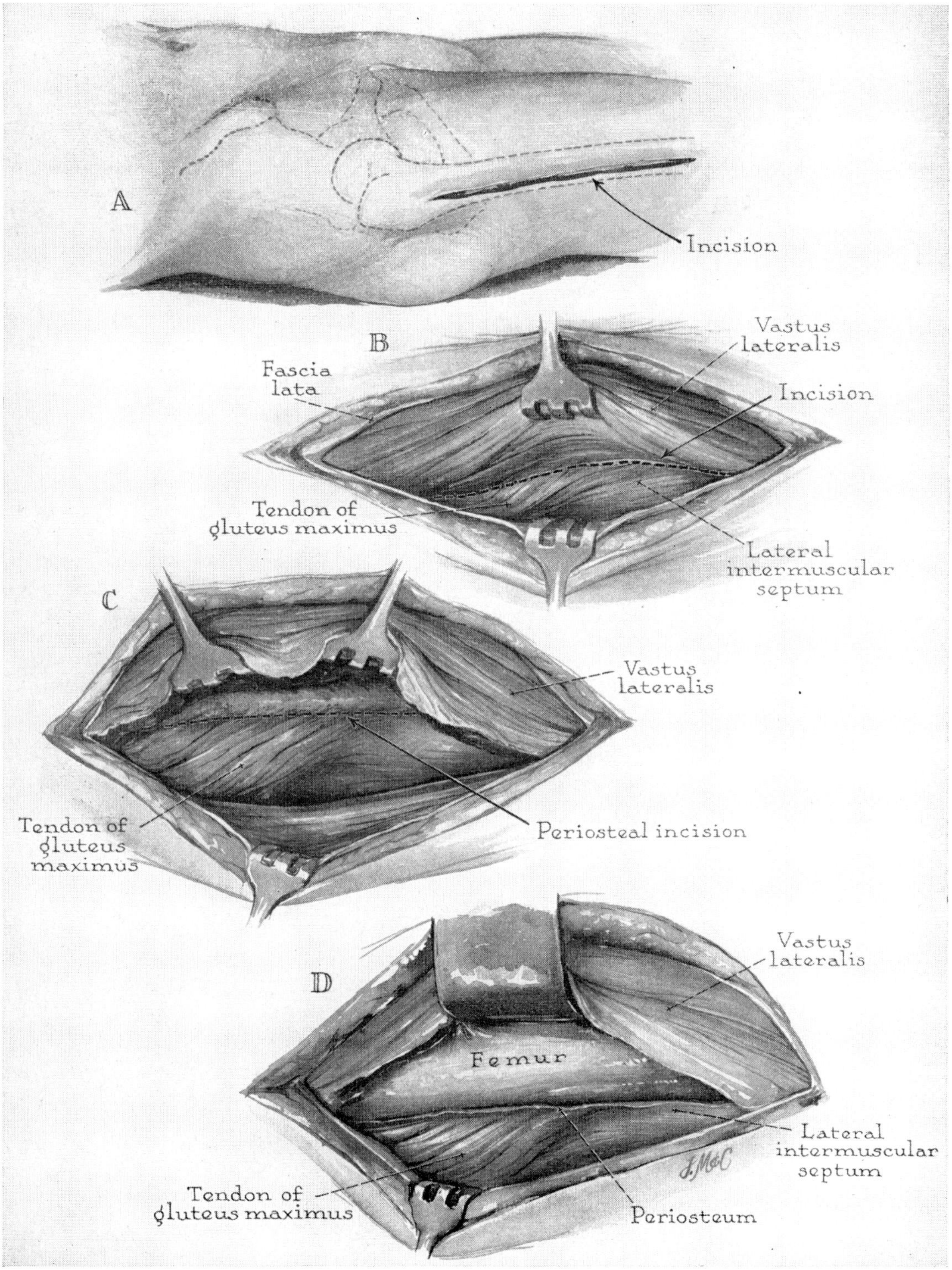

Exposure of the proximal third of the shaft of the femur through a posterior lateral incision

EXPOSURE OF THE MIDDLE TWO-THIRDS OF THE SHAFT OF THE FEMUR THROUGH AN ANTERIOR LATERAL INCISION

Indications: 1. Open Reduction of Acute Fractures

2. Treatment of Un-united and Mal-united Fractures

3. Resection of New Growths

Plate 122: Description of Procedure

A An incision, some 10 inches long, begins at the flare of the lateral condyle of the femur and then extends upward, paralleling the lateral margin of the rectus femoris muscle.

B The skin flaps are undermined, and the deep fascia is opened in line with the skin incision to expose the junction of the rectus femoris and vastus lateralis muscles. The junction may be recognized by a line of fat stretching lengthwise of the wound.

C The vastus lateralis muscle is separated from the rectus muscle by blunt dissection above and, if necessary, with the aid of a scalpel, distally. Care must be taken to isolate and protect the nerves and blood vessels which enter the vastus lateralis at the proximal end of the dissection. These structures cross the incision obliquely downward and laterally, and then descend along the deep surface of the muscle not far from the margin which has been separated from the rectus femoris muscle.

The rectus femoris and vastus lateralis muscles are retracted to expose the vastus intermedius muscle, which is easily recognized by its glistening white surface and the unusual manner in which it surrounds the anterior two-thirds of the shaft of the femur.

D The anterior surface of the femur is exposed by incising the vastus medialis muscle and periosteum in the midline and retracting the margins. Exposure of the entire circumference of the femur is effected by subperiosteal stripping of the soft tissues posteriorly and from the linea aspera. This incision will give an excellent exposure of the femur.

NOTE: Care must be exercised to do as little injury as possible to the quadriceps apparatus. The disadvantage of this incision is the formation of adhesions between the individual muscles and between the muscles and the femur which delimit flexion and extension of the knee joint. Suppurative lesions of the midportion of the femur are best treated through a posterolateral incision. If the lesion must be approached medially, an anteromedial incision can be made.

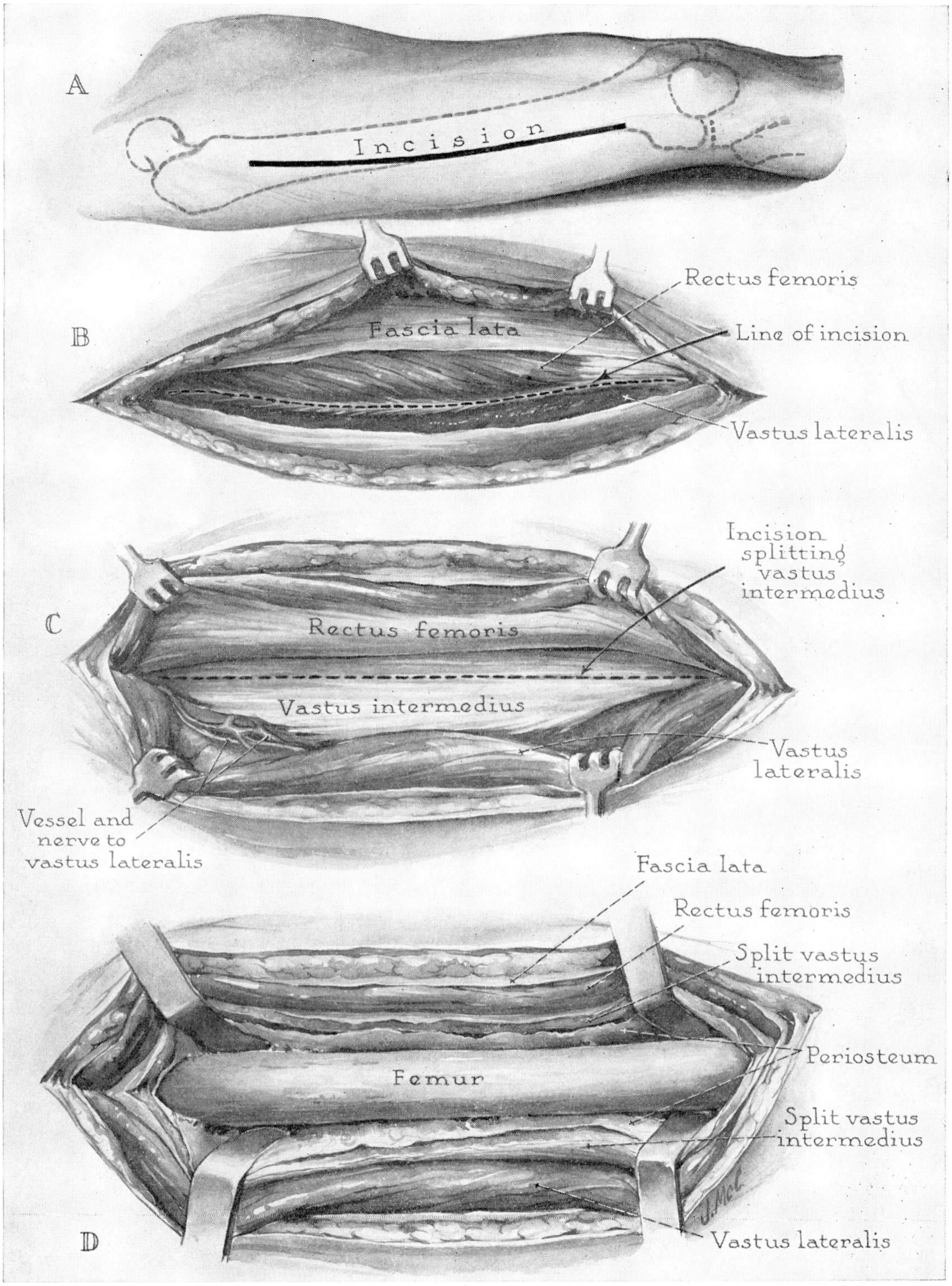

Exposure of the middle two-thirds of the shaft of the femur through an anterior lateral incision

EXPOSURE OF THE DISTAL HALF OF THE FEMUR THROUGH A LATERAL INCISION, REFLECTING THE VASTUS LATERALIS MUSCLE FORWARD

Indications: 1. Open Reduction of Recent Fractures

2. Treatment of Un-united Fractures

3. Partial Ostectomy for Chronic Osteomyelitis

4. Resection of Benign and Malignant Tumors

5. Correction of Deformities by Osteotomy of the Femur

Plate 123: Description of Procedure

A The skin incision is made over the posterior lateral aspect of the thigh; it commences at the flare of the lateral femoral condyle and from there extends upward for approximately 8 inches.

B The fascia is incised and dissected from the underlying muscle.

C The vastus lateralis muscle is raised from the inner aspect of the lateral flap of the fascia lata. The lateral intermuscular septum is followed by blunt dissection to the lateral lip of the linea aspera of the femur. Two or more branches of the perforating arteries may be encountered here as they pass upward through the lateral intermuscular septum to supply the vastus lateralis muscle; these may be ligated if necessary.

D The entire circumference of the femur may be exposed by incising the periosteum at the linea aspera and then reflecting all the muscles away from the bone subperiosteally.

NOTE: This is the safest procedure for exposure of the distal end of the femur. It is preferable to the anterolateral incision, because it leaves the extensor apparatus of the knee undisturbed and does not expose the vastus lateralis muscle to injury.

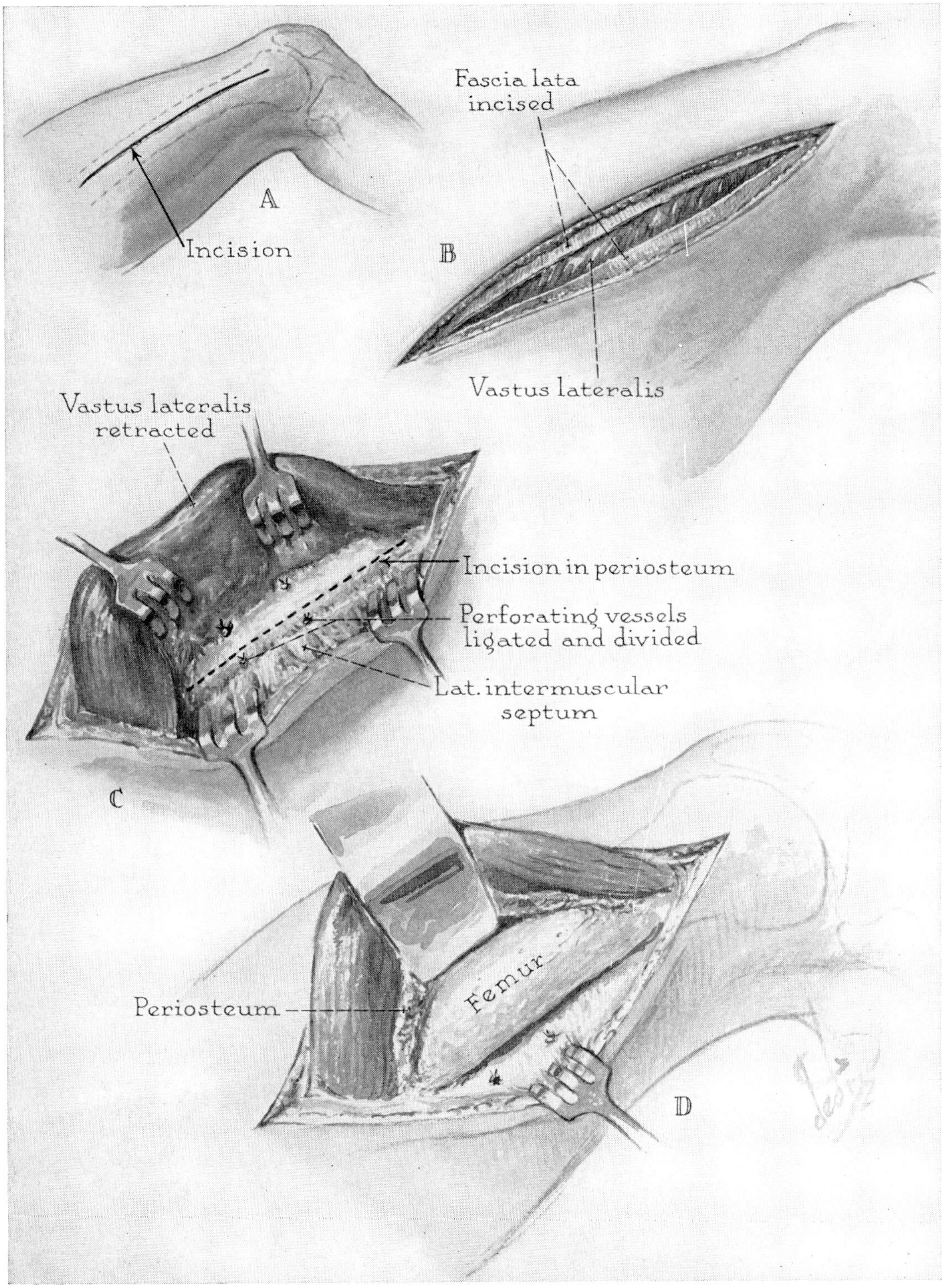

Exposure of the distal half of the femur through a lateral incision, reflecting the vastus lateralis muscle forward

EXPOSURE OF THE MIDDLE TWO-THIRDS OF THE SHAFT OF THE FEMUR THROUGH AN ANTERIOR MEDIAL INCISION

Indications: 1. Resection of Benign Tumors along the Medial Aspect of the Femur

2. Partial Ostectomy for Chronic Osteomyelitis Which Cannot be Reached Through a Posterior Lateral Incision

Plate 124: Description of Procedure

A The incision begins at the level of the flare of the medial femoral condyle and extends upward along the inner margin of the rectus femoris muscle to a point approximately 5 inches distal to the inguinal ligament.

B The fascia lata is incised in line with the skin incision. The interval between the rectus femoris and the vastus medialis muscles is developed.

C The white glistening surface of the vastus intermedius will be seen as the two muscles just mentioned are separated and retracted to either side. The dissection, high in the wound, must be done carefully, for the branches of the femoral nerve which supply the rectus femoris, the vastus lateralis and the vastus intermedius muscles must be identified and protected from injury.

D The next incision is made through the aponeurotic surface of the vastus intermedius muscle, somewhat medial to its midline. The muscle is separated longitudinally and the medial and lateral portions are retracted to their respective sides of the wound, as the femur is exposed subperiosteally.

NOTE: The femoral artery is located beneath the sartorius and directly medial to the vastus medial muscle in the upper portion of the wound; it must not be injured.

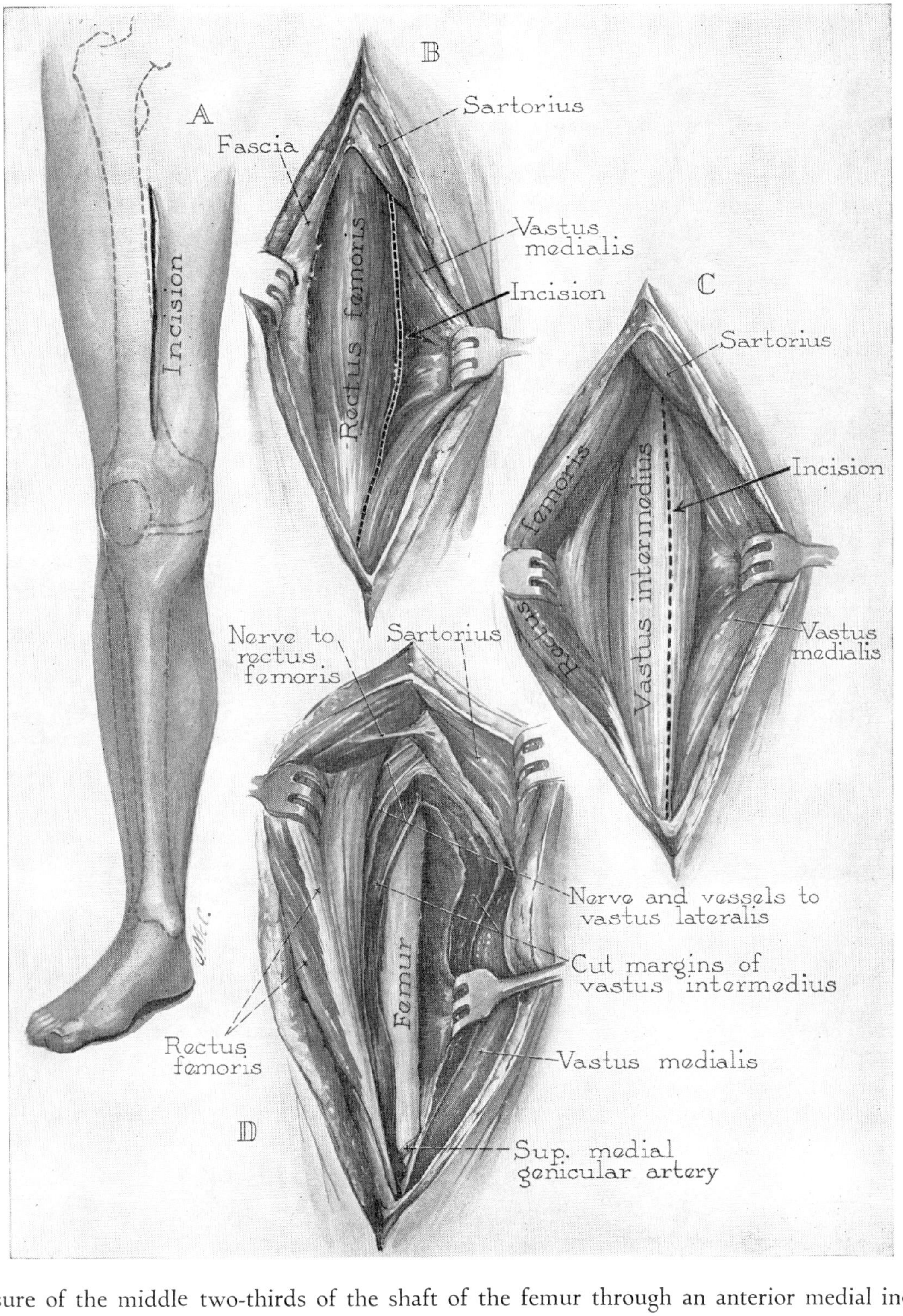

Exposure of the middle two-thirds of the shaft of the femur through an anterior medial incision

EXPOSURE OF THE MIDDLE THIRD OF THE FEMUR THROUGH AN ANTERIOR MEDIAL INCISION

Indications: 1. Partial Ostectomy for Chronic Osteomyelitis

2. Resection of Benign Tumors Occupying the Medial or Posterior Medial Aspect of the Middle Third of the Femur

Plate 125: Description of Procedure

A A skin incision approximately 6 inches long begins about 3 inches above the medial aspect of the superior pole of the patella, and extends upward in line with the medial margin of the rectus femoris muscle. The fascia lata is incised in line with the skin incision.

B The junction between the vastus medialis and the rectus femoris muscles is identified, and the two structures are separated by sharp dissection. The vastus medialis muscle is retracted toward the midline, and the rectus femoris muscle is reflected laterally. It will be noted that the aponeurotic undersurface of the rectus femoris muscle and the surface of the vastus intermedius muscle are both shiny white.

C The vastus intermedius muscle is split longitudinally in line with its fibers by means of a scalpel.

D The femur is exposed by stripping each portion of the divided muscle from the bone subperiosteally, and then retracting the portions to their respective sides. If necessary, the subperiosteal dissection can be continued around the entire circumference of the femur.

NOTE: The 5 inches of exposure of the femur which this incision provides is excellent, for it permits ready access to the medial aspect of this bone. Attempts to obtain the same exposure by lateral approaches are much more difficult.

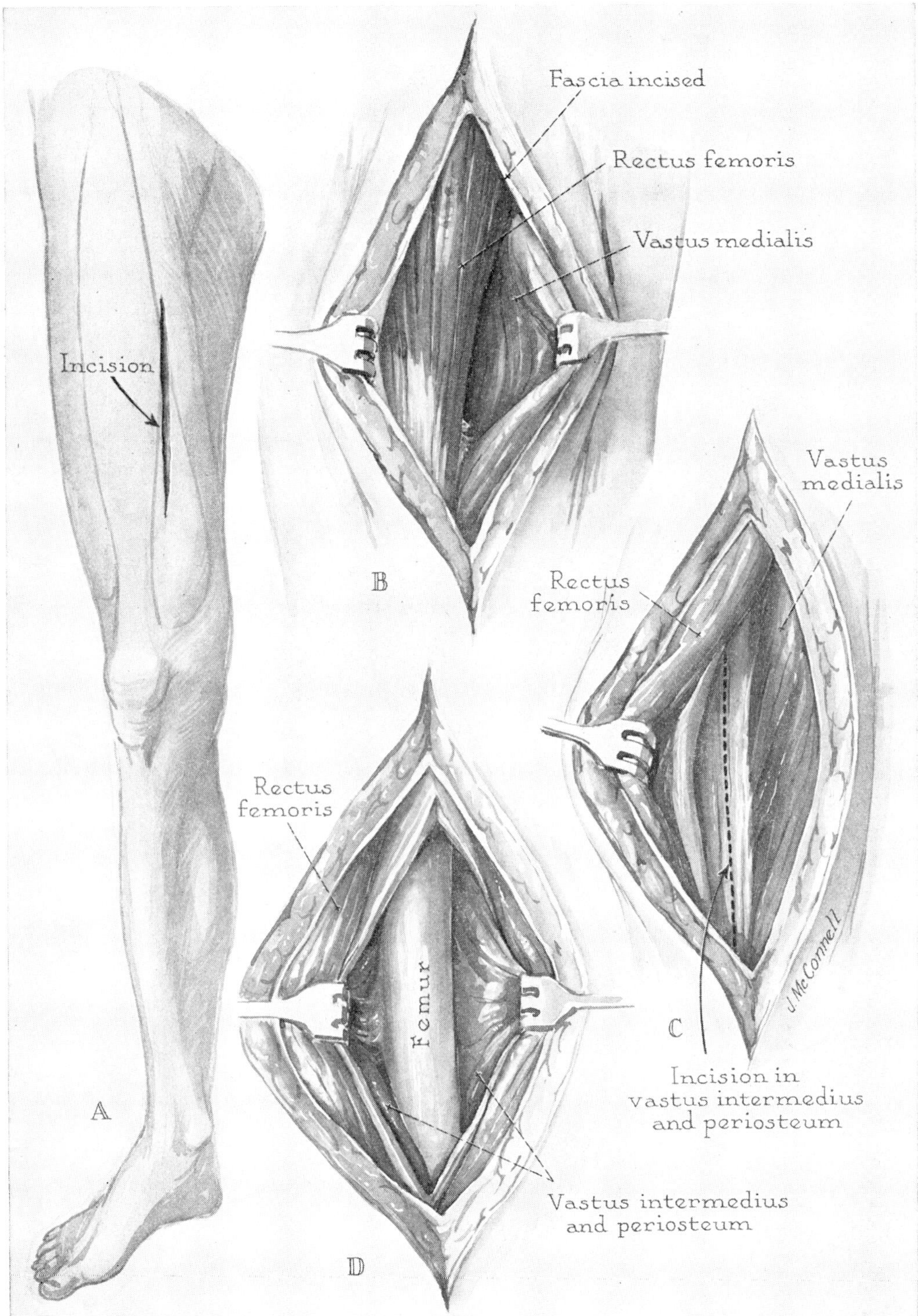

Exposure of the middle third of the femur through an anterior medial incision

EXPOSURE OF THE DISTAL THIRD OF THE SHAFT OF THE FEMUR THROUGH AN ANTERIOR MEDIAL INCISION

Indications: 1. Partial Ostectomy for Chronic Osteomyelitis

2. Resection of Benign Tumors Occupying the Medial and Posterior Medial Aspects of the Distal Third of the Shaft of the Femur

Plate 126: Description of Procedure

A The incision, approximately 5 inches long, is centered over the junction of the anterior margin of the vastus medialis and the tendon of the rectus femoris muscle, which can be located by palpation. The incision begins at the superior medial aspect of the patella and extends vertically upward.

B The skin margins are undercut and retracted. The fascia lata is opened in line with the skin incision. The vastus medialis is easily recognized by the downward and medial direction of its fibers. The vastus medialis is now separated from the rectus femoris muscle proximally, and from its tendon distally as far as the patella. (Procedure continued on Plate 127.)

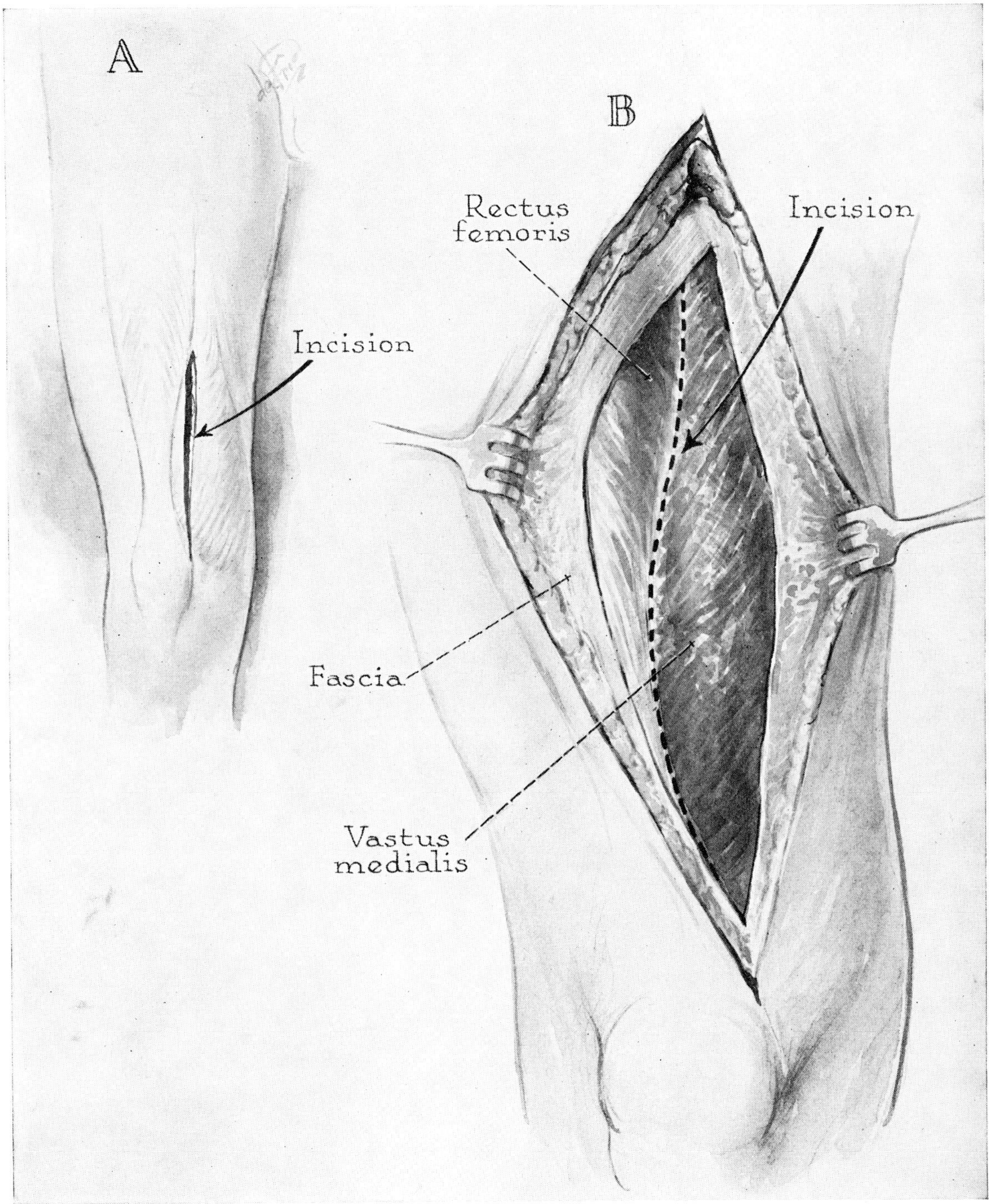

Exposure of the distal third of the femur through an anterior medial incision

EXPOSURE OF THE DISTAL THIRD OF THE SHAFT OF THE FEMUR THROUGH AN ANTERIOR MEDIAL INCISION *(Continued)*

Plate 127: Description of Procedure

C The rectus femoris muscle and tendon are retracted laterally, while the vastus medialis muscle is pulled medially. The undersurface of the rectus femoris muscle has a white aponeurotic structure, as does the presenting surface of the vastus intermedius muscle which is now exposed in the bottom of the wound. The next incision extends the length of the vastus intermedius muscle, as indicated by the broken line in the illustration. The incision should be made along the medial third rather than along the midline.

D The margins of the vastus intermedius muscle are retracted with rake retractors to expose the underlying periosteum. The final incision is made through the periosteum to the femur, which then is exposed subperiosteally as far as necessary. The wound can be extended upward to the junction of the middle and proximal thirds of the shaft of the femur, or distally into the knee joint, by opening the capsule and synovia.

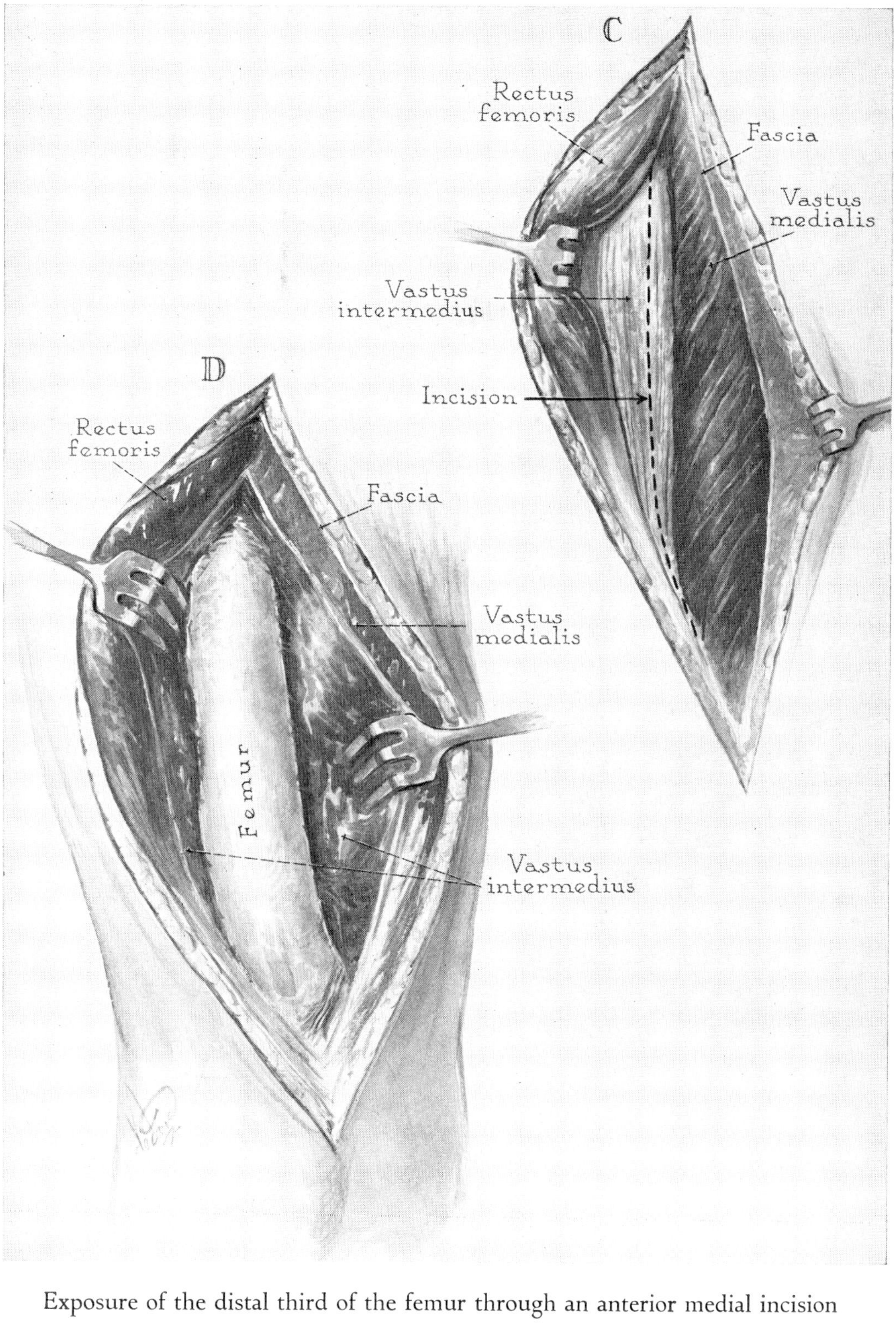

Exposure of the distal third of the femur through an anterior medial incision

EXPOSURE OF THE DISTAL THIRD OF THE FEMUR THROUGH A MEDIAL INCISION, REFLECTING THE VASTUS MEDIALIS MUSCLE FORWARD

Indications: 1. Resection of Benign Tumors of the Femur

2. Partial Ostectomy for Osteomyelitis

3. Resection of Tumors of the Vastus Medialis Muscle

Plate 128: Description of Procedure

A The medial epicondyle of the femur is located by palpation to serve as the starting point for the skin incision which extends upward in a straight line for a distance of 5 inches.

B The deep fascia is incised to expose the vastus medialis muscle.

C This muscle then is lifted upward and laterally by means of rake retractors, to facilitate dissection between it and the medial intermuscular septum. An incision is made through the periosteum between the attachment of the septum and the side of the vastus medialis muscle.

D Exposure of the femur is effected by subperiosteal elevation of the vastus medialis muscle from the bone; it can be extended completely around this bone.

NOTE: The incision affords adequate exposure, and is simple and safe. It should be used whenever possible, in preference to an anterior incision which involves the separation of the vastus medialis muscle from the rectus femoris muscle.

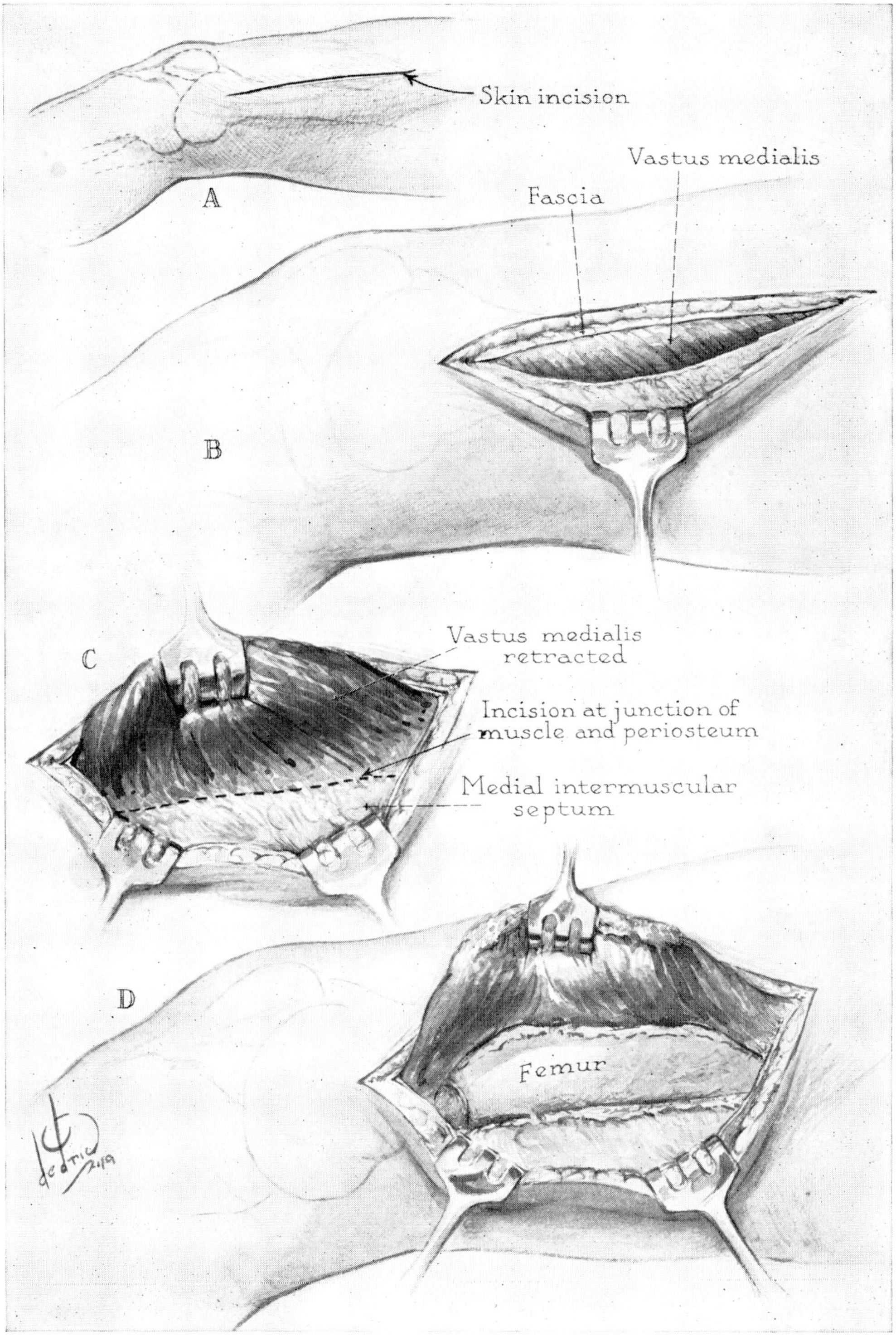

Exposure of the distal third of the femur through a medial incision, reflecting the vastus medialis muscle forward

EXPOSURE OF THE LESSER TROCHANTER REGION OF THE FEMUR THROUGH A POSTERIOR LATERAL INCISION, REFLECTING THE GLUTEUS MAXIMUS MUSCLE

Indications: 1. Resection of Benign Tumors

2. Partial Ostectomy for Chronic Infections

Plate 129: Description of Procedure

A The operation is performed with the patient lying on the table in the prone position. The skin incision extends vertically downward from the posterior aspect of the tip of the greater trochanter for a distance of 3 1/2 inches.

B The skin, and especially the medial flap, is widely mobilized. The gluteus maximus muscle is easily identified, for it is the only muscle exposed in the field; its fibers are inserted into the fascia lata. This muscle is mobilized by sectioning the fascia along its lateral extremity. (Procedure continued on Plate 130.)

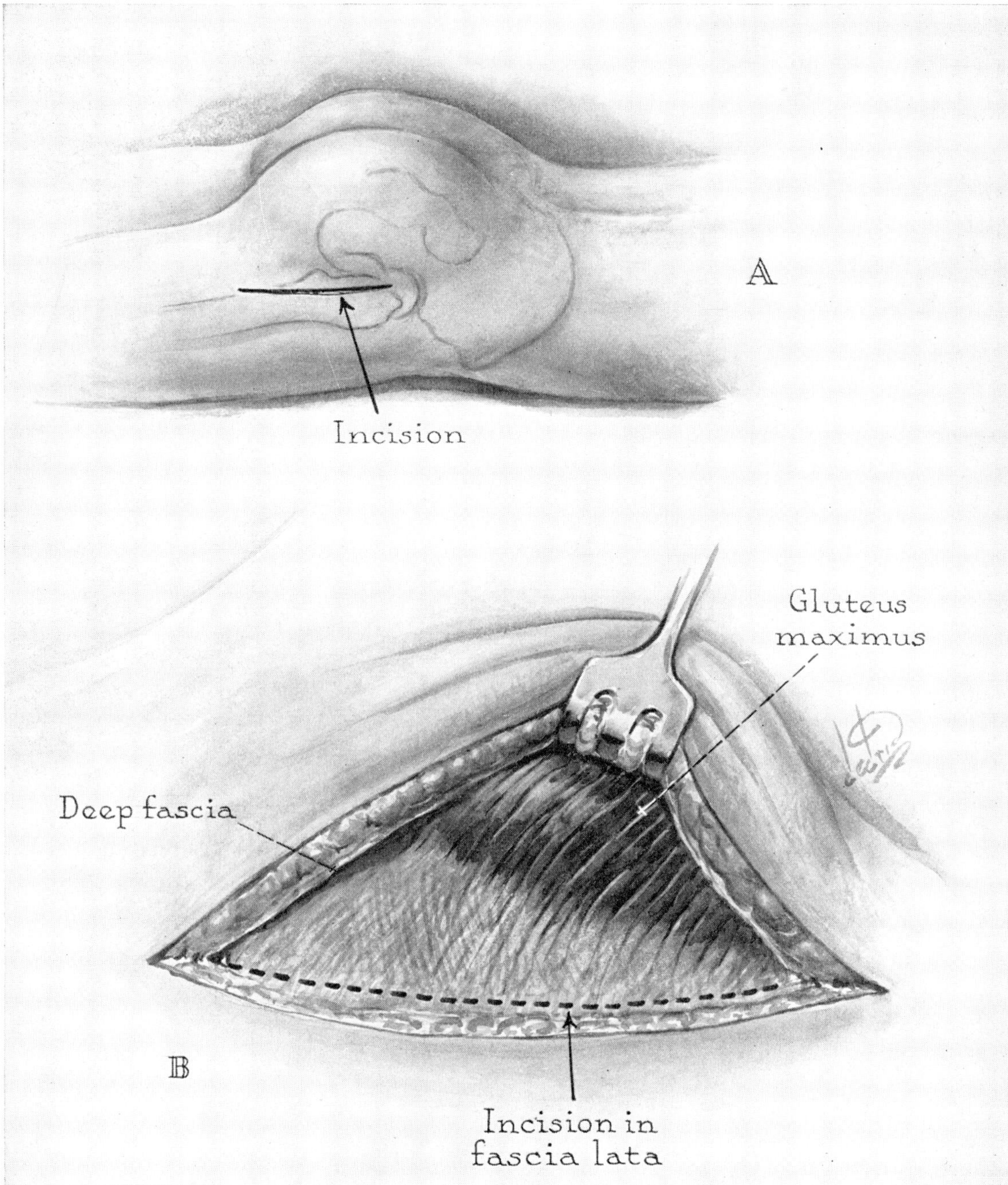

Exposure of the lesser trochanter region of the femur through a posterior lateral incision, reflecting the gluteus maximus muscle

EXPOSURE OF THE LESSER TROCHANTER REGION OF THE FEMUR THROUGH A POSTERIOR LATERAL INCISION REFLECTING THE GLUTEUS MAXIMUS MUSCLE *(Continued)*

Plate 130: Description of Procedure

C The gluteus maximus muscle is dissected from the underlying structures to which it is attached by loose areolar tissue. It then is pulled medially, and the sciatic nerve is isolated beneath it. This nerve must be protected from injury.

D The floor of the wound contains the quadratus femoris muscle. This muscle can in part be retracted superiorly by sectioning the lower third of its lateral margin and lifting the lower edge. The posterior surface of the femur at the level of the lesser trochanter is exposed subperiosteally.

E Still further extension of the incision along the lateral margin of the quadratus femoris muscle will permit a correspondingly increased exposure of the lesser trochanter and the femur. The iliopsoas tendon can be seen at its attachment to the lesser trochanter. The adjacent posterior surface of the proximal portion of the shaft of the femur may be exposed by subperiosteal stripping of the adductors and the long head of the biceps muscle.

NOTE: The incision is relatively avascular. No important nerves are encountered, moreover, excepting the sciatic nerve, which is identified easily in the surgical field and with proper care should remain undamaged.

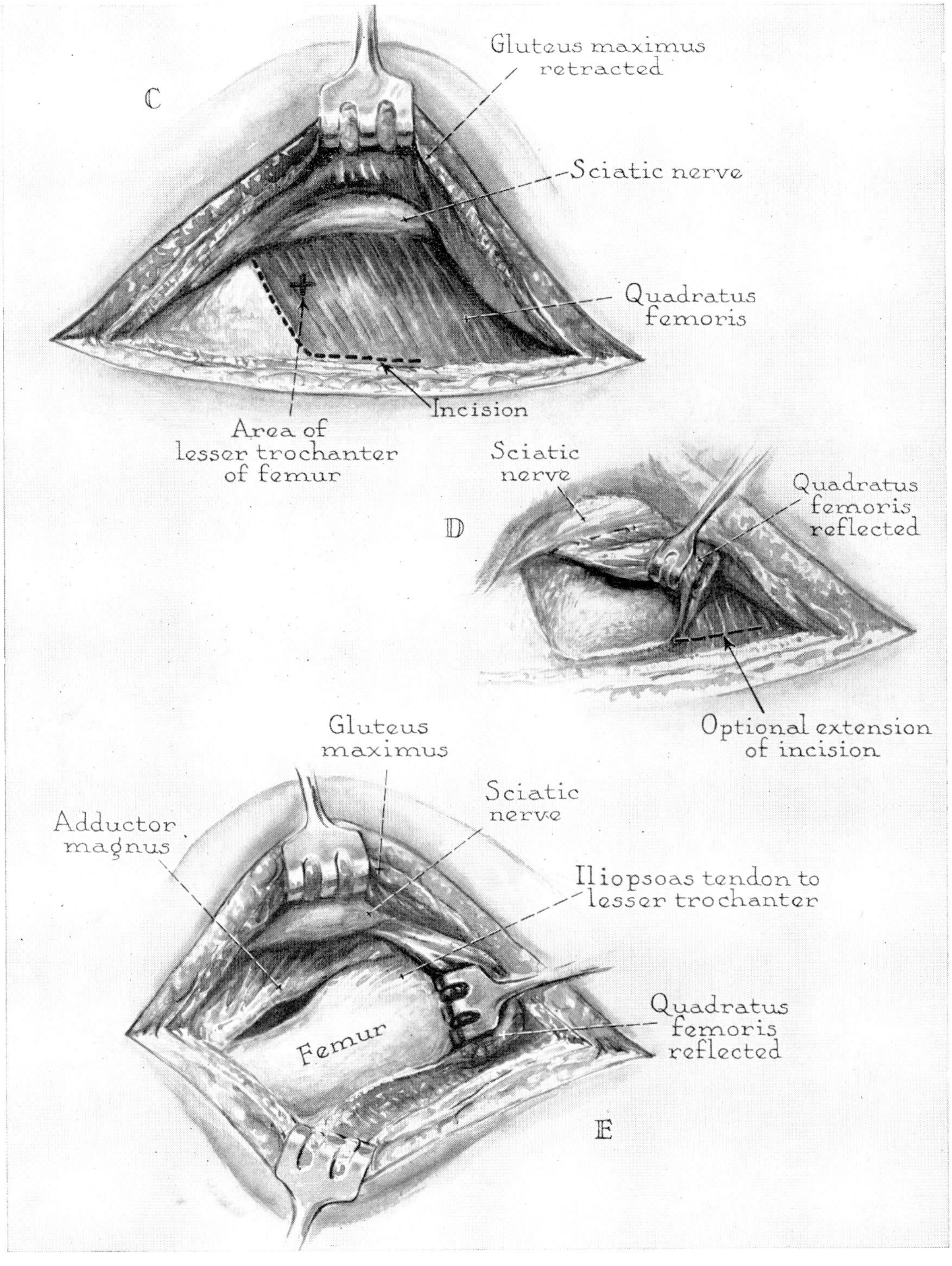

Exposure of the lesser trochanter region of the femur through a posterior lateral incision, reflecting the gluteus maximus muscle

EXPOSURE OF THE PROXIMAL HALF OF THE SHAFT OF THE FEMUR THROUGH A POSTERIOR LONGITUDINAL INCISION, WITH REFLECTION OF THE LONG HEAD OF THE BICEPS MUSCLE MEDIALLY

Indications: 1. Partial Ostectomy for Chronic Osteomyelitis Which Cannot Be Exposed Adequately through a Posterior Lateral Incision

2. Removal of Benign Tumors

Plate 131: Description of Procedure

A The incision is placed just lateral to the midline of the thigh, as illustrated. It extends straight downward from the inferior margin of the gluteus maximus muscle for the desired distance.

B The deep fascia must be incised with care to avoid injury to the posterior cutaneous nerve of the thigh.

C The long head of the biceps muscle is now visible in the wound. The muscle is pulled toward the midline and is then separated laterally from the posterior surface of the lateral intermuscular septum. A linear incision is next made through the periosteum, and the underlying bone is exposed.

D The dissection can be carried around the femur by raising the adjacent muscles subperiosteally.

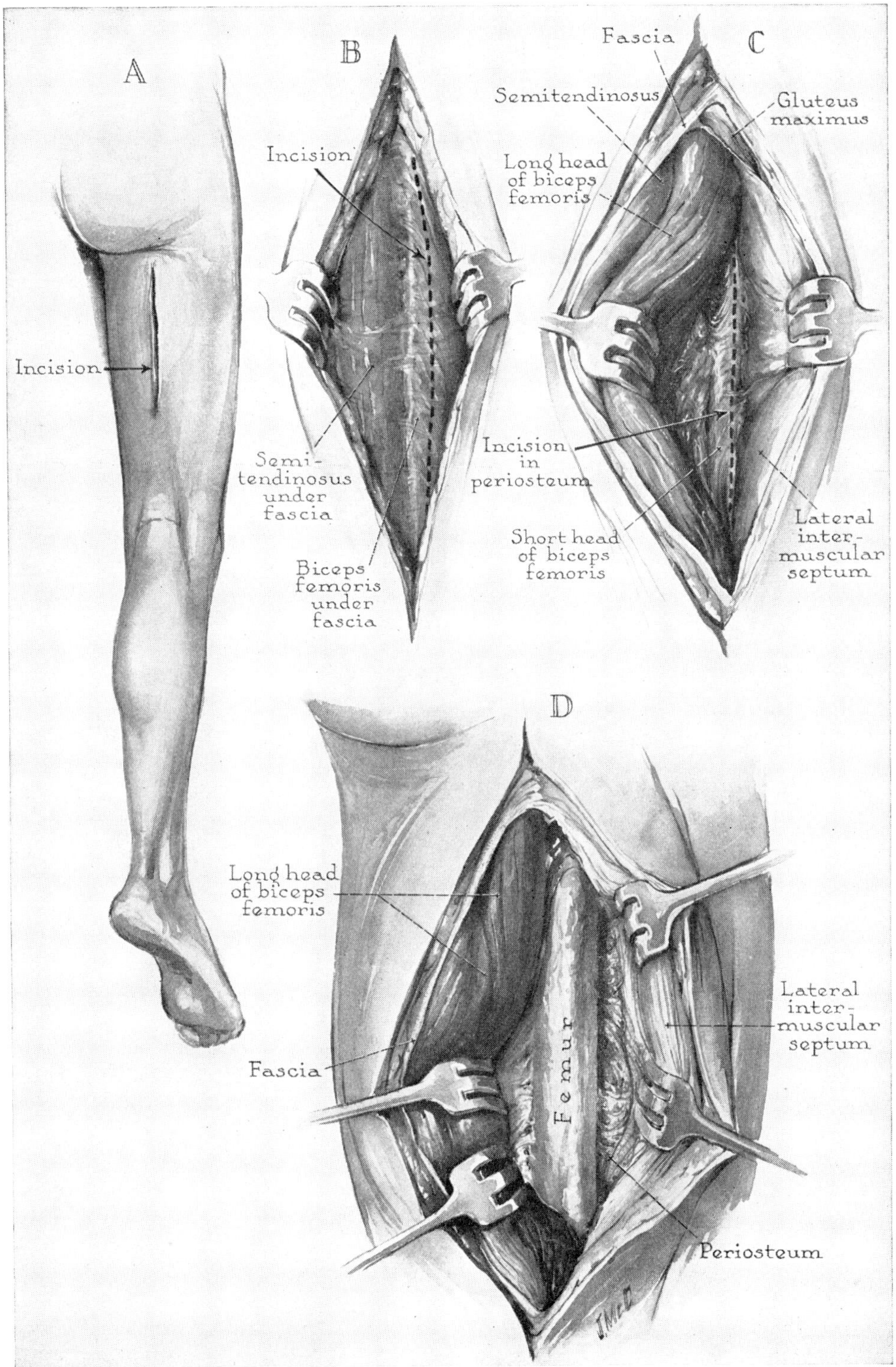

Exposure of the proximal half of the shaft of the femur through a posterior longitudinal incision with reflection of the long head of the biceps muscle medially

EXPOSURE OF THE MIDDLE TWO-THIRDS OF THE SHAFT OF THE FEMUR THROUGH A POSTERIOR LONGITUDINAL INCISION, REFLECTING THE BICEPS MUSCLE MEDIALLY

Indications: 1. Partial Ostectomy for Chronic Osteomyelitis Which Cannot Be Exposed Adequately through a Posterior Lateral Incision

2. Removal of Benign Tumors

Plate 132: Description of Procedure

A An incision approximately 12 inches long is made straight down the midline of the thigh, starting from the inferior margin of the gluteal fold.

B The skin margins are mobilized, and the posterior cutaneous nerve of the thigh is protected as the deep fascia is opened.

C The lateral flap of fascia is strongly retracted to give access to the posterior surface of the lateral intermuscular septum and permit separation therefrom of the biceps muscle. The long and short heads of this muscle are mobilized from the underlying bone and retracted toward the midline.

D An incision through the periosteum will expose the femur. The nerve supply of the biceps muscle which enters by way of its posterior and medial surfaces is not endangered if the dissection just described is done carefully. The sciatic nerve coursing in the midline of the thigh between the biceps and medial hamstring muscles is adequately protected from injury.

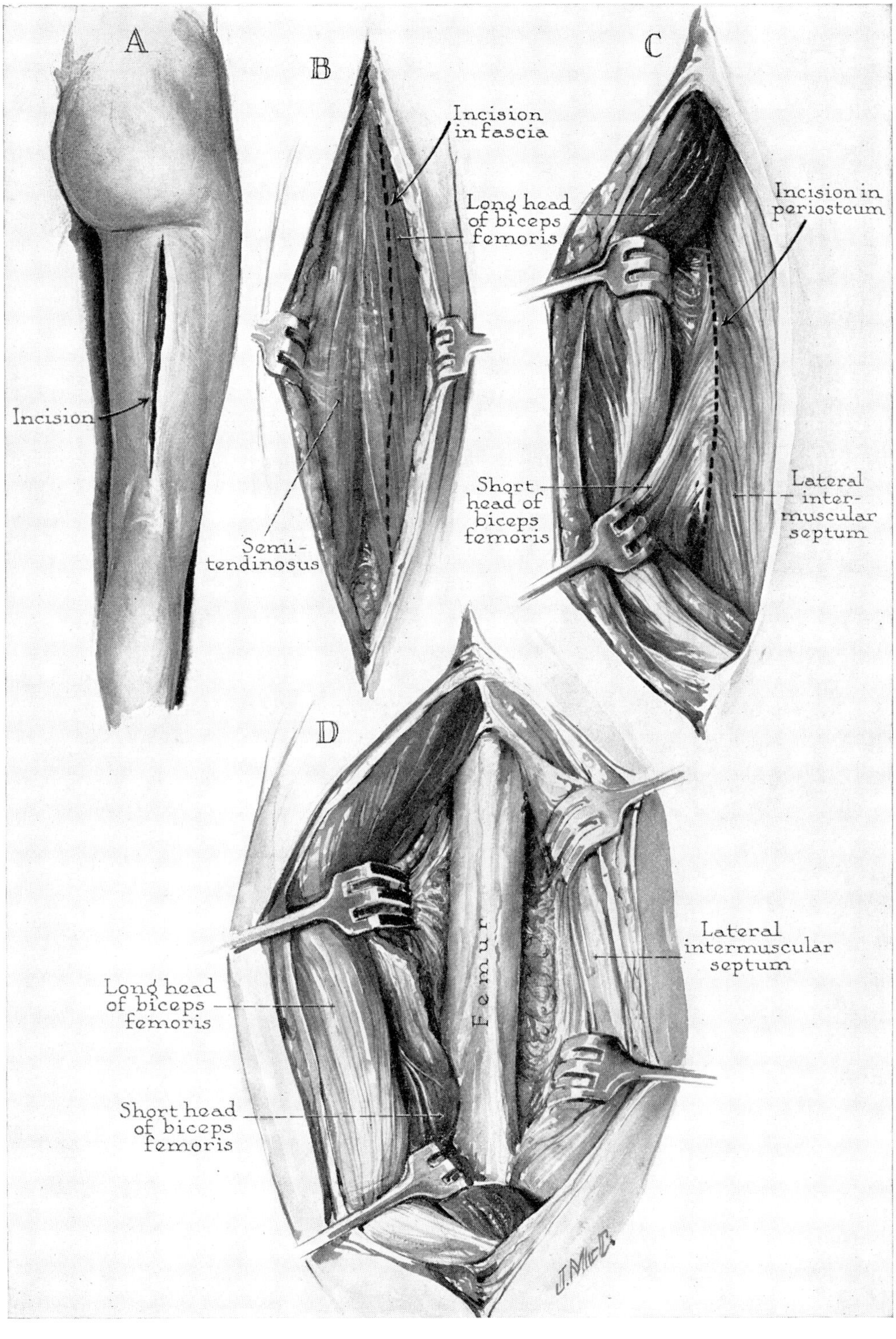

Exposure of the middle two-thirds of the shaft of the femur through a posterior longitudinal incision reflecting the biceps muscle medially

EXPOSURE OF THE FEMORAL NERVE IN THE THIGH

Indications: 1. Neurolysis of the Femoral Nerve

2. Suture of Lacerations of the Femoral Nerve

Plate 133: Description of Procedure

A The incision starts about 1 inch medial to the inner side of the anterior superior iliac spine, and extends obliquely downward along the medial margin of the sartorius muscle for one-third of the length of the thigh. The skin is undercut and retracted to open the wound.

B The fascia lata is incised in line with the skin incision and the sartorius muscle beneath it is exposed. The iliopsoas muscle is seen beneath its own fascia, just medial to the sartorius. The latter muscle now is retracted laterally and the medial fascial flap is pulled inward.

C The femoral nerve is seen at the bottom of the wound after its emergence from the pelvis. This nerve gives off numerous branches to the surrounding muscles before it continues distally in the adductor canal.

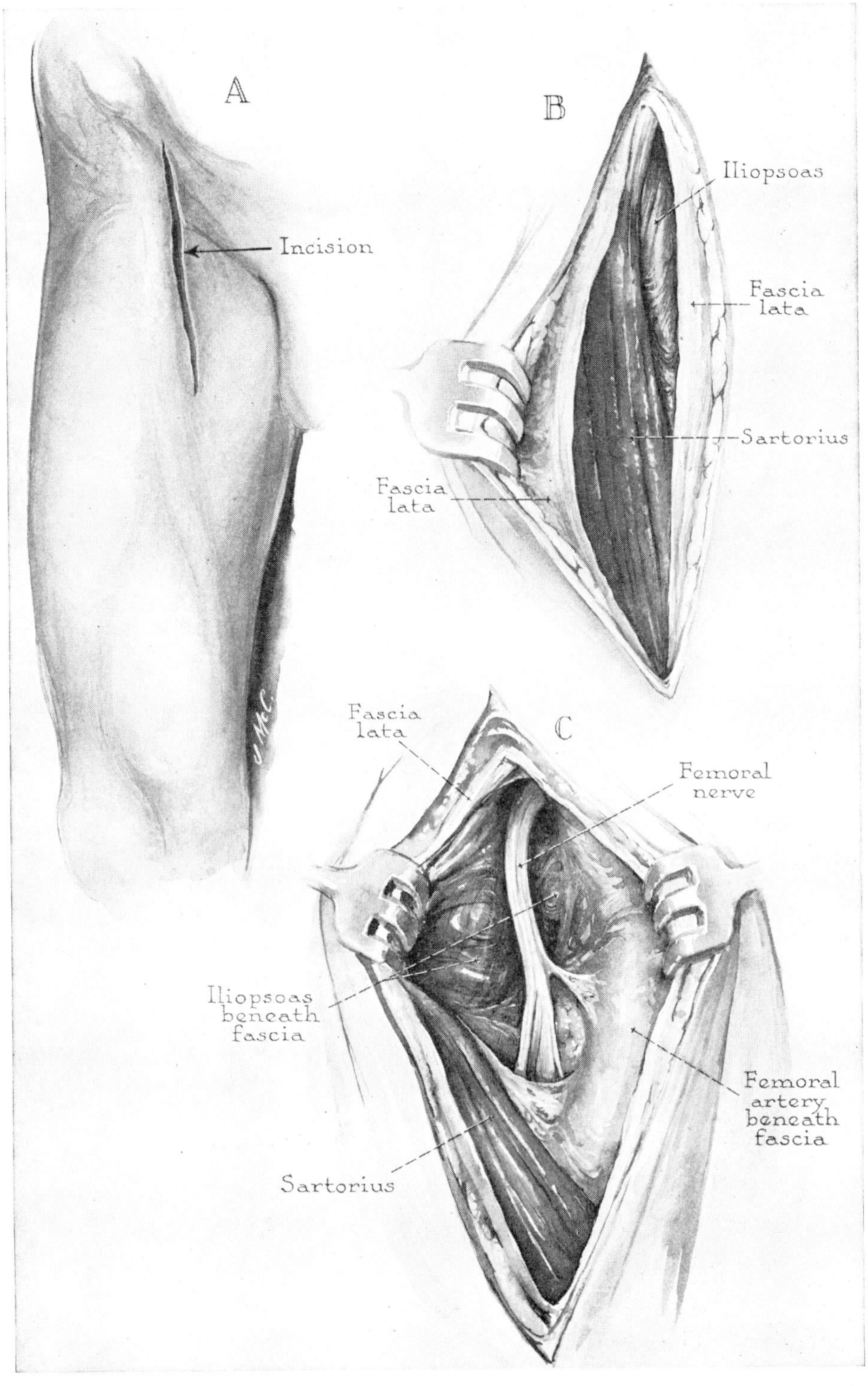

Exposure of the femoral nerve in the thigh

EXPOSURE OF THE SCIATIC NERVE IN THE THIGH THROUGH A POSTERIOR LONGITUDINAL INCISION

Indications: 1. Neurolysis of the Sciatic Nerve

2. Repair of Lacerations of the Sciatic Nerve

Plate 134: Description of Procedure

A The incision is placed in the midline of the thigh. It may extend from the popliteal area upward to the gluteal fold, and the wound can then be enlarged proximally by skirting the lateral and superior margins of the gluteus maximus muscle. The latter is then retracted medially to expose the portion of the sciatic nerve which lies beneath it.

B The fascia is opened carefully so as to protect the posterior femoral cutaneous nerve of the thigh beneath it from injury.

C The semitendinosus muscle is separated from the biceps and the dissection is continued deep between the semimembranosus and biceps muscles.

D The sciatic nerve located in this interval is surrounded by loose areolar tissue and fat. Branches of the sciatic nerve to the hamstring muscles must not be cut. Division of the sciatic nerve into the posterior tibial and peroneal nerves takes place in the thigh at levels which may vary.

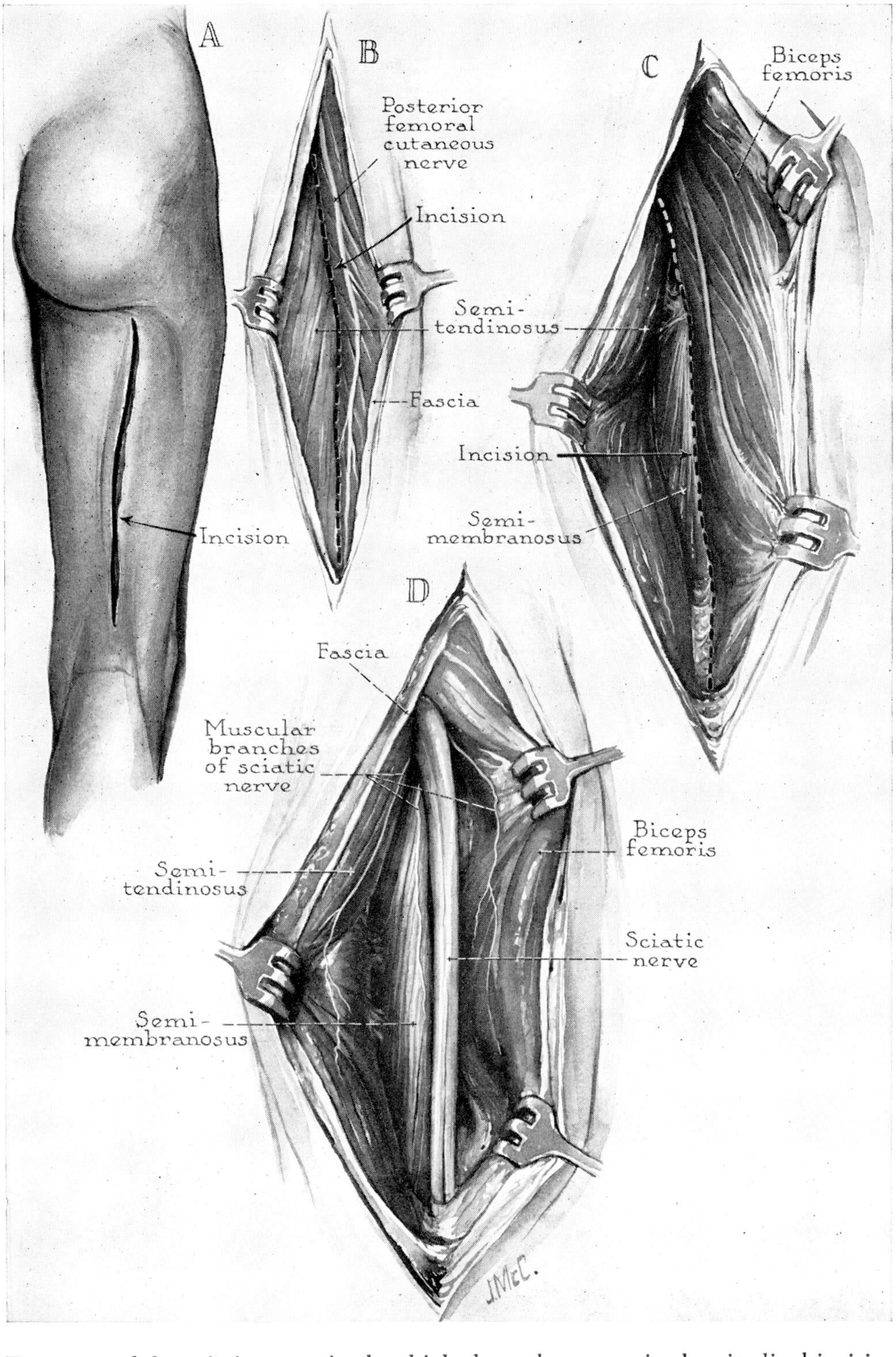

Exposure of the sciatic nerve in the thigh through a posterior longitudinal incision

EXPOSURE OF THE COMMON FEMORAL ARTERY

Indications: I. Exposure of the Femoral Artery

1. Embolectomy
2. Sling control for surgery upon the superficial femoral artery
3. Ligation

II. Exposure of the Femoral Vein

1. Ligation
2. Ligation of the saphenous vein for varicosities
3. Venotomy and thrombectomy

Plate 135: Description of Procedure

A The skin incision for the exposure of the femoral artery is indicated by the line a–a_1; it may, if necessary, be continued across the inguinal fold to a_2. In some instances, the angular incision, a to a_1 to a_3, as illustrated, may prove advantageous. The location of the incision is determined by the maximal pulsations. If no pulsations are palpable, the incision may be made along a line running from the middle of Poupart's ligament to the proximal inner aspect of the medial condyle of the femur. This same incision will expose the femoral vein and the saphenofemoral junction, except that the cut is made slightly more medially for the latter exposure. Some surgeons prefer the incision indicated by the line b–b_1 for exposure of the saphenofemoral junction and it is the one generally utilized in obese individuals, in whom it is placed about 1/2 inch below and parallel to the inguinal crease.

B The incision is carried through the superficial fascia beneath which is found the long saphenous vein. The latter enters the femoral vein, passing through an opening in the cribriform fascia. Tributaries of the saphenofemoral junction may enter either the long saphenous vein or the femoral vein itself. Shown in the illustration are the superficial circumflex iliac and the superficial external pudendal veins. In the particular specimen here illustrated, the superficial inferior epigastric vein formed a common stem with the superficial circumflex iliac, but it may join directly the long saphenous or the femoral vein.

C For exposure of the femoral artery, it is usually necessary to sever the lateral venous tributaries before making a vertical incision in the deep fascia (fascia lata) of the thigh. Its profunda femoral branch arises about 1 1/2 inches distal to Poupart's ligament and dips abruptly downward and somewhat laterally, beneath the medial border of the sartorius muscle. The superficial femoral artery is the continuation of the common femoral artery. The femoral branch of the genitofemoral nerve (not shown in the illustration) may lie on the artery in its uppermost aspect beneath Poupart's ligament.

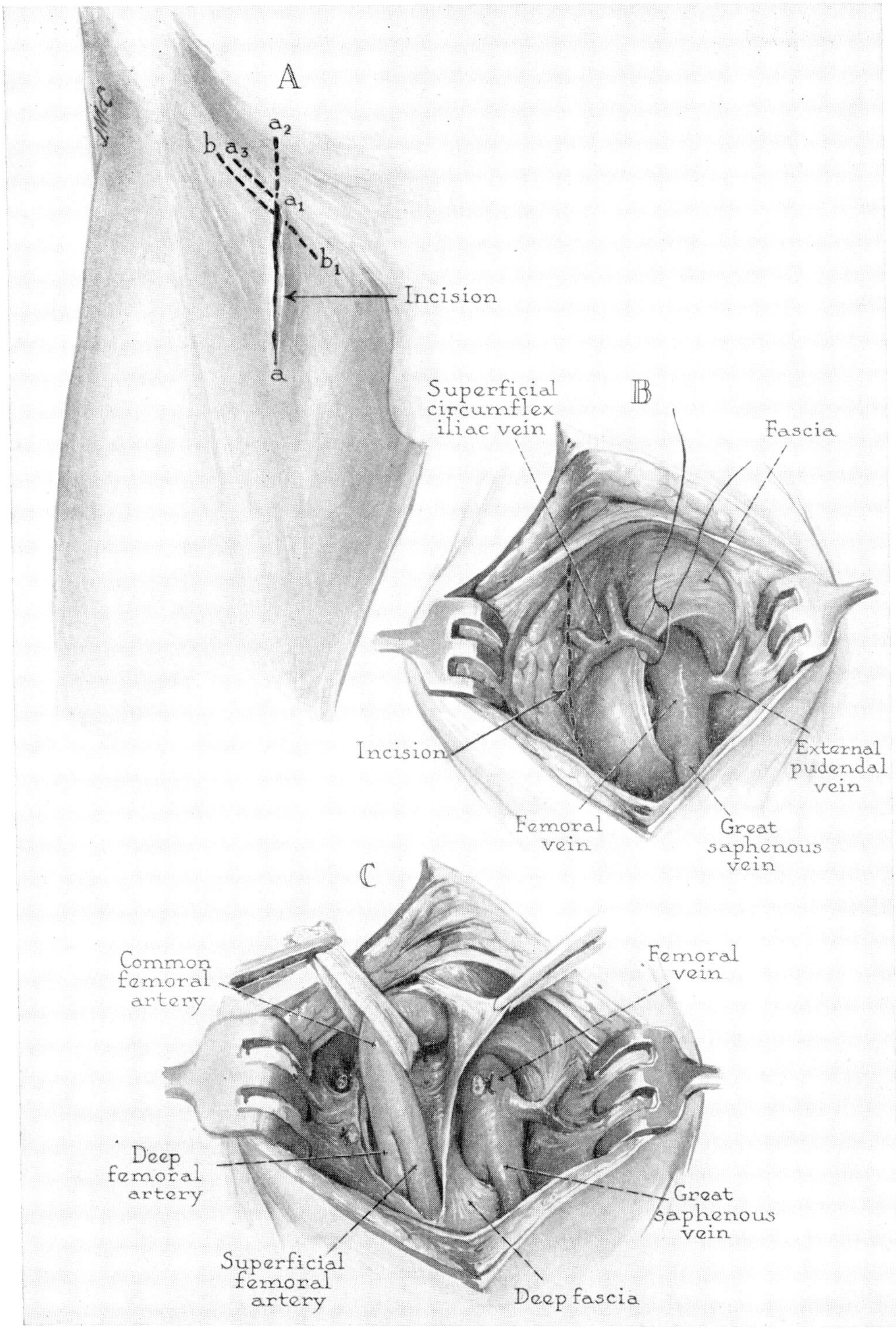

Exposure of the common femoral artery

EXPOSURE OF THE SUPERFICIAL FEMORAL ARTERY IN THE ADDUCTOR (HUNTER'S) CANAL

Indications: 1. Embolectomy

2. Ligation

Plate 136: Description of Procedure

A A skin incision, 4 to 5 inches long, is made parallel to the inferior border of the sartorius muscle, with the extremity placed in external rotation. The skin margins are mobilized and retracted.

B The fascia lata is incised and the sartorius muscle identified and retracted laterally. The gracilis muscle may occasionally have to be pulled over medially, to afford better exposure. The roof of the adductor canal, formed by an extension of the fascia lata, is now seen in the wound. It is incised, under direct vision, as far medially as possible to permit the opening up of the adductor canal. Here are located the femoral artery and vein, and also some branches of the femoral nerve.

C The artery is imbedded in dense fascial tissue superficial to the vein with which it is in close approximation. Separation by dissection of the two vessels must be done with the utmost care to prevent damage.

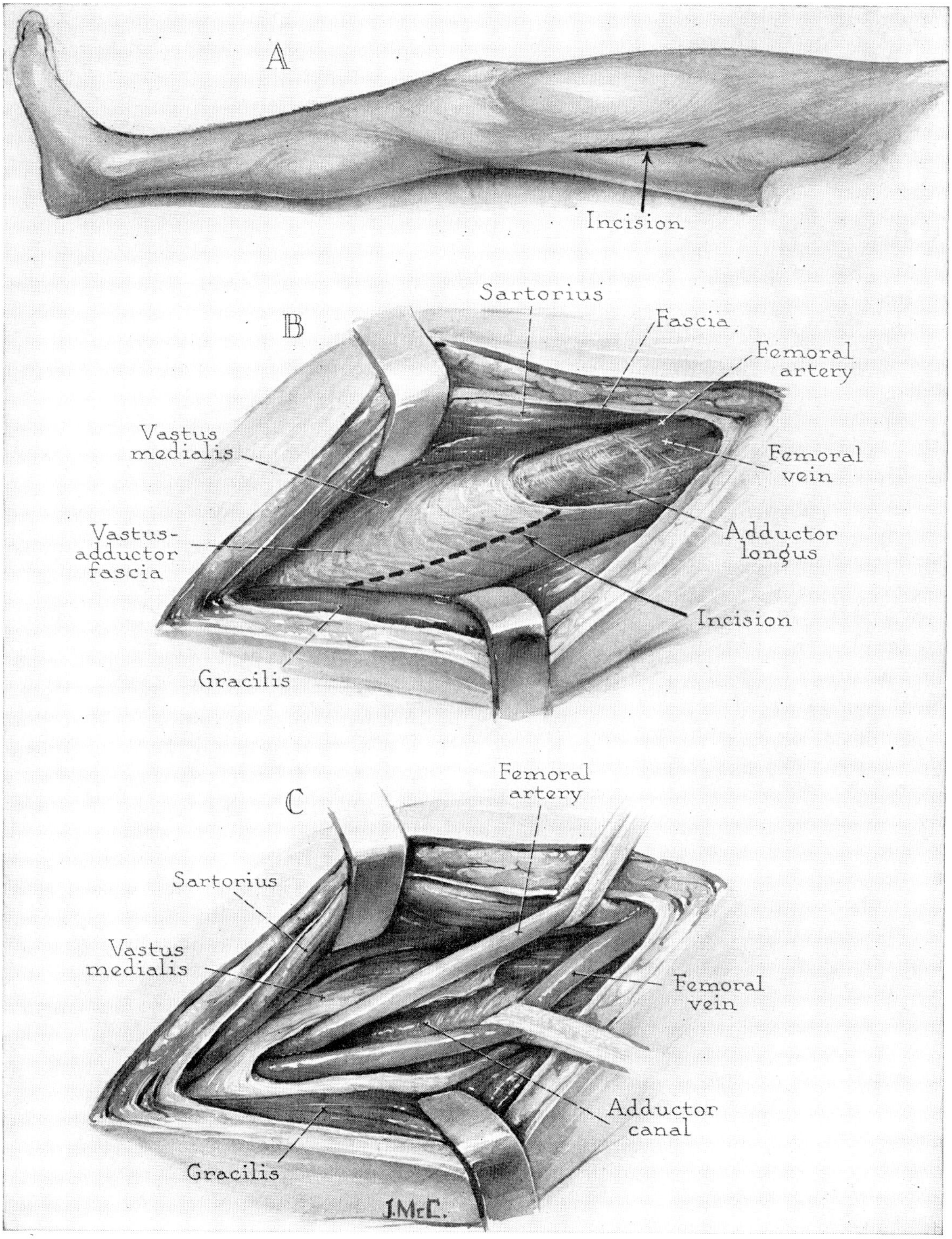

Exposure of the superficial femoral artery in the adductor (Hunter's) canal

EXPOSURE OF THE TENDON OF THE RECTUS FEMORIS MUSCLE THROUGH AN ANTERIOR MIDLINE INCISION

Indications: 1. Repair of Acute Lacerations and Auvlsions of the Quadriceps Tendon

2. Tendoplasties of the Quadriceps Tendon

Plate 137: Description of Procedure

A The skin incision, about 4 inches in length, begins at the superior margin of the patella and extends proximally along the midline for the desired distance. If necessary, the incision can be extended further at either end.

B The deep fascia is incised, and the skin flaps are reflected.

C The rectus femoris muscle and tendon can be mobilized by parallel incisions which will separate these two structures from the vastus lateralis laterally, and the vastus medialis medially. The vastus intermedius muscle lies beneath the rectus femoris. The quadriceps bursa, which represents an upward extension of the knee joint, is located directly proximal to the patella and below the tendon

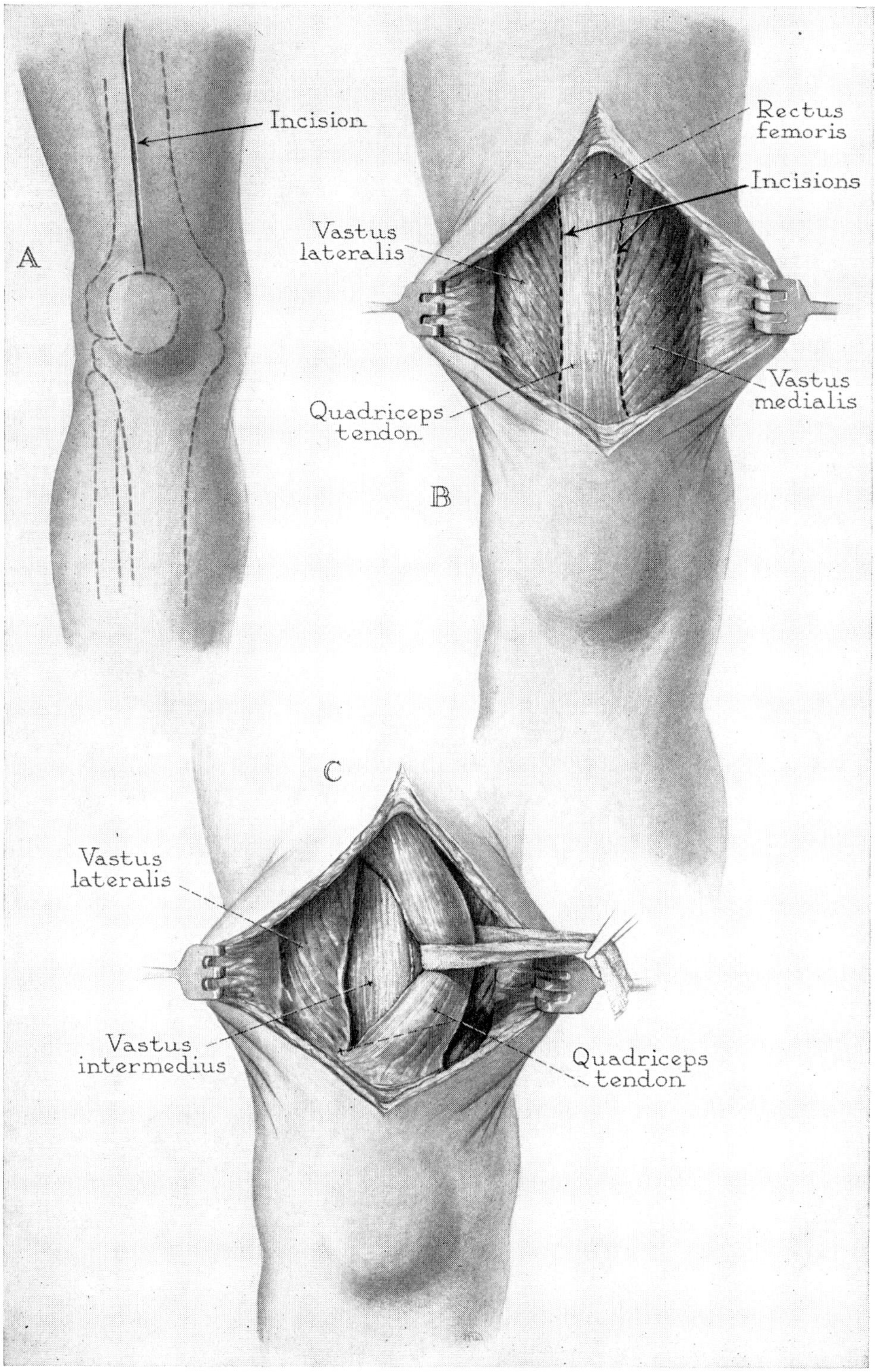

Exposure of the tendon of the rectus femoris muscle through an anterior midline incision

Section IX

Region of the Knee Joint

EXPOSURE OF THE DISTAL FOURTH OF THE SHAFT OF THE FEMUR, INCLUDING THE KNEE JOINT, THROUGH AN ANTERIOR LATERAL INCISION

Indications: 1. Open Reduction of Comminuted Fractures of the Distal End of the Femur

2. Resection of Benign and Malignant Tumors

Plate 138: Description of Procedure

A The incision is made between the rectus femoris tendon and the anterior edge of the vastus lateralis muscle. It extends from the lower third of the femur to the patella, where it curves laterally onto the adjacent portion of the knee joint. The incision is approximately 5 1/2 inches long. The skin flaps are mobilized and retracted.

B The fascia lata is incised in line with the skin incision, and the knee joint is opened in the distal portion of the wound by cutting through the capsule and synovial membrane. The vastus lateralis muscle is now separated by sharp dissection from the tendon of the rectus muscle, to permit retraction of these structures to their respective sides of the wound.

C The vastus intermedius muscle which covers the front of the femur is split longitudinally to expose the periosteum. A periosteal incision, which curves distally around the articular margin of the lateral femoral condyle, then permits access to the bone.

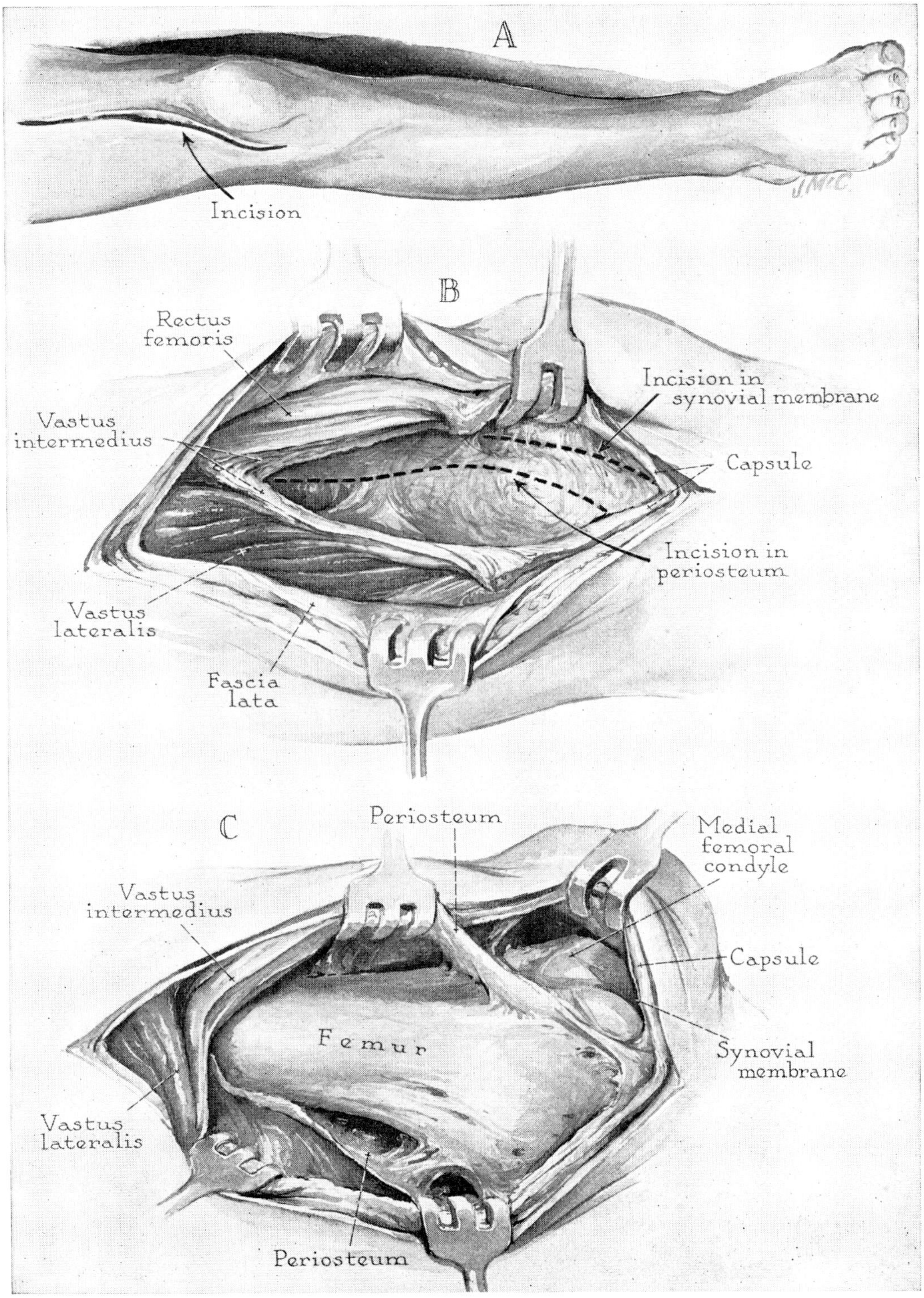

Exposure of the distal fourth of the shaft of the femur, including the knee joint, through an anterior lateral incision

EXPOSURE OF THE DISTAL FOURTH OF THE SHAFT OF THE FEMUR, INCLUDING THE KNEE JOINT, THROUGH AN ANTERIOR MEDIAL INCISION

Indications: 1. Open Reduction of Comminuted Fractures of the Distal End of the Femur Which Extend into the Knee Joint

2. Resection of Benign and Malignant Tumors

Plate 139: Description of Procedure

A An incision, approximately 5 1/2 inches long, is placed over the junction between the rectus femoris tendon and the anterior margin of the vastus medialis muscle. The dissection extends distally onto the proximal half of the medial capsule of the knee joint. The skin flaps are mobilized and retracted. The fascia lata is incised in line with the skin incision.

B The capsule is opened in the distal portion of the wound. The interval is developed proximally between the vastus medialis muscle and the tendon of the rectus femoris. Distally the incision separates the vastus medialis and the quadriceps tendons down to the patella. The rectus femoris and quadriceps tendons are retracted outward, and the vastus medialis muscle is pulled inward. The vastus intermedius is split longitudinally.

C The synovial membrane is incised to open the knee joint. The next cut is placed through the periosteum over the anterior medial aspect of the shaft and medial condyle just proximal to the articular margin to expose the bone subperiosteally.

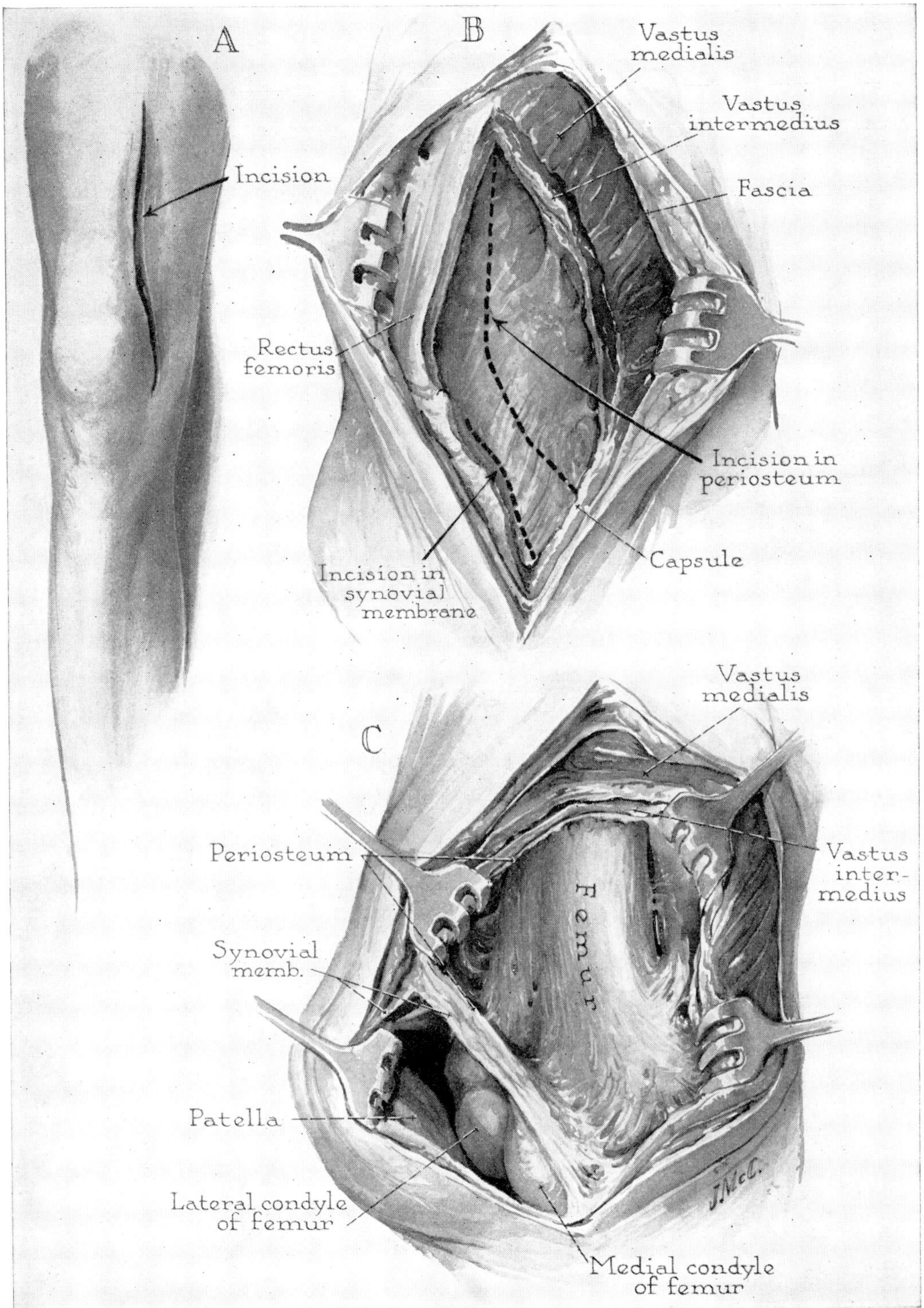

Exposure of the distal fourth of the shaft of the femur, including the knee joint, through an anterior medial incision

EXPOSURE OF THE KNEE JOINT THROUGH A MEDIAL PARAPATELLAR INCISION REFLECTING THE PATELLA LATERALLY

Indications: 1. Synovectomy of the Knee Joint

2. Removal of Loose Bodies

3. Excision of Benign Tumors of the Synovia

4. Débridement for Degenerative Arthritis

5. Removal of Semilunar Cartilage

Plate 140: Description of Procedure

A The incision begins over the medial aspect of the rectus femoris tendon about 1 1/2 inches above the patella, and extends downward to a level of the proximal pole of the latter, where it curves gently along the medial aspect of the joint to end at the tibia near the tubercle.

B The skin margins are mobilized and the capsule is opened in line with the skin incision. The rectus femoris tendon is separated from the vastus medialis to expose the quadriceps expansion (pouch) of the joint cavity below.

C The synovia is incised to expose the interior of the joint. The patella is dislocated from the femoral groove and retracted to the lateral aspect of the lateral condyle of the femur.

NOTE: The authors rarely use this incision. They prefer the medial parapatellar, bilateral capsular incision for synovectomies and débridement of the knee joint. The semilunar cartilage can be removed adequately through a short medial or lateral parapatellar incision. A transverse skin incision, with bilateral parapatellar capsular openings into the joint, offers adequate exposure when both semilunar cartilages are to be removed.

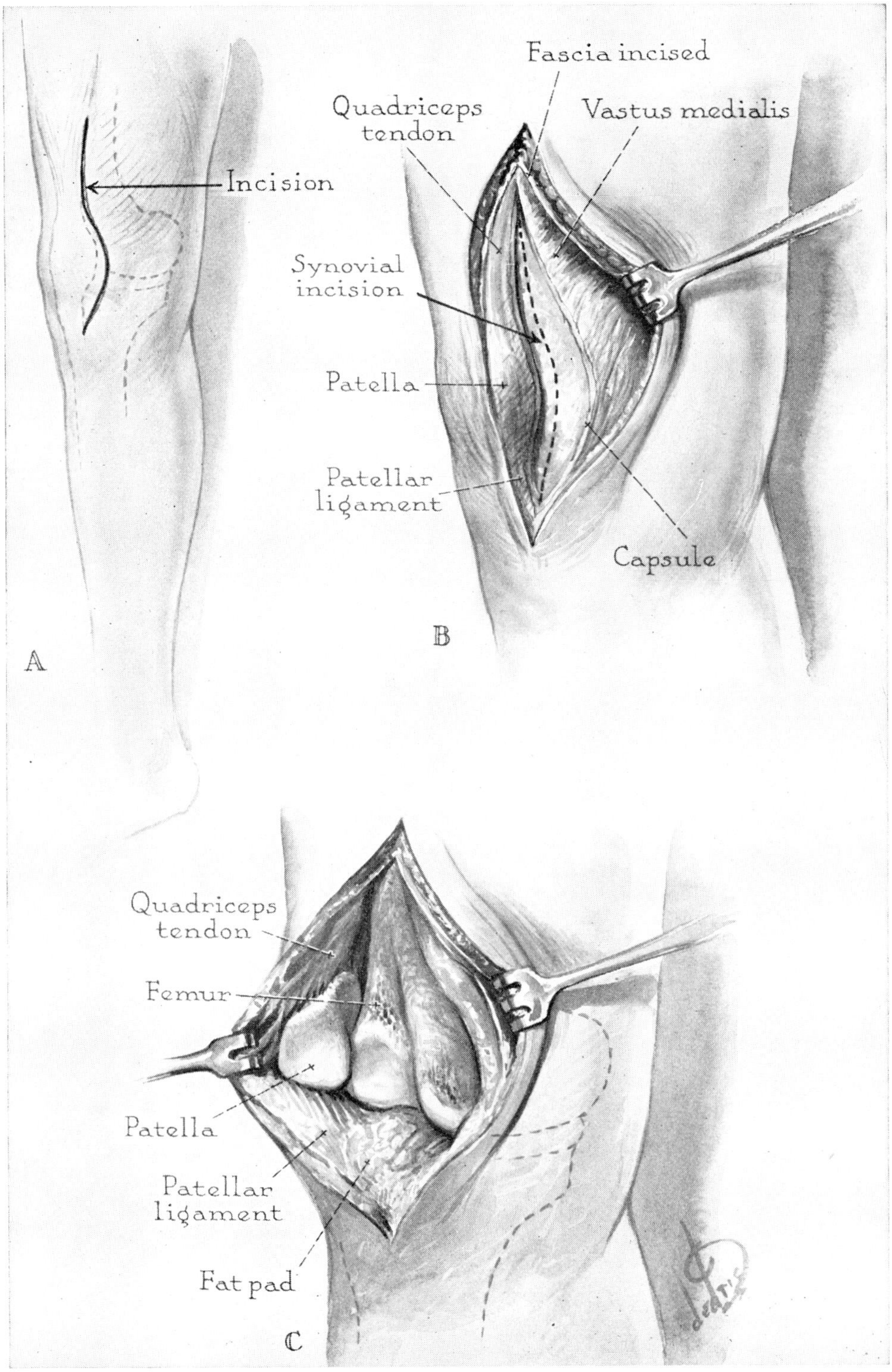

Exposure of the knee joint through a medial parapatellar incision, reflecting the patella laterally

EXPOSURE OF THE KNEE JOINT THROUGH A MEDIAL SKIN AND BILATERAL PARAPATELLAR CAPSULAR INCISION

Indications: 1. Excision of the Medial and Lateral Semilunar Cartilages

2. Synovectomy of the Knee Joint

3. Débridement of the Knee Joint for Degenerative Arthritis

4. Release of Intracapsular Adhesions Causing Fibrous Ankylosis of the Knee

Plate 141: Description of Procedure

A The incision begins at the inner aspect of the tibial tubercle and extends upward along the medial side of the joint, to end 1 or 2 inches proximal to the patella over the line of junction of the rectus femoris and vastus medialis muscles.

B Both flaps are undermined, and especially the lateral one, to expose the lateral capsule of the knee. The dissection should be kept close to the surface of the capsule to avoid injury to the sensory nerves which are located in the subcutaneous fat. The skin has a good blood supply so that the lateral flap will not necrose.

C The medial side of the joint is opened by an incision through the capsule and synovia, and the suprapatellar pouch is exposed by sharp dissection along the junction of the rectus femoris tendon and the vastus medialis muscle in the upper end of the incision. This portion of the incision provides a good exposure of the pouch, the medial condyle of the femur, the patella, the medial semilunar cartilage and the synovia in the medial half of the front of the knee. (Procedure continued on Plate 142.)

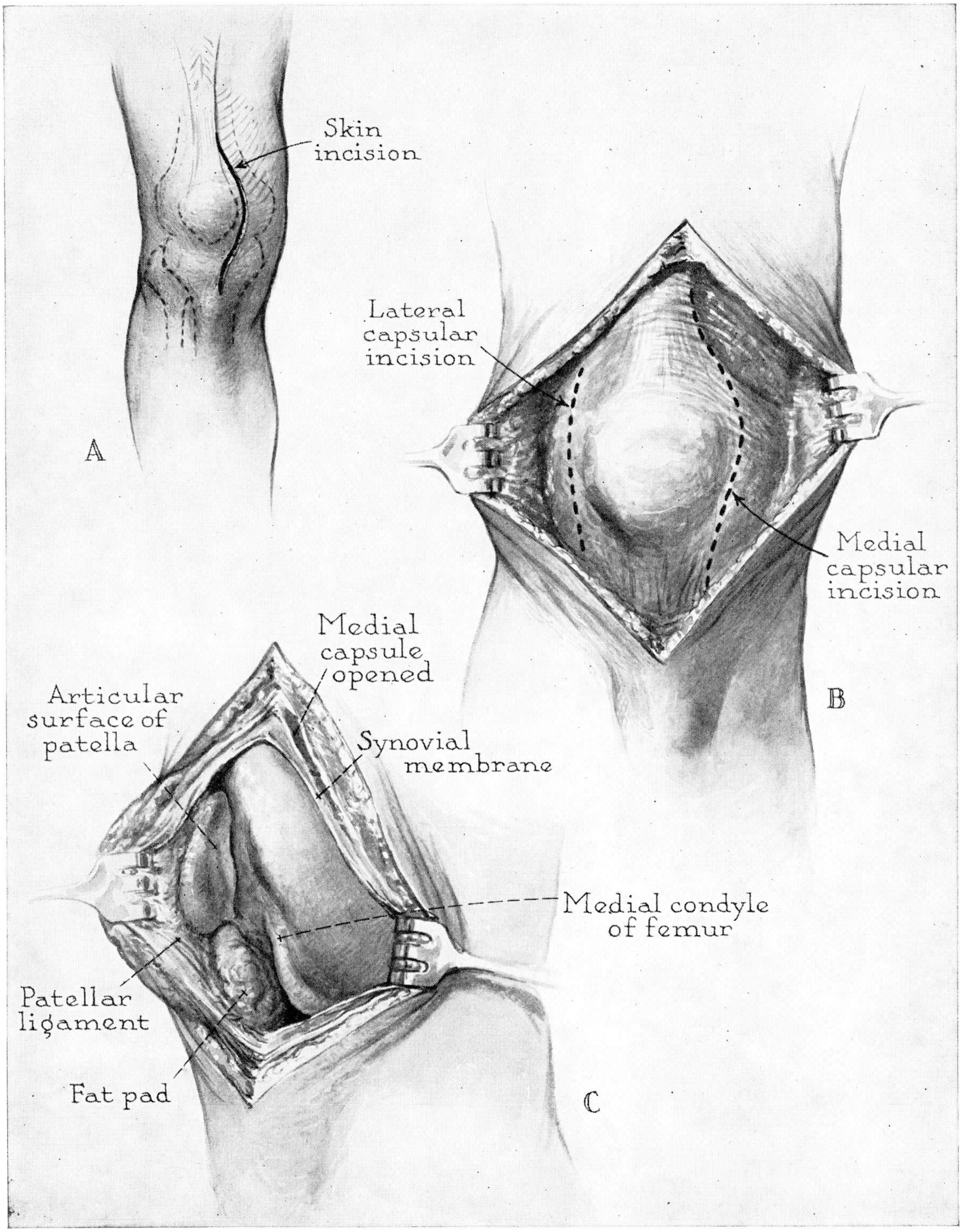

Exposure of the knee joint through a medial skin and bilateral parapatellar capsular incision

EXPOSURE OF THE KNEE JOINT THROUGH A MEDIAL SKIN AND BILATERAL PARAPATELLAR CAPSULAR INCISION *(Continued)*

Plate 142: Description of Procedure

D The lateral side of the joint is opened by an incision in the corresponding portion of the capsule and synovial membrane. This incision must be slightly farther away from the patella than the medial capsular incision.

E The synovia in the lateral anterior half of the joint, the lateral condyle of the femur and the lateral semilunar cartilage are all readily accessible. Maximal exposure of the knee joint is obtained by displacing the patella first to one and then to the other side.

NOTE: This incision is deserving of wider usage. It offers a better exposure of the lateral portion of the joint than is obtained by the long medial parapatellar incision in which the patella is dislocated to the lateral side of the knee. Both sides of the knee joint can be exposed in a similar manner through a transverse skin incision. The access to the patellar pouch is more difficult, but the incision has the advantage of not requiring cutting into the quadriceps apparatus.

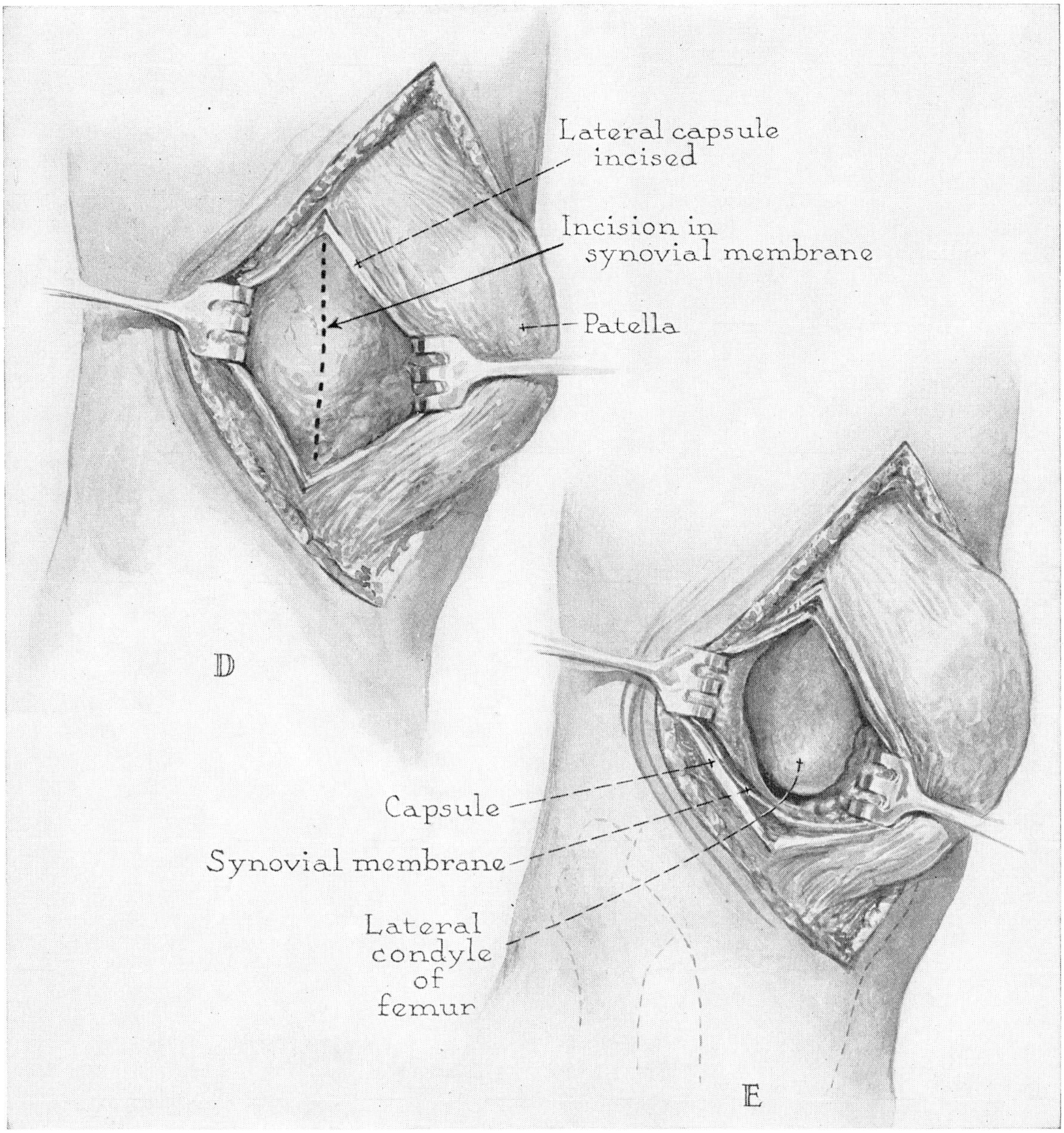

Exposure of the knee joint through a medial skin and bilateral parapatellar capsular incision

EXPOSURE OF THE KNEE JOINT THROUGH A LATERAL PARAPATELLAR INCISION

Indications: 1. Removal of the Lateral Semilunar Cartilage

2. Removal of Loose Bodies and Benign Tumors

Plate 143: Description of Procedure

A The skin incision is centered over the lateral aspect of the joint and extends from the top of the patella to the upper margin of the tibia, paralleling the lateral margin of the patella. The skin is retracted and the deep fascia is opened in line with the skin incision.

B The capsule is incised, as illustrated, to expose the synovial membrane.

C The lateral half of the knee joint is entered by incising the synovial membrane and retracting the wound.

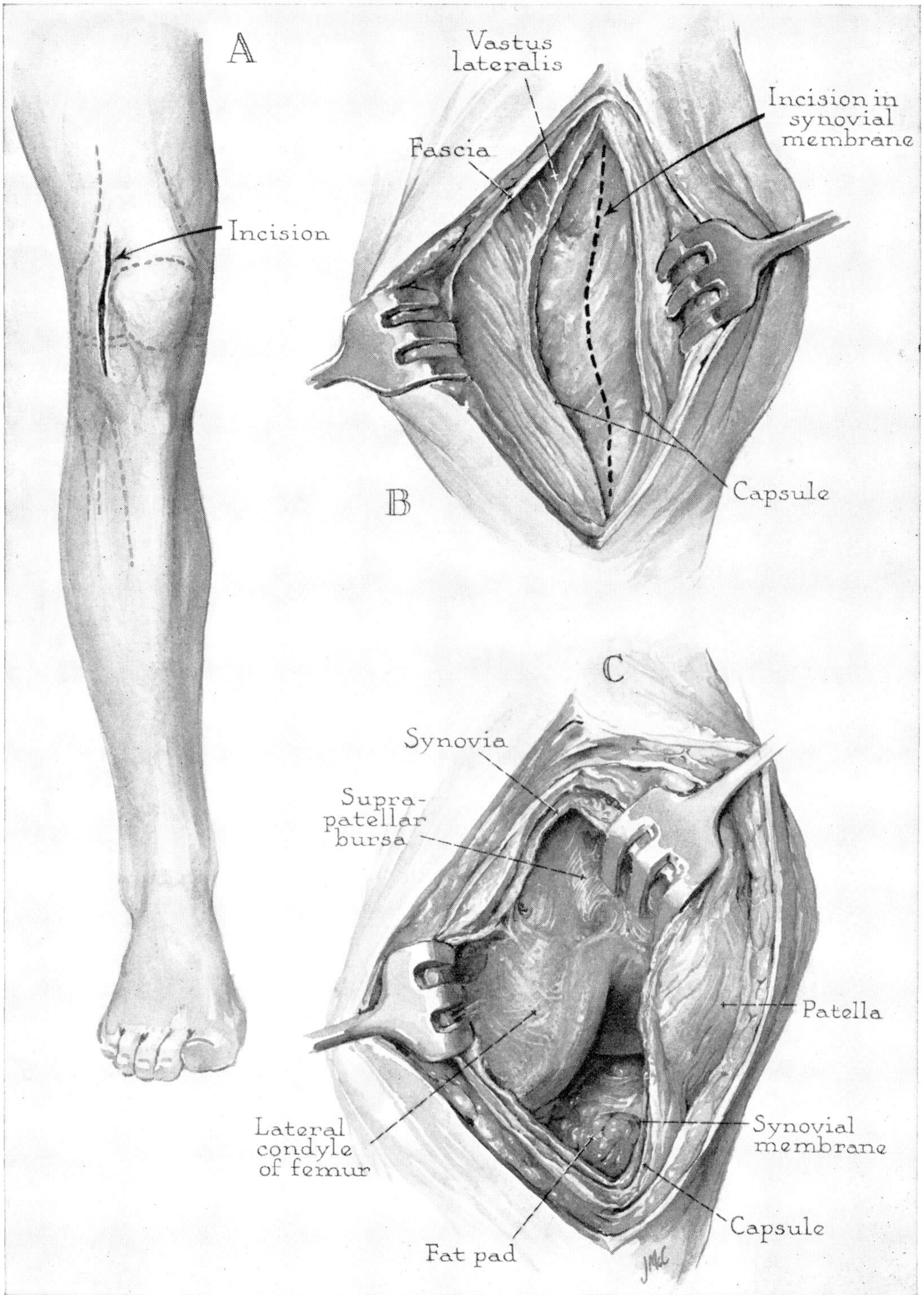

Exposure of the knee joint through a lateral parapatellar incision

EXPOSURE OF THE KNEE JOINT THROUGH A U-SHAPED INCISION WITH TRANSECTION OF THE PATELLAR LIGAMENT

Indications: 1. Arthrodesis of the Knee Joint

2. Arthroplasty of the Knee Joint

Plate 144: Description of Procedure

A The incision begins in the region of the medial epicondyle of the femur and extends across the knee joint in a U-shaped manner, as illustrated. The two ends of the incision may be prolonged proximally for a more extended exposure.

B The skin flaps—and especially the proximal one—are mobilized and retracted. The local blood supply is sufficient to prevent necrosis.

C A second incision, with its two ends placed somewhat closer to the patella, cuts the capsule and the patellar ligament. The incision is carried further down through the synovial membrane and fat pad, and the interior of the joint is widely exposed as the margins of the wound are strongly retracted.

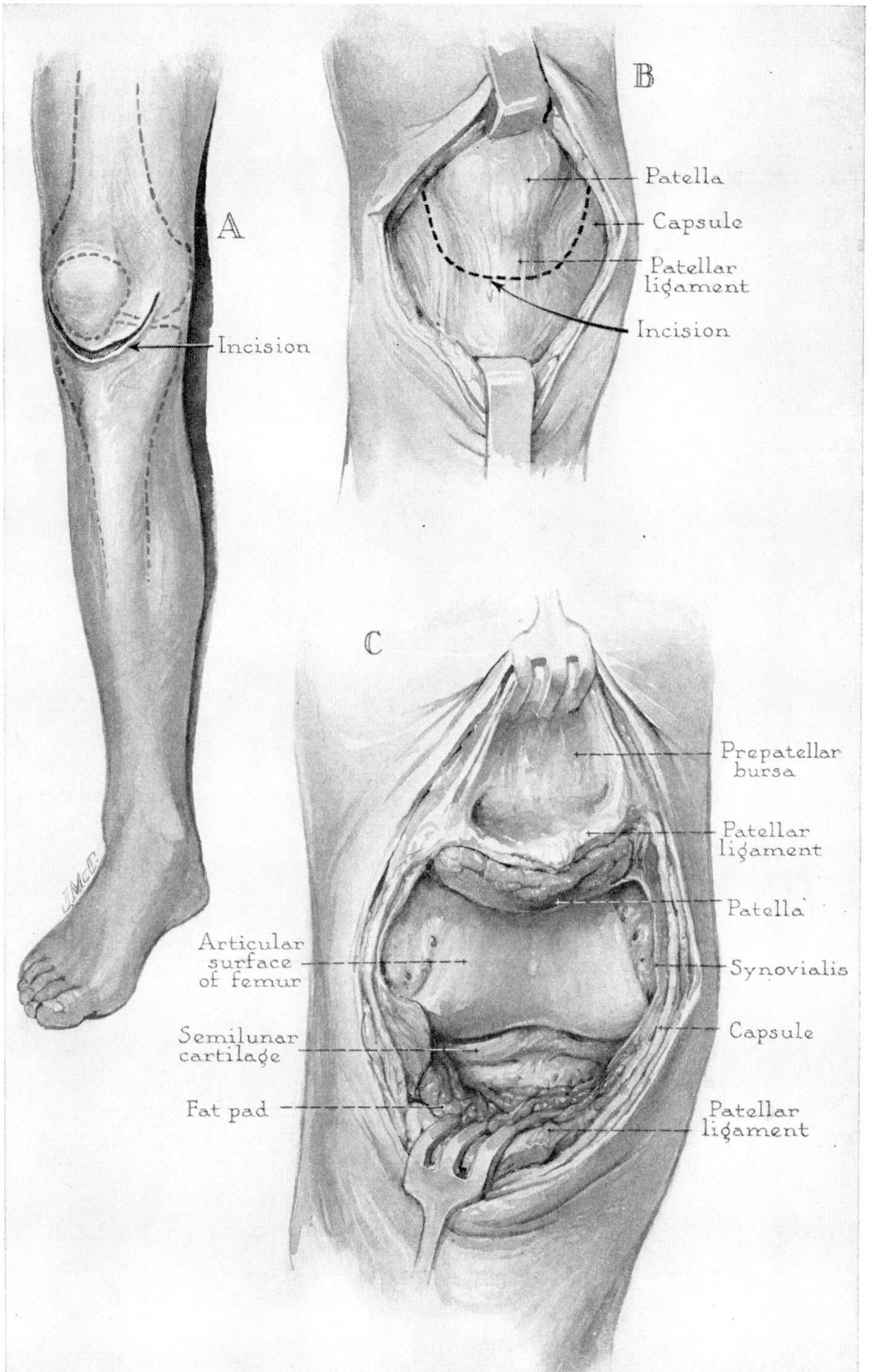

Exposure of the knee joint through a U-shaped incision, with transection of the patellar ligament

EXPOSURE OF THE KNEE JOINT THROUGH A POSTERIOR MEDIAL INCISION

Indications: 1. Excision of the Posterior Portion of the Medial Semilunar Cartilage

2. Removal of Loose Bodies and Benign Tumors from the Knee Joint

3. Removal of Benign Lesions from the Posterior Medial Aspect of the Medial Condyle of the Femur

Plate 145: Description of Procedure

A The incision begins at the upper end just posterior to the medial epicondyle of the femur and extends downward in a slightly curved manner as far as the proximal end of the tibia.

B The deep fascia is opened and the sartorius muscle and tendon are identified and retracted posteriorly.

C The dissection is carried through the areolar tissue between the capsule of the knee joint and the medial head of the gastrocnemius muscle, which is pulled posteriorly. A linear incision through the capsule exposes the interior of the joint.

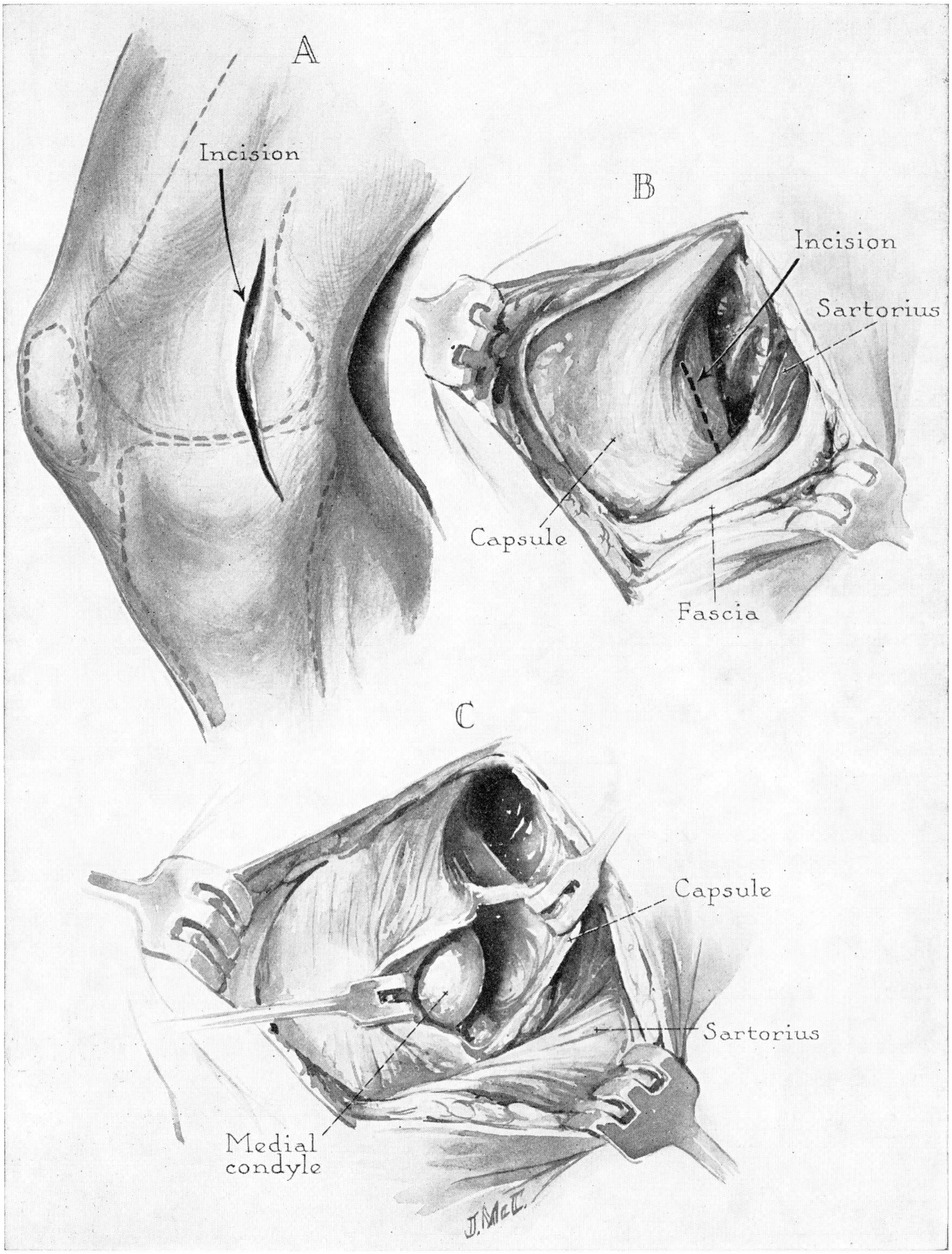

Exposure of the knee joint through a posterior medial incision

EXPOSURE OF THE POSTERIOR LATERAL COMPARTMENT OF THE KNEE JOINT THROUGH A POSTERIOR LATERAL INCISION

Indications: 1. Removal of Loose Bodies

2. Excision of the Posterior Portion of the Lateral Semilunar Cartilage

Plate 146: Description of Procedure

A The skin incision, about 4 1/2 inches long, begins at the level of the lateral condyle of the tibia and curves upward paralleling the posterior margin of the iliotibial tract. The dissection then proceeds in the interval between the lateral intermuscular septum and the tendon of the biceps muscle, as shown in the illustration. The peroneal nerve lies along the inferior margin of the biceps tendon and need not be exposed, although its proximity to the dissection must not be lost sight of.

B The iliotibial band is retracted upward and the biceps muscle downward, thus exposing the lateral head of the gastrocnemius muscle and the popliteal fat. The lateral superior geniculate artery crosses the field and is ligated. The lateral collateral ligament of the knee is located by palpation, for it extends from the lateral epicondyle of the femur to the head of the fibula. The lateral head of the gastrocnemius muscle is separated from the capsule of the knee joint which it covers.

C The capsule is opened by an incision which parallels the posterior margin of the lateral collateral ligament, as illustrated. The tendon of the popliteus muscle can be seen inside the joint along the inner aspect of the collateral ligament, where it runs obliquely downward and backward before emergence from the joint to enter the leg. Care must be exercised not to injure this tendon while incising the synovial membrane. The contents of the popliteal space lie medially to the dissection and are protected by the fatty tissue which separates them from the operative field.

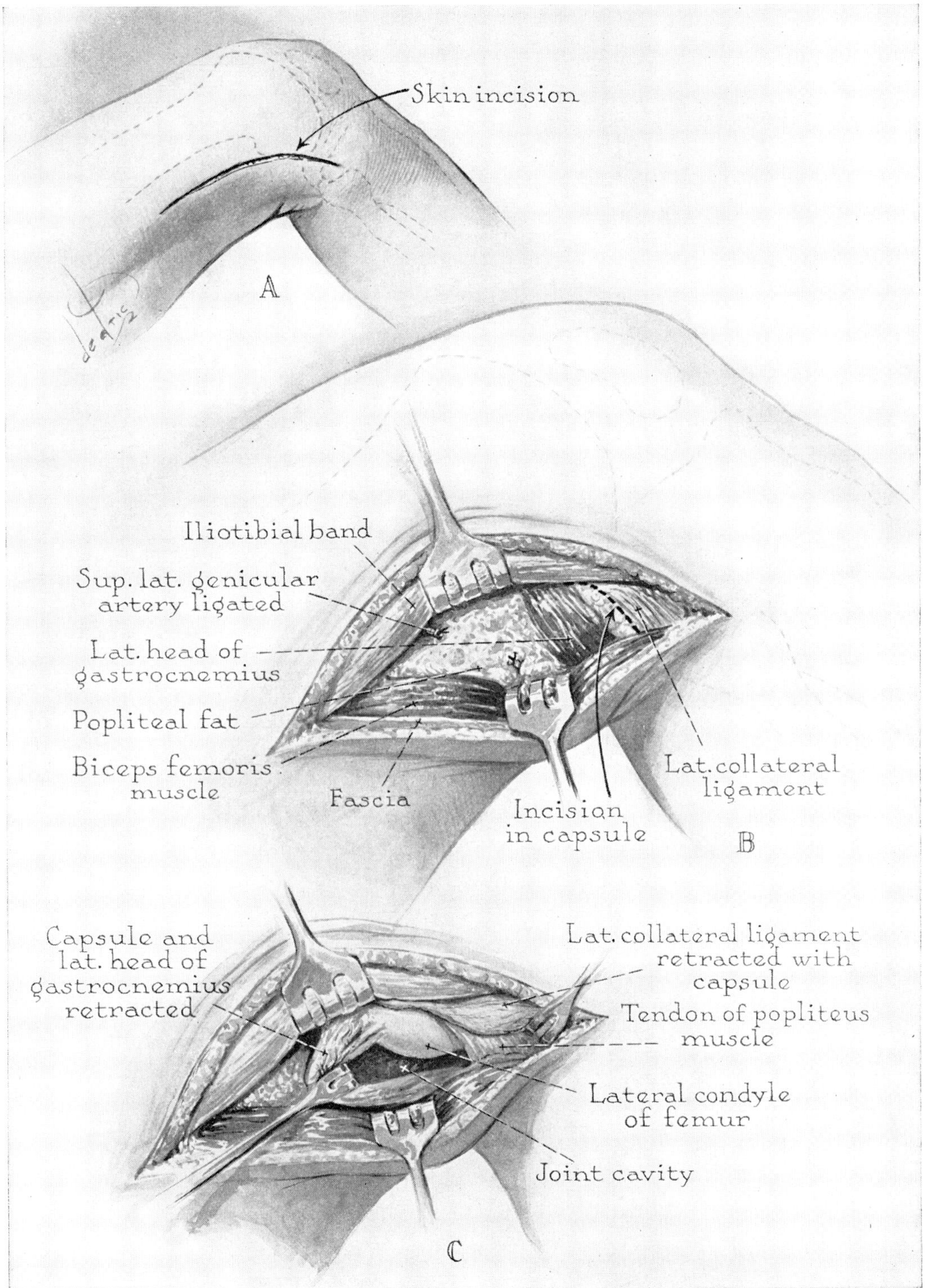

Exposure of the posterior lateral compartment of the knee joint through a posterior lateral incision

EXPOSURE OF THE KNEE JOINT THROUGH A POSTERIOR POPLITEAL INCISION

Indications: 1. Removal of Loose Bodies or Tumors in the Posterior Compartment of the Knee Joint Which Cannot Be Approached through a Posterior Medial or a Posterior Lateral Incision

2. Open Reduction of Fractures in the Posterior Medial Articular Portion of the Femur or Tibia

3. Removal of Benign Tumors of the Posterior Surface of the Medial Condyle of the Tibia

Plate 147: Description of Procedure

A The skin incision is first directed downward at a place just posterior to the biceps tendon; it then is extended horizontally across the popliteal space in a flexion crease, and finally is continued distally between the tendon of the semitendinosus and the medial head of the gastrocnemius for several inches. The deep fascia is cut in line with the incision. The small saphenous vein which is exposed in the wound may be ligated or retracted as might be indicated.

B The interval is developed through the areolar tissue between the tendon of the semitendinosus and the medial head of the gastrocnemius, and then is continued distally along the medial margin of the gastrocnemius and soleus muscles.

C The semitendinosus and semimembranosus are retracted medially. The gastrocnemius then is pulled laterally to expose the posterior aspect of the capsule of the knee joint. The joint cavity is opened by an appropriate incision in the capsule. The wound may be extended distally to the proximal portion of the tibia. The medial semilunar cartilage should not be detached from the tibia unless it is to be excised.

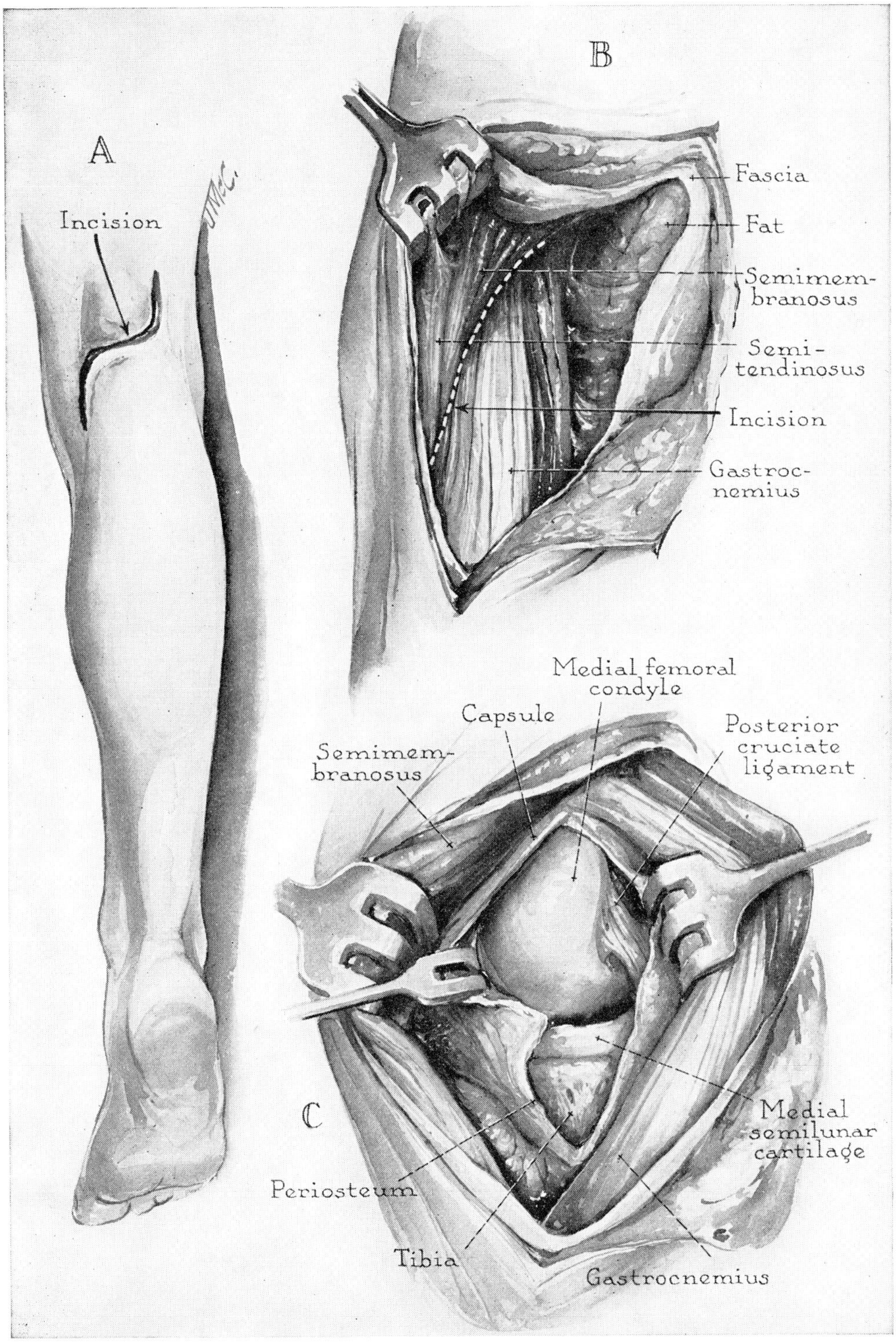

Exposure of the knee joint through a posterior popliteal incision

EXPOSURE OF THE PERONEAL NERVE IN THE POPLITEAL REGION

Indications: 1. Neurolysis of the Peroneal Nerve

2. Repair of Lacerations of the Peroneal Nerve

Plate 148: Description of Procedure

A A roughly S-shaped skin incision is made, with its central portion running transversely across the popliteal space by following a flexion crease, as illustrated. The proximal end of the incision extends upward for several inches over the hamstring tendons, and the distal end downward over the adjacent fibula.

B The deep fascia is opened just posterior to the biceps tendon, and the dissection is carried further downward in the wound over the fibula. The fascial margins are retracted and the tendon of the biceps muscle is identified.

C The peroneal nerve is located just posterior to the biceps tendon; it can be traced distally to the neck of the fibula where it curves anteriorly and then disappears in the adjacent muscles. The peroneal nerve gives off the lateral sural nerve in the popliteal region, and also supplies branches to the peroneal muscles at the level of the head of the fibula.

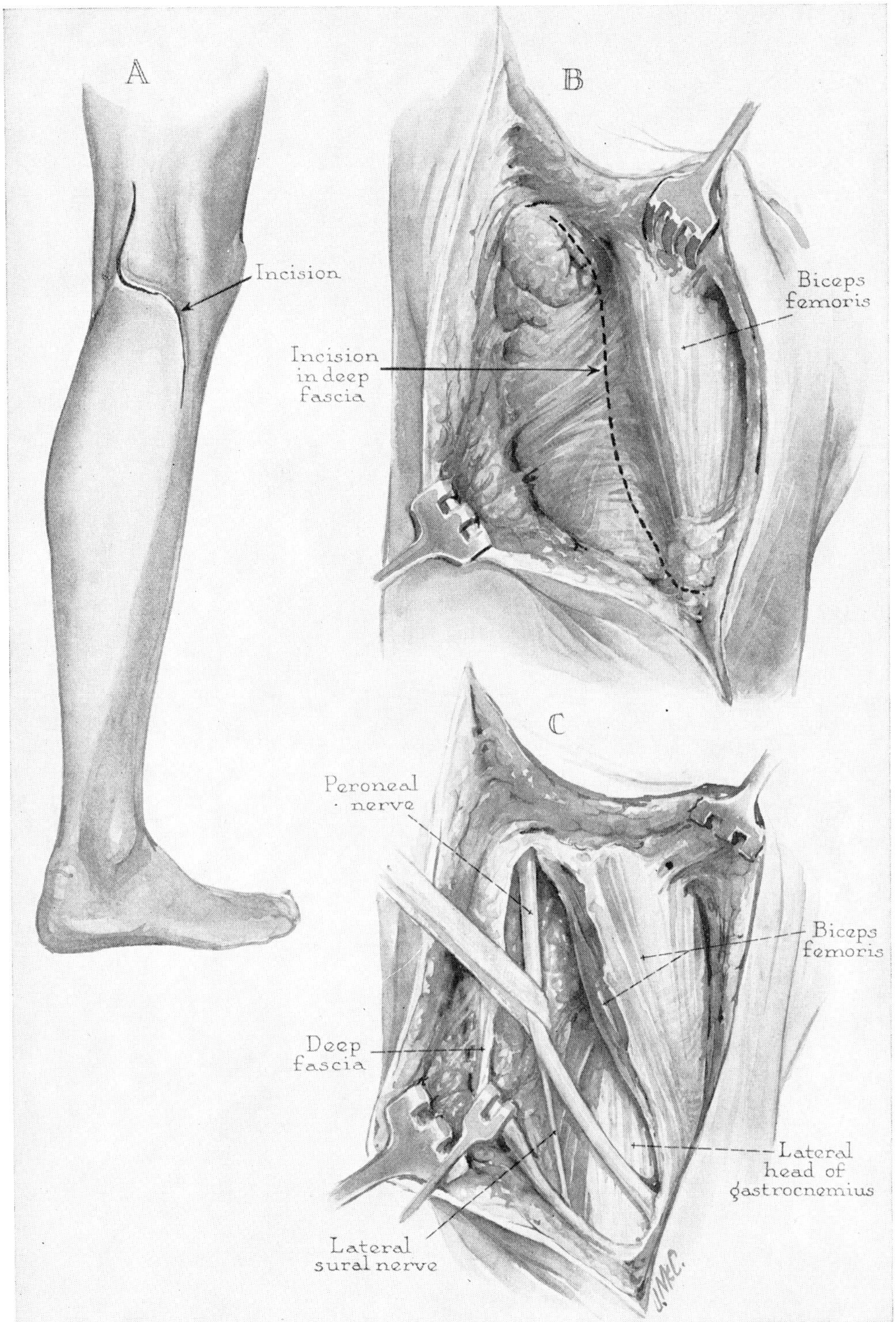

Exposure of the peroneal nerve in the popliteal region

EXPOSURE OF THE POPLITEAL ARTERY

Indications: 1. Embolectomy

2. Ligation of the Popliteal Artery

3. Sling Control of the Popliteal Artery

Plate 149: Description of Procedure

A The incision is made as a flattened S curve, as illustrated. It begins in the region of the semimembranosus-semitendinosus area, swings laterally in line with the skin folds of the popliteal space, and then turns downward over the lateral head of the gastrocnemius muscle.

B A vertical incision is made in the deep fascia. It usually passes just lateral to the point of exit of the short saphenous vein. This vein requires ligation in most cases.

C The semimembranosus and semitendinosus muscles are separated from the biceps proximally, while distally the medial and lateral heads of the gastrocnemius are pulled to their respective sides of the wound. The peroneal nerve may be seen as it skirts the posterior margin of the lowest portion of the biceps muscle; it must be protected from injury. The popliteal vein is exposed and retracted laterally. The popliteal artery is located behind and medial to the vein. The posterior tibial nerve is lateral to the popliteal vein, as illustrated.

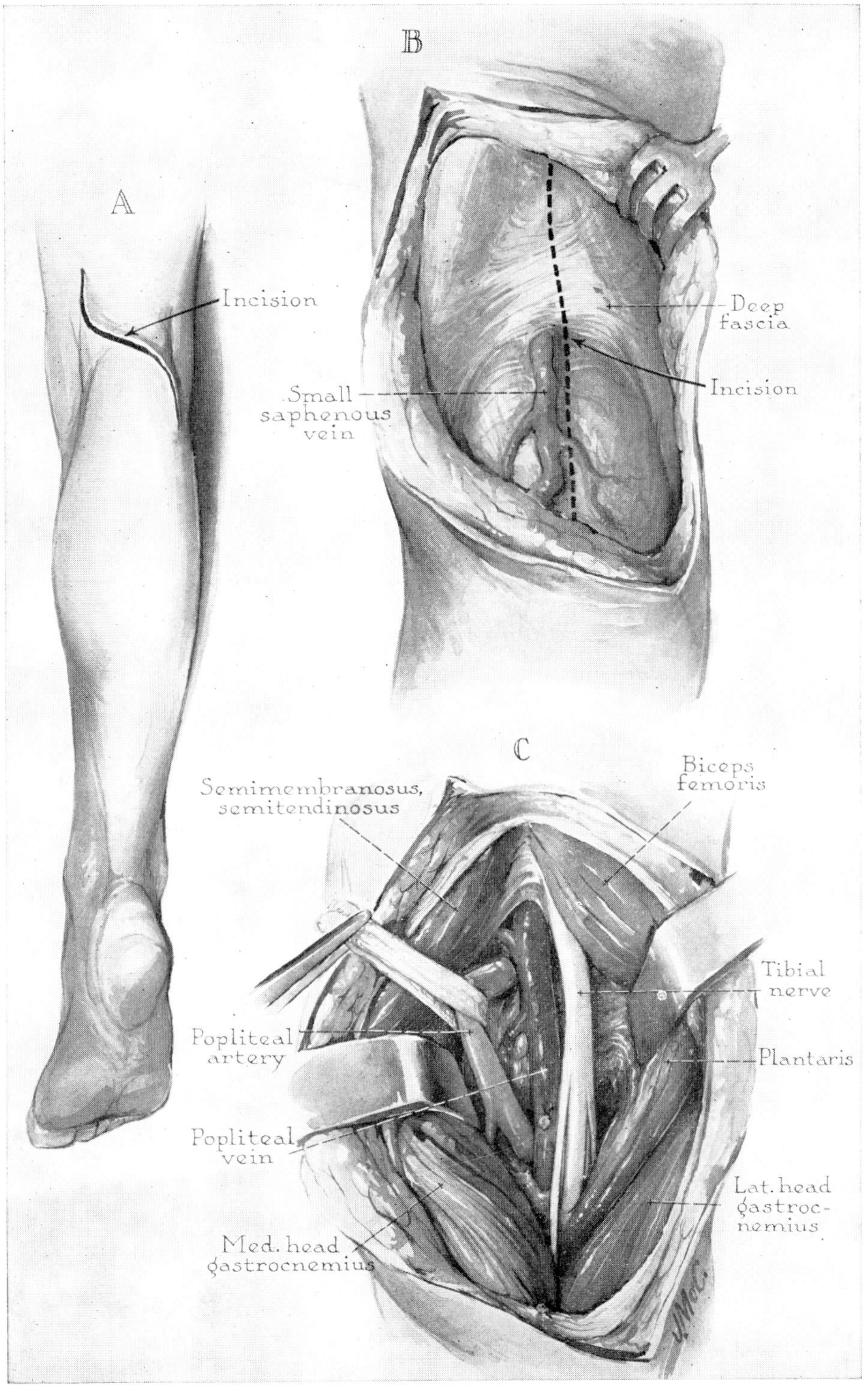

Exposure of the popliteal artery

Section X

Region of the Tibia and Fibula

EXPOSURE OF THE KNEE JOINT, THE LATERAL CONDYLE AND THE ADJACENT PORTION OF THE MEDIAL SURFACE OF THE TIBIA THROUGH A LATERAL KNEE, ANTERIOR TIBIAL INCISION

Indication: 1. Open Reduction of Plateau Fractures of the Lateral Condyle of the Tibia

Plate 150: Description of Procedure

A A curved incision, approximately 6 1/2 inches long, begins over the midlateral aspect of the knee joint level with the top of the patella. The incision first runs straight downward, and then extends across the lateral condyle of the tibia and continues along the anterior margin of the flare of the condyle, to end over the medial surface of the tibia. The incision may be extended as far distally over the tibia as necessary.

B The lateral compartment of the knee joint is opened by cutting through the capsule and synovial membrane. The periosteum is incised along the anterior margin of the lateral condyle and the medial surface of the tibia.

C The anterior tibial muscle is reflected subperiosteally from the lateral surface of the condyle and shaft of the tibia. The dissection is extended distally to expose as much of the medial surface of the tibia as necessary.

D The lateral semilunar cartilage (frequently torn) is removed to obtain an unobstructed view of the articular surface of the lateral condyle of the tibia.

NOTE: No important nerves or blood vessels are encountered in this operation. The peroneal nerve, which is located along the lateral surface of the anterior tibial muscle, will not be injured if this muscle is mobilized subperiosteally. The anterior tibial artery enters the anterior compartment of the leg high in the interval between the tibia and fibula, and must not be injured when the anterior tibial muscle is peeled off from the posterior part of the lateral surface of the tibial condyle. A window cut into the cortex of the medial surface of the tibia will permit access to the interior of the tibia for reduction of the depressed fracture, and the cortical bone can be used as a support beneath the reduced fragments.

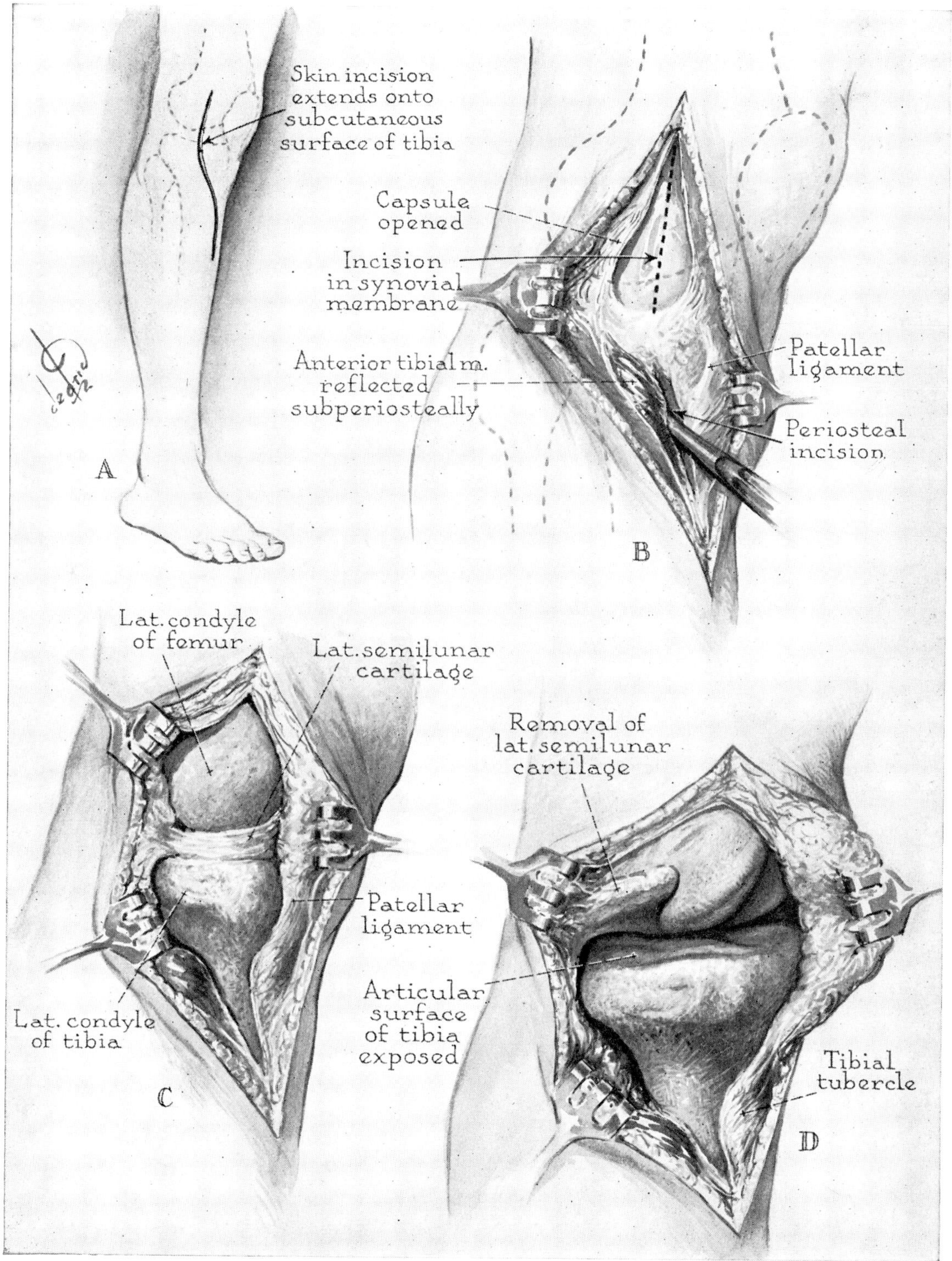

Exposure of the knee joint, the lateral condyle and adjacent portion of the medial surface of the tibia through a lateral knee, anterior tibial incision

EXPOSURE OF THE KNEE JOINT AND THE MEDIAL CONDYLE OF THE TIBIA THROUGH A MEDIAL KNEE AND TIBIAL INCISION

Indication: 1. Open Reduction of Fractures
of the Medial Tibial Condyle

Plate 151: Description of Procedure

A The incision begins at the level of the top of the patella and extends downward over the medial aspect of the knee joint to the tibia, where it gently curves laterally over the condyle and ends on the medial surface of the tibia. The skin margins are developed and retracted.

B The next incision extends through the capsule of the knee joint, across the fascia over the medial condyle of the tibia; it continues distally through the expansions of the tendons of the sartorius, gracilis, semimembranosus and semitendinosus muscles to expose the underlying bursa, and then ending over the adjacent tibia.

C The anterior and medial aspects of the condyle and the adjacent shaft of the tibia are exposed subperiosteally by an incision through the posterior wall of the bursa and the periosteum beneath it.

D The synovial membrane of the knee joint is incised, as illustrated, to expose the interior of the knee joint. The medial semilunar cartilage should not be separated from the capsule unless the cartilage is to be removed. The incision may be extended downward on the tibia, as desired.

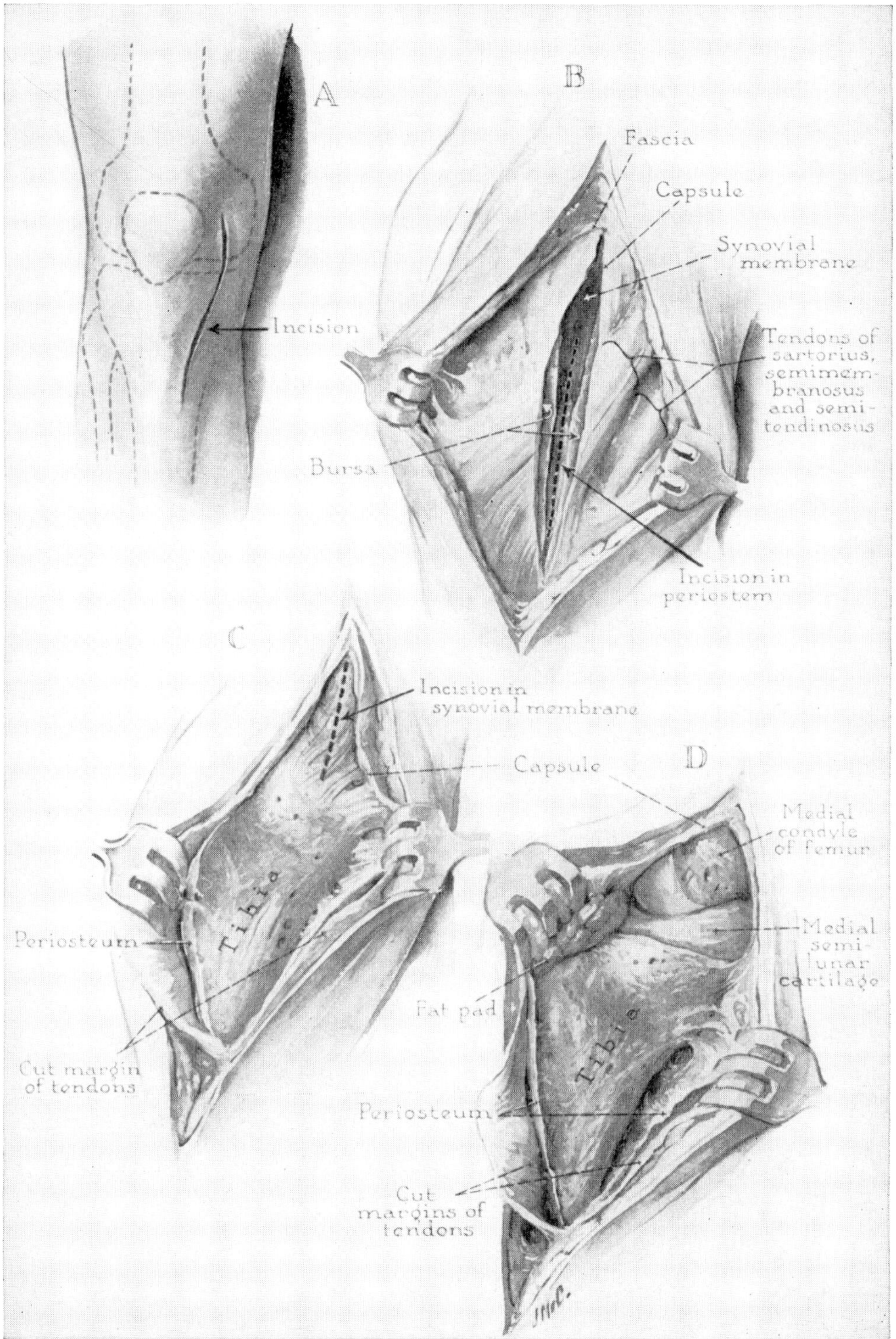

Exposure of the knee joint and the medial condyle of the tibia through a medial knee and tibial incision

EXPOSURE OF THE LATERAL CONDYLE OF THE TIBIA

Indications: 1. Removal of Benign Tumors

2. Partial Ostectomy for Osteomyelitis

Plate 152: Description of Procedure

A A skin incision about 4 inches long begins near the lateral margin of the tibia at the level ot the knee joint and extends in a curved manner distally over the lateral condyle onto the anterior crest of the tibia. The skin margins are mobilized and retracted.

B An incision is made through the periosteum medial to the attachment to the tibia of the deep fascia which covers the anterior tibial muscle. The latter structure is located just lateral to the tibia, from which it in part originates.

C The anterior and lateral surfaces of the condyle and the adjacent portion of the shaft of the tibia are exposed by reflecting the periosteum and the adjacent soft tissues.

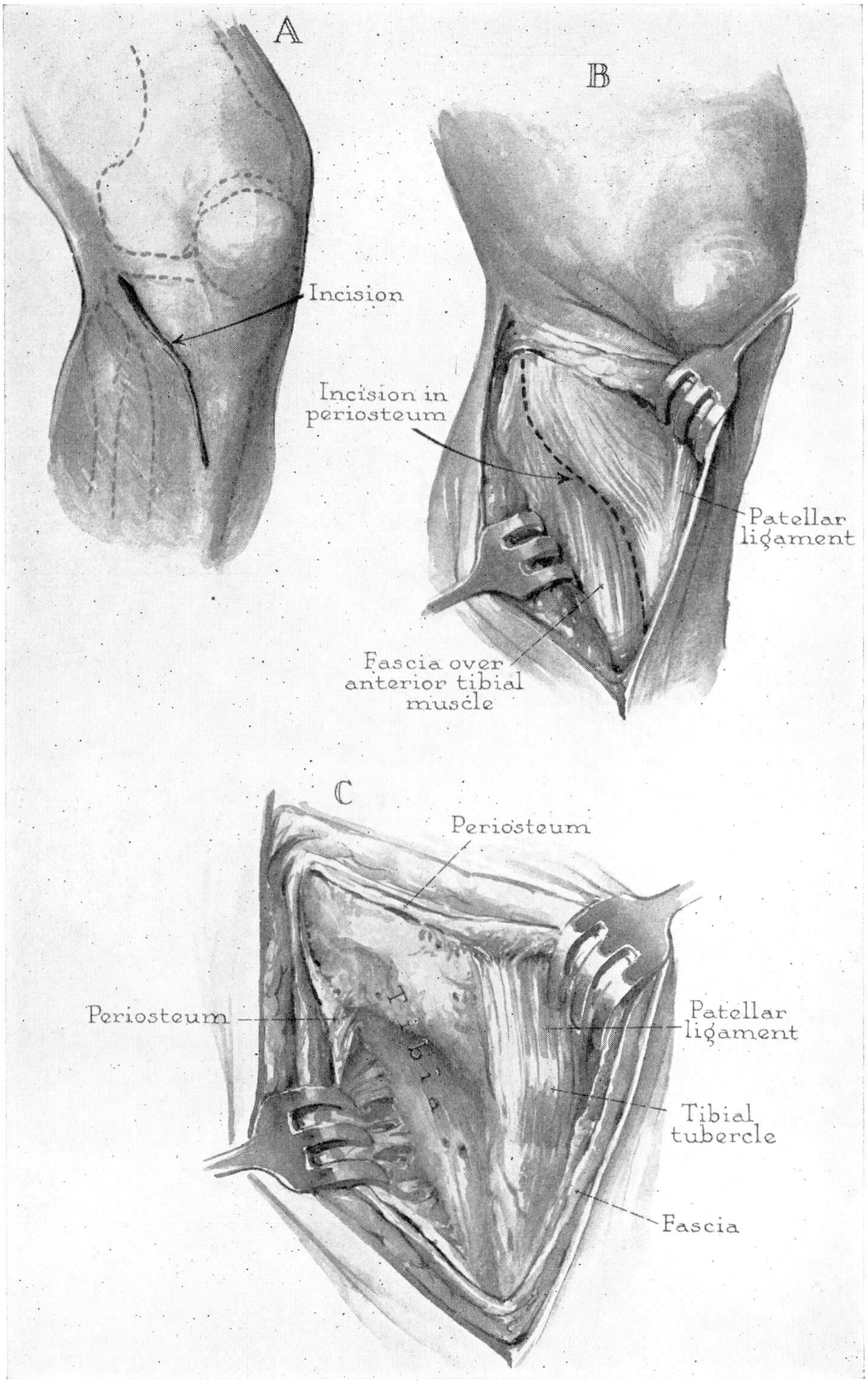

Exposure of the lateral condyle of the tibia

EXPOSURE OF THE MEDIAL (SUBCUTANEOUS) SURFACE OF THE PROXIMAL PORTION OF THE TIBIA THROUGH A CURVED INCISION

Indications: 1. Open Reduction of Recent Fractures of the Tibia

2. Treatment of Un-united Fractures of the Tibia

3. Osteotomy for Mal-united Fractures and Other Deformities

4. Partial Ostectomy for Osteomyelitis

5. Resection of Tumors, Benign and Malignant

6. Removal of Cortical Bone for the Purpose of Transplantation

Plate 153: Description of Procedure

A An arched incision begins at the level of the knee joint, medial to the patellar tendon, and extends downward parallel with the anterior margin of the tibia for the required distance, and then swings inward again across the tibia to end at its medial margin.

B The skin flaps are elevated to give sufficient exposure of the medial surface of the tibia. The veins which cross the field are ligated. The saphenous vein and nerve must be protected from injury.

C The tibia is exposed subperiosteally by an incision along the midline of its medial surface. Proximally, the dissection is carried across the tendons of the sartorius, the gracilis and the semitendinosus muscles as well as the underlying anserinal bursa, to give access to the bone beneath. This subperiosteal exposure of the tibia will be facilitated by elevating the anterior tibial muscle from the lateral surface of the bone.

NOTE: An incision through the skin, fascia and periosteum will give exposure of any desired segment or of the whole medial subcutaneous surface of the tibia.

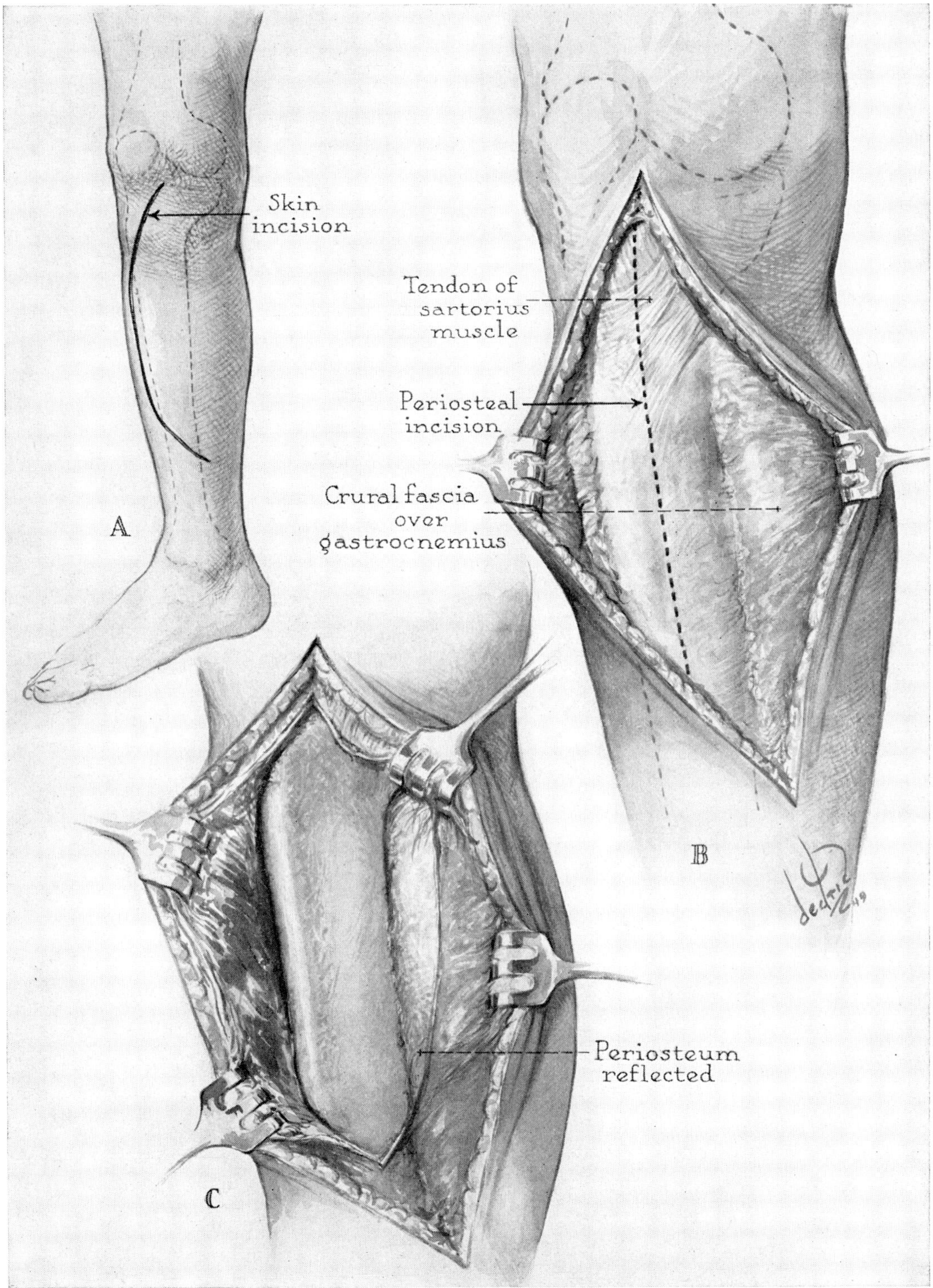

Exposure of the medial (subcutaneous) surface of the proximal portion of the tibia through a curved incision

EXPOSURE OF THE ANTERIOR AND LATERAL SURFACE OF THE DISTAL END OF THE TIBIA THROUGH A LATERAL INCISION

Indications: 1. Removal of Benign Tumors

2. Exposure of the Talofibular Junction

3. Partial Ostectomy for Osteomyelitis

Plate 154: Description of Procedure

A A skin incision, approximately 3 inches long, is made along and parallel with the anterior margin of the distal end of the fibula.

B The deep fascia including the transverse crural ligament is cut the length of the wound. The margin of the peroneus tertius muscle is isolated and retracted medially from the interrosseous membrane.

C The lateral surface of the tibia is now in view. The anterior and lateral surfaces of the bone are exposed subperiosteally by incising the periosteum along the lateral aspect of the tibia. The anterior tibial artery and the deep branch of the peroneal nerve lie directly on the surface of the tibia and must be identified before the periosteal incision is made.

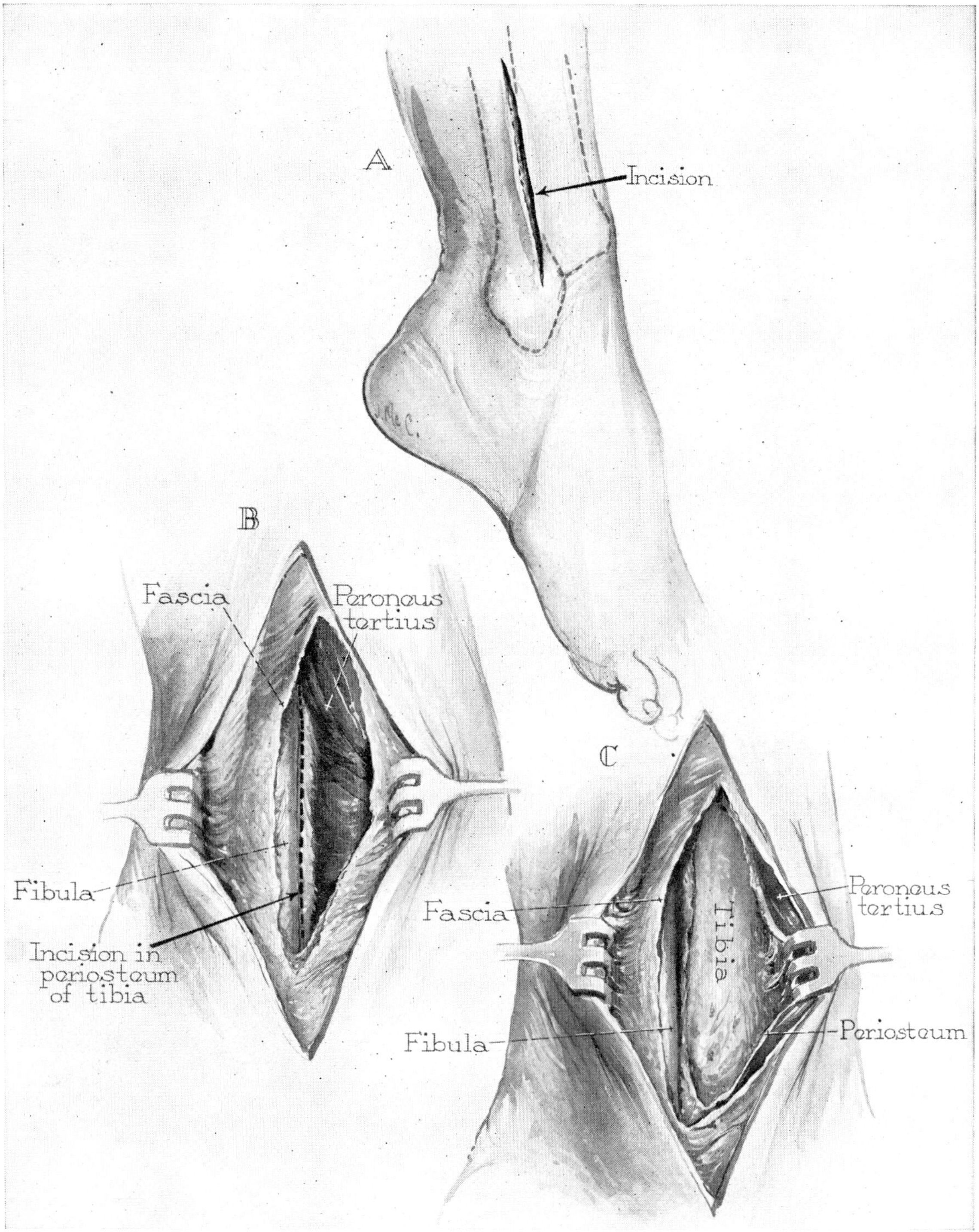

Exposure of the anterior and lateral surface of the distal end of the tibia through a lateral incision

EXPOSURE OF THE PROXIMAL THIRD OF THE FIBULA THROUGH A LINEAR INCISION

Indications: 1. Resection of Benign and Malignant Tumors

2. Partial Resection for Osteomyelitis

Plate 155: Description of Procedure

A An incision, about 4 1/2 inches long, begins 1 inch proximal to the head of the fibula and extends distally over the posterior margin of this bone for the remaining distance. The skin flaps are undermined and retracted.

B The fascia is opened at the distal end of the wound and the incision is extended proximally over a groove director to avoid injury to the peroneal nerve.

C The peroneal nerve, in the proximal end of the wound, is isolated as it emerges from the posterior margin of the biceps muscle approximately 1 inch above the head of the fibula. The nerve is separated from the head and neck of the fibula by being dissected from above downward. Branches of the nerve are given off to the peroneal muscles, as it passes around the head of the fibula. The main portion of the nerve disappears anteriorly into the adjacent muscles.

D With this nerve kept constantly in view, and the peroneus longus and the proximal portion of the peroneus brevis muscle lifted forward, an incision is made through the periosteum to permit subperiosteal exposure of the fibula. Located posteriorly to the attachment of the fascia which overlies the peroneal muscles are the lateral portions of the gastrocnemius and soleus muscles. These muscles are located within a fascial compartment and are not usually seen.

NOTE: It is dangerous to expose the proximal end of the fibula without dissecting out the peroneal nerve and all of its local branches.

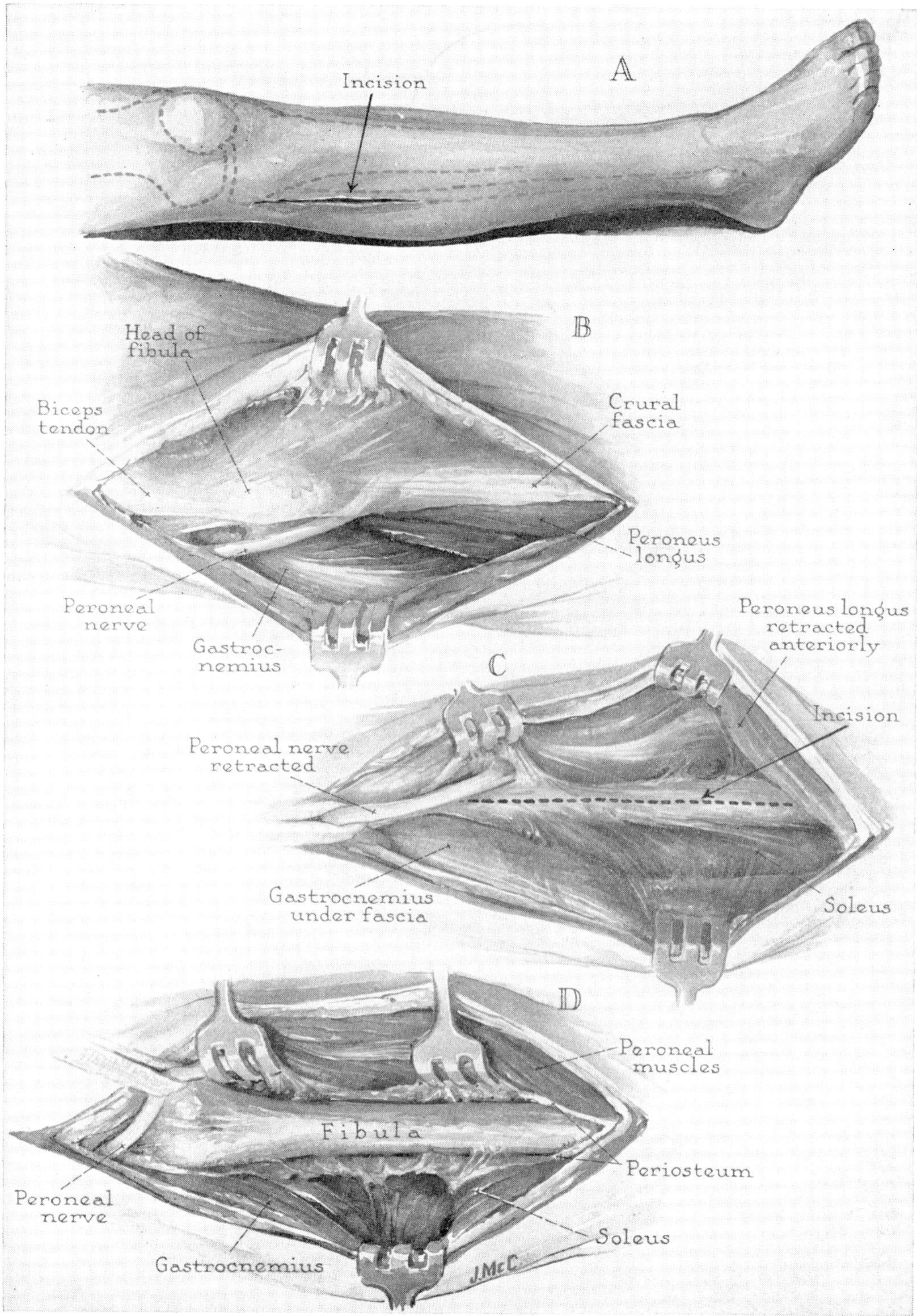

Exposure of the proximal third of the fibula through a linear incision

EXPOSURE OF THE DISTAL THIRD OF THE FIBULA THROUGH A LINEAR INCISION

Indications: 1. Removal of Benign Tumors

2. Partial Ostectomy for Chronic Osteomyelitis

3. Open Reduction of Fractures

Plate 156: Description of Procedure

A The incision begins directly distal to the tip of the lateral malleolus and extends upward in a straight line, centering on the bone for the desired distance. The skin margins are developed and retracted. The deep fascia is incised and retracted with the skin.

B The peroneal tendons and muscles are visible through the deep fascia posteriorly, and are identified. The transverse crural ligament can be recognized anteriorly in the fascia as a thickening. The peroneus tertius muscle is found beneath the fascia in front of the fibula.

C An incision is next made through the periosteum, and the fibula is exposed subperiosteally for the required distance. The anterior lateral malleolar ligament can be seen attached to the anterior margin of the lateral malleolus. The peroneal tendons and the superior peroneal retinaculum must be identified and preserved at the posterior and inferior aspects of the malleolus.

NOTE: No important nerves or vessels are encountered in this incision.

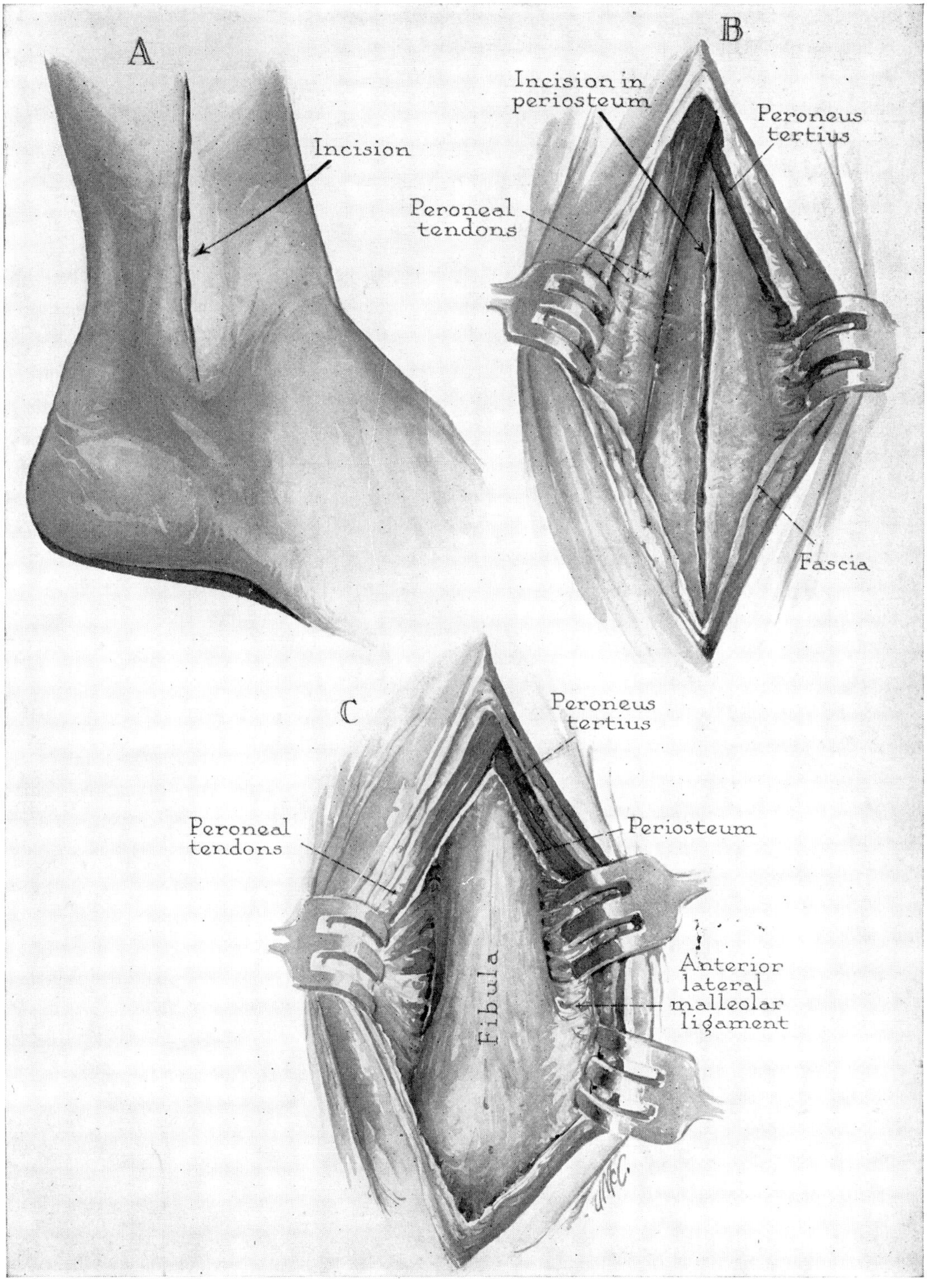

Exposure of the distal third of the fibula through a linear incision

EXPOSURE OF THE PROXIMAL FOURTH OF THE POSTERIOR SURFACE OF THE TIBIA THROUGH A TRANSVERSE POPLITEAL, MEDIAL LEG INCISION

Indications: 1. Excision of Benign Tumors

2. Partial Ostectomy for Osteomyelitis

3. Treatment of Non-union of the Tibia When the Anterior Approach Is Not Possible

Plate 157: Description of Procedure

A The operation is performed in the prone position. The incision runs transversely along the flexion crease of the knee, from the lateral side, and then turns gently downward to continue along the medial side of the calf for 3 1/2 inches or more.

B The distal flap of skin is mobilized and reflected, and the deep fascia is incised and opened along the skin incision. The fascia over the midportion of the popliteal space is thin and must be handled carefully.

C The tendon of the semitendinosus muscle and the medial head of the gastrocnemius are identified by palpation, and the dissection is continued between these two muscles. The semitendinosus then is retracted upward and medially, and the gastrocnemius and soleus (the latter muscle lies beneath the gastrocnemius) are pulled over to the opposite side. The floor of the wound is occupied by the popliteus and flexor digitorum longus muscles.

D The posterior surface of the proximal fourth of the tibia is exposed by elevating the flexor digitorum longus muscle subperiosteally and then reflecting it downward and laterally. The popliteus muscle may be lifted away from the bone and retracted upward in a similar manner.

NOTE: The incision can be enlarged distally along the medial side of the calf by keeping the dissection in the same muscle planes. The posterior tibial nerve and artery are located beneath the soleus and must be a primary concern because of their proximity to the operative field.

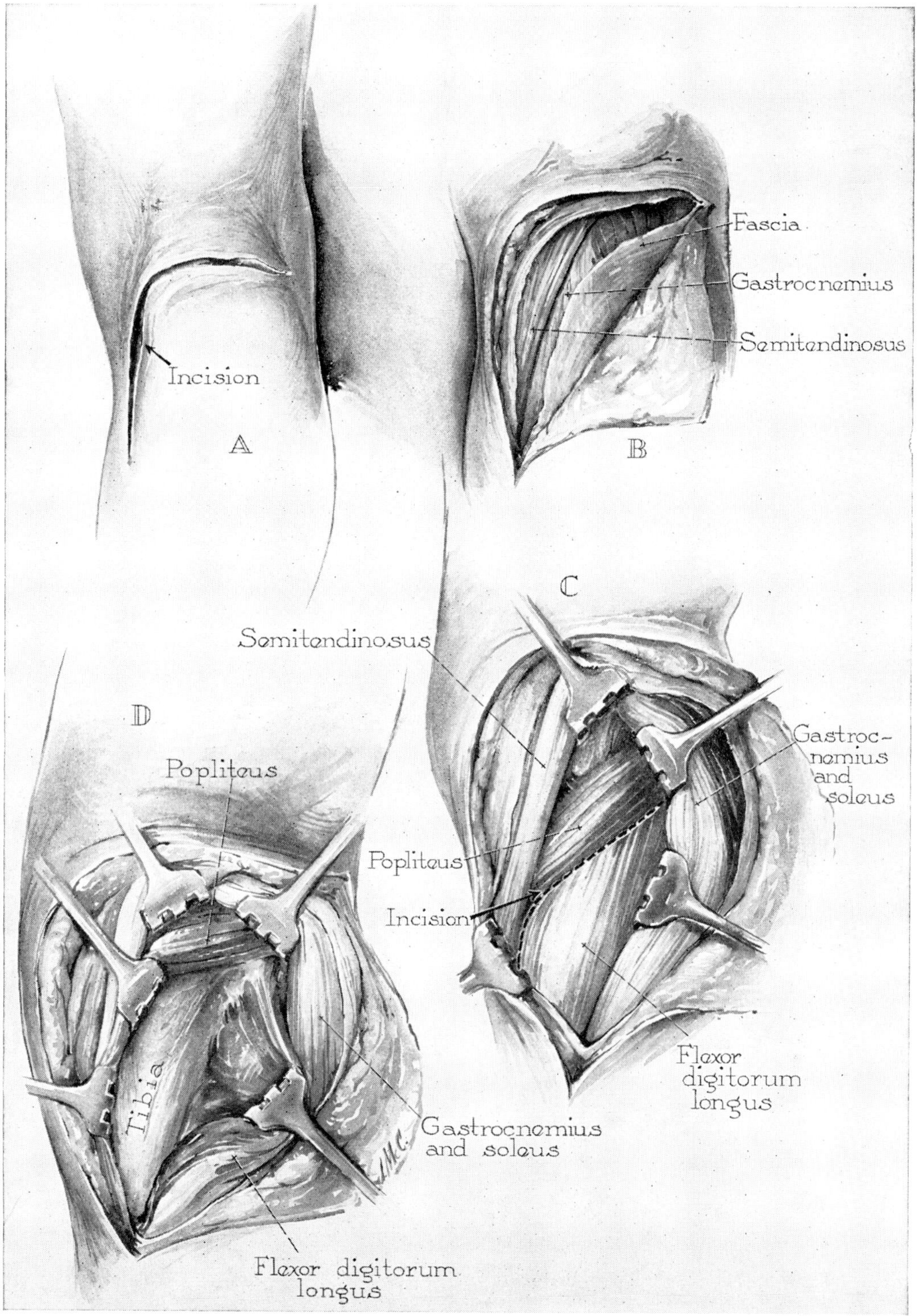

Exposure of the proximal fourth of the posterior surface of the tibia through a transverse popliteal medial leg incision

EXPOSURE OF THE POSTERIOR SURFACE OF THE TIBIA THROUGH A MEDIAL LONGITUDINAL INCISION

Indications: 1. Removal of Benign Tumors

2. Partial Ostectomy for Osteomyelitis

Plate 158: Description of Procedure

A An incision of appropriate length is made over the medial margin of the shaft of the tibia, centering on the lesion.

B The skin flaps are retracted and the fascia is incised the length of the wound.

C The medial margin of the tibia is identified and the periosteum is sectioned directly anterior to it.

D The remainder of the dissection, that is, the exposure of the posterior surface of the tibia, is done subperiosteally. No muscles are exposed in the wound. The gastrocnemius and soleus are situated beneath the fascia in the medial portion of the wound, while the flexor digitorum longus is separated subperiosteally from the posterior surface of the tibia, together with the periosteum.

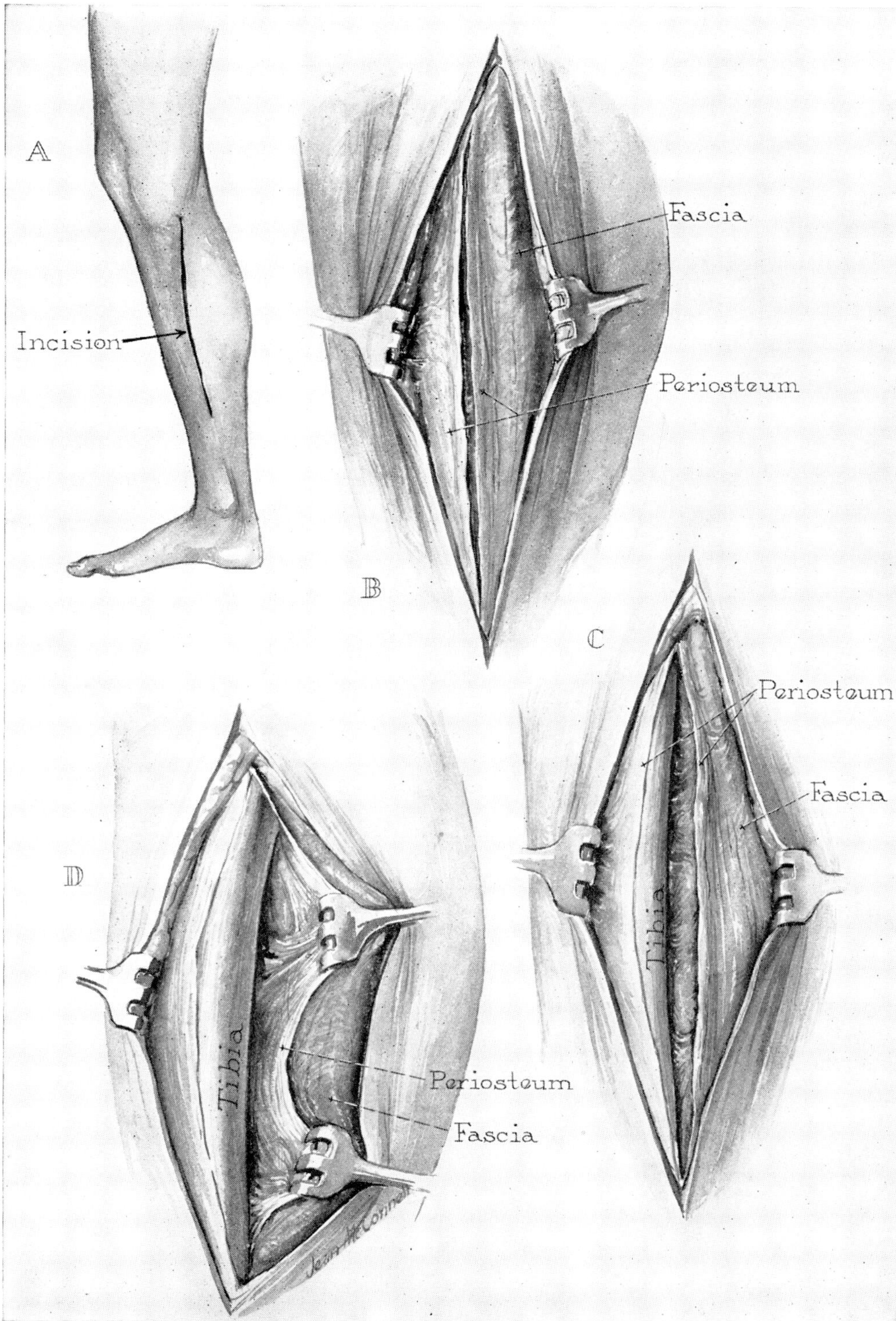

Exposure of the posterior surface of the tibia through a medial longitudinal incision

EXPOSURE OF THE POSTERIOR SURFACE OF THE DISTAL END OF THE TIBIA THROUGH A LINEAR INCISION LATERAL TO THE ACHILLES TENDON

Indications: 1. Open Reduction of Fractures of the Posterior Aspect of the Distal End of the Tibia (Posterior Malleolus)

2. Resection of Benign Tumors

3. Partial Ostectomy for Osteomyelitis Which Cannot Be Treated Through an Anterior incision

Plate 159: Description of Procedure

A The patient is placed on the operating table in the prone position, with a sandbag beneath the ankle so that the foot can be extended. The skin incision begins at the level of the lateral malleolus and extends upward for approximately 3 1/2 inches, midway between the Achilles tendon and the fibula.

B The fascia is incised longitudinally and retracted adequately together with the skin. Next, a longitudinal incision is made directly behind the peroneal tendons through the fascia which covers the flexor hallucis longus muscle.

C The distal portion of this muscle is then brought into view by reflecting the fascia toward the Achilles tendon.

D An incision is made through the lateral fibers of the flexor hallucis longus and the periosteum of the tibia. The bone is exposed subperiosteally, as the flexor hallucis longus, the soleus muscle and the Achilles tendon are retracted medially. The posterior capsule of the ankle joint may be opened, if necessary, but the posterior tibiofibular ligament must not be cut.

NOTE: No motor nerves are encountered in this incision. Care must be exercised, however, while dissecting the subcutaneous tissues, to protect branches of the sural nerve from injury.

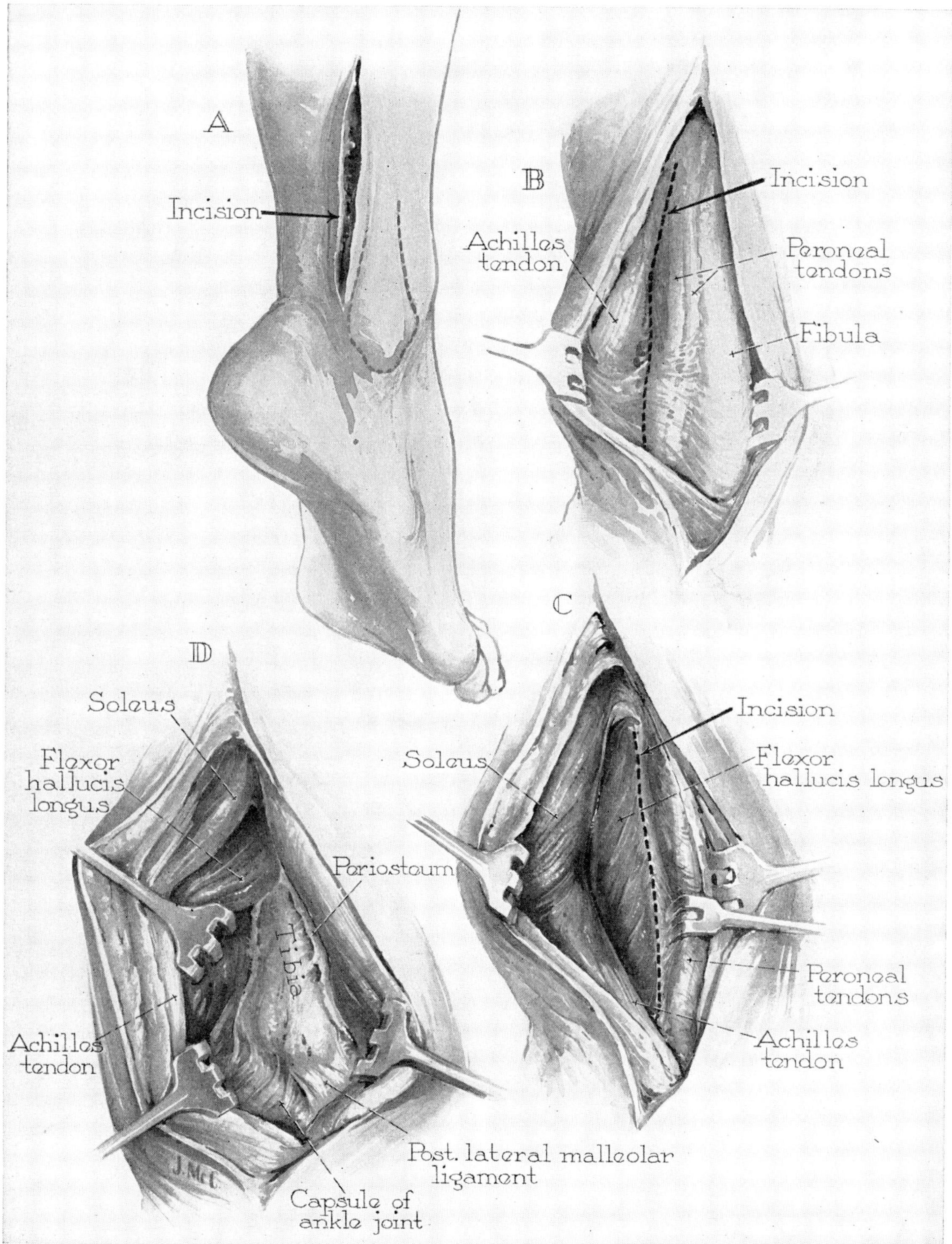

Exposure of the posterior surface of the distal end of the tibia through a linear incision lateral to the Achilles tendon

EXPOSURE OF THE POSTERIOR TIBIAL NERVE THROUGH A TRANSVERSE POPLITEAL, MEDIAL LEG INCISION

Indications: 1. Neurolysis of the Posterior Tibial Nerve

2. Suture of Lacerations of the Posterior Tibial Nerve

Plate 160: Description of Procedure

A The patient is placed upon the operating table in the prone position. An inverted L incision is made along the flexion crease of the knee and then downward along the medial side of the calf, for the desired distance. The incision can be extended upward along the outer aspect of the thigh, for exploration of the nerve at a higher level.

B The fascia is incised and the interval between the semitendinosus tendon and the gastrocnemius muscle is opened to expose the popliteus and soleus muscles.

C The soleus is mobilized from the popliteus above, and from the flexor digitorum longus lying deep below.

D Both the soleus and the gastrocnemius muscles are then firmly retracted laterally to expose the posterior tibial nerve. The posterior tibial artery is situated medially to the nerve and must not be injured.

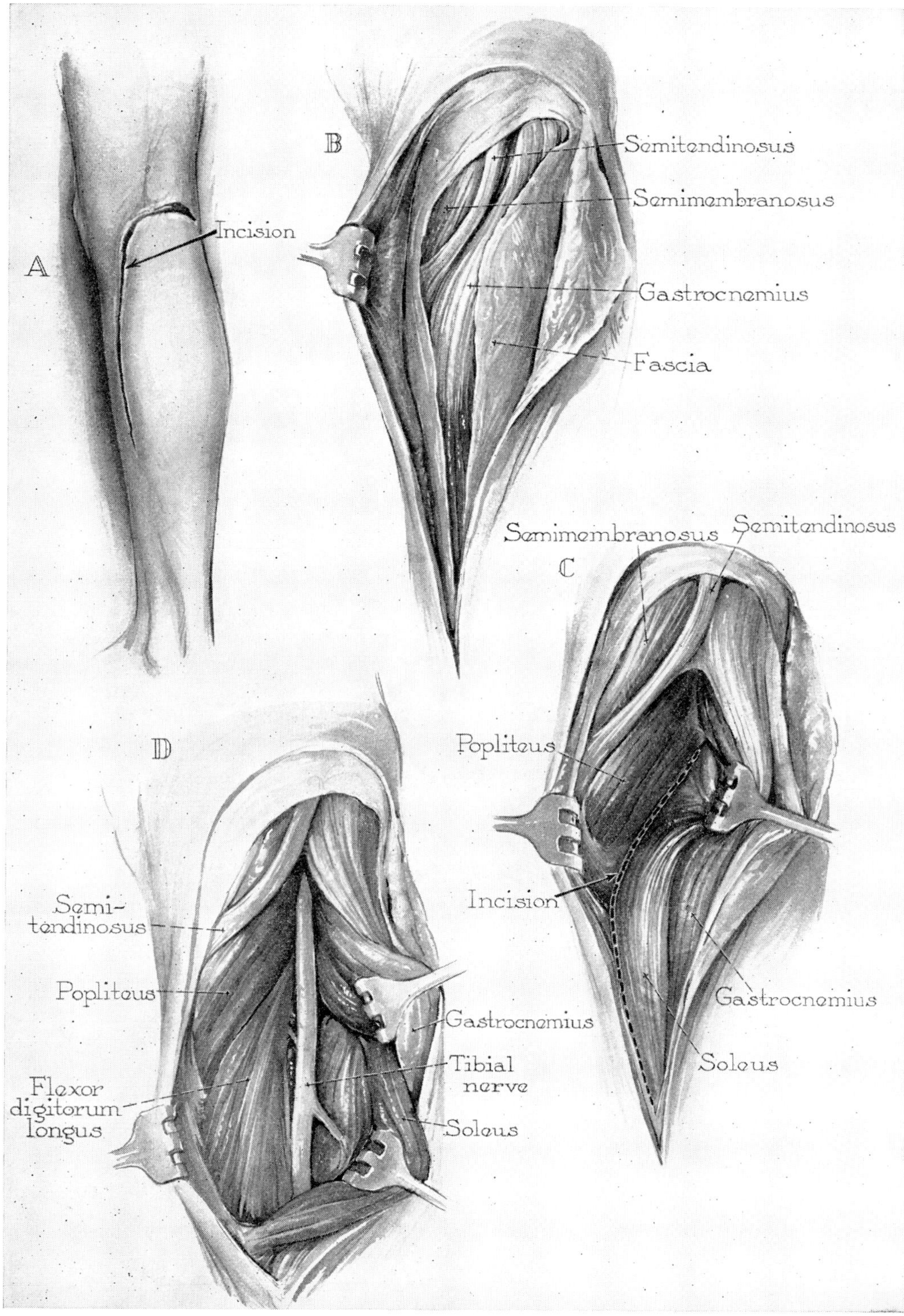

Exposure of the posterior tibial nerve through a transverse popliteal, medial leg incision

EXPOSURE OF THE ANTERIOR TIBIAL ARTERY

Indication: 1. Ligation of the Anterior Tibial Artery

Plate 161: Description of Procedure

A A vertical incision, some 3 or 4 inches in length, as illustrated, is made along the junction between the anterior tibial muscle and the extensor digitorum longus muscle. This space can be palpated before the incision is made.

B The incision is carried through the crural fascia in line with the skin wound.

C The anterior tibial muscle is then separated from the extensor hallucis longus to expose the anterior tibial artery and the veins alongside it. The deep peroneal nerve lies lateral to the artery. The veins may be small and densely adherent to the artery, and can be ligated together with it.

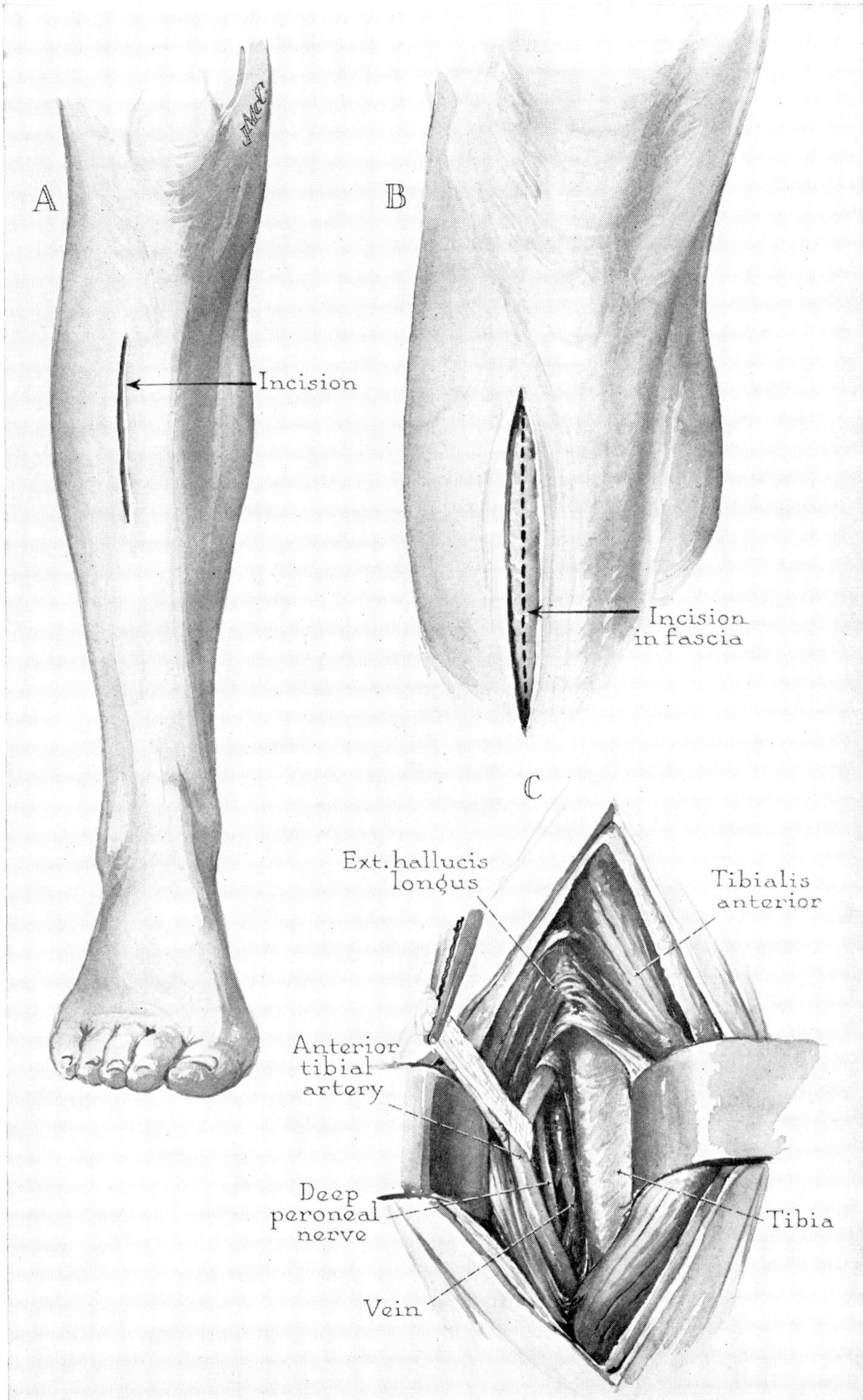

Exposure of the anterior tibial artery

EXPOSURE OF THE POSTERIOR TIBIAL ARTERY

Indications: 1. Ligation of the Posterior Tibial Artery

Plate 162: Description of Procedure

A A longitudinal incision is made in the midportion of the leg along the medial border of the gastrocnemius muscle, as illustrated.

B The long saphenous vein usually is situated immediately beneath and anterior to the locale of this skin incision. The dense fascia overlying the gastrocnemius muscle is then incised in line with the wound and the wound and this muscle are retracted.

C The fibers of the soleus muscle are similarly cut and retracted.

D Both the soleus and gastrocnemius muscles are drawn away from the bone to expose the posterior tibial artery. The posterior tibial vein lies immediately beneath the artery and is in close approximation to it. The tibial nerve is on the lateral side of the artery.

E In incising the thick fibrous sheath overlying the artery, care must be taken not to injure this vessel. A sling is placed about the artery to facilitate its handling.

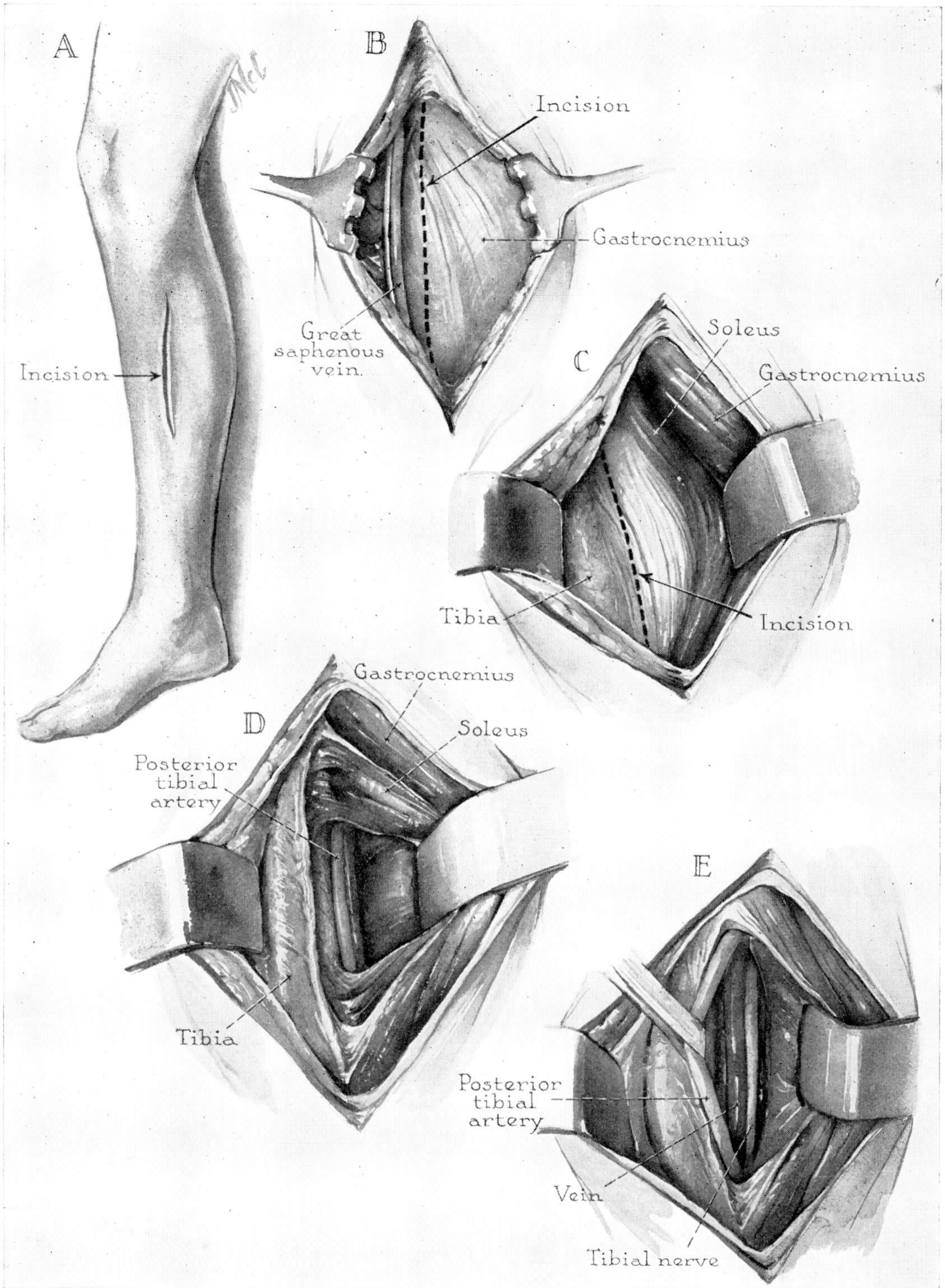

Exposure of the posterior tibial artery

Section XI

Region of the Ankle Joint and Foot

EXPOSURE OF THE ANKLE JOINT THROUGH AN ANTERIOR LATERAL INCISION

Indications: 1. Arthrodesis of the Ankle Joint

2. Removal of Loose Bodies

3. Open Reduction of Fractures of the Distal Anterior Articular Portion of the Tibia

Plate 163: Description of Procedure

A The skin incision, some 4 1/2 inches long, extends along the lateral margin of the peroneus tertius muscle and tendon and ends 1 1/2 inches distal to the ankle joint.

B The skin flaps are elevated, and the veins crossing the field are ligated. The sensory nerves which are encountered must be protected by retraction to one side of the wound. The deep fascia is opened, and so are the transverse crural ligament in the proximal portion and the cruciate crural ligament in the distal extremity of the wound. These ligaments must be resutured accurately when closing the wound to prevent spanning of the extensor tendons during dorsiflexion motion of the foot. The peroneus tertius muscle is identified and its lateral margin is raised by use of a rake retractor and blunt dissection, to give access to the tibia beneath it. More distally, the tendon of the peroneus muscle is pulled medially to make the anterior surface of the ankle joint accessible.

C A vertical incision, the length of the wound, is made through the periosteum and the anterior capsule of the ankle. The fleshy tissues and the tendons of the peroneus tertius, the extensor digitorum longus, the extensor hallucis longus and the anterior tibial muscles, respectively, are firmly retracted to the medial side to facilitate the subperiosteal exposure of the anterior surface of the tibia. The capsule is detached from the adjacent tibia and talus, to permit access to the ankle joint. The lateral flap is developed to expose the distal anterior tibiofibular ligament and the lateral malleolus.

NOTE: The anterior tibial artery and the deep branch of the peroneal nerve are located between the anterior tibial and extensor hallucis longus muscles and tendons. The artery and nerve pass directly in front of the supra-articular end of the tibia and must be identified before the periosteum is incised, to avoid their being injured. This incision gives complete access to the frontal portion of the ankle joint. Adequate space for the unhampered removal of the articular cartilage of the medial malleolus is rather difficult to obtain in this incision. However, the same difficulty is encountered laterally when the surgical approach is made from a site near the anterior tibial tendon.

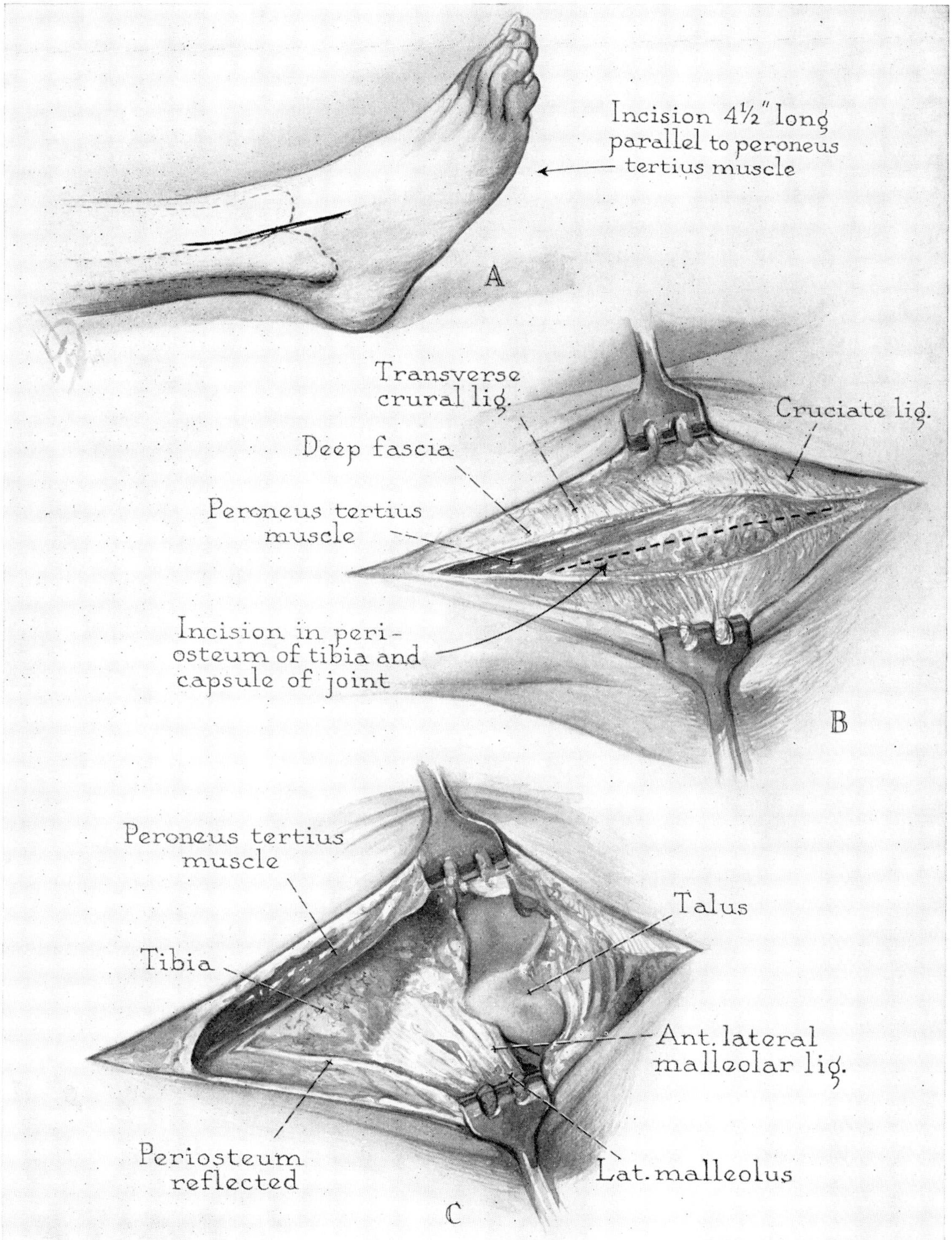

Exposure of the ankle joint through an anterior lateral incision

EXPOSURE OF THE TALOTIBIAL, TALONAVICULAR, TALOCALCANEAL AND CALCANEOCUBOID JOINTS THROUGH AN ANTEROLATERAL LEG AND FOOT INCISION

Indication: 1. Panastragalar Arthrodesis for Instability Due to Muscle Paralysis, or for Pain Following Injury

Plate 164: Description of Procedure

A The proximal portion of the incision is identical with the one previously described for the exposure of the ankle joint through an anterolateral approach. The incision is extended distally onto the foot by approximately 1 1/2 inches. It is recalled that the deep fascia and the transverse crural ligament were cut proximally to expose the peroneus tertius muscle. The incision now is continued distally by cutting the deep fascia and the cruciate ligament of the foot, to uncover the fat in the sinus tarsi and expose the extensor digitorum brevis muscle.

B Likewise, the peroneus tertius muscle and its tendon are retracted medially and an incision is made through the periosteum of the tibia and the capsule of the ankle joint. The periosteum and capsule are reflected to both sides of the wound to expose the anterior surface of the tibia and the interior of the ankle joint.

C The fat is removed from the sinus tarsi to permit exposure of the talocalcaneal joint. The extensor digitorum brevis is separated from the calcaneus and the capsule of the calcaneocuboid joint, and is retracted downward.

D A linear incision now is made along the inferior lateral surface of the neck and head of the talus. The underlying bone is exposed subperiosteally. The capsule of the talonavicular joint is stripped from the adjacent portion of the talus and navicular bones to expose their articular surtaces. The calcaneocuboid joint is opened in a similar manner. The peroneal tendons are retracted downward (not shown in the illustration).

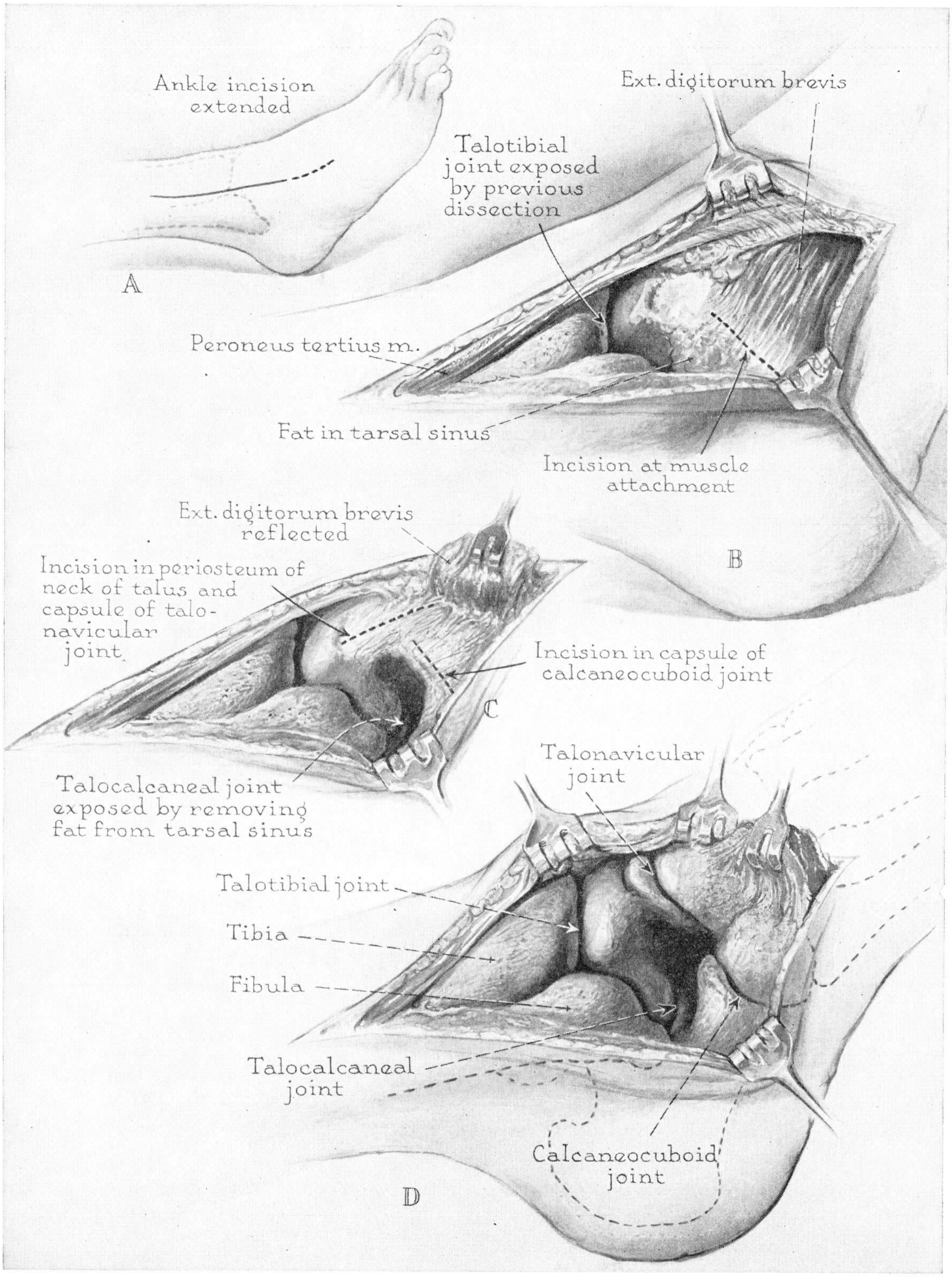

Exposure of the talotibial, talonavicular, talocalcaneal and calcaneocuboid joints through an anterior lateral leg and foot incision

EXPOSURE OF THE ANKLE JOINT THROUGH A LATERAL TRANS-FIBULAR INCISION

Indication: 1. Arthrodesis of the Ankle Joint

Plate 165: Description of Procedure

A The incision begins 1 inch distal to the tip of the lateral malleolus and extends upward for 5 inches, centering on the fibula. The skin margins are mobilized and retracted to their respective sides. The deep fascia is incised in line with the skin incision and retracted.

B The distal third of the fibula is now exposed subperiosteally after a linear incision has been made through it.

C An osteotomy is performed at the distal fourth of the fibula in an obliquely medial and downward direction, leaving a bevelled surface on the proximal fragment of the fibula. The fibular fragment is then rotated outward as the distal anterior lateral malleolar and anterior talofibular ligaments are being severed. The fragment is still further rotated externally to permit exposure and transection of the posterior lateral malleolar and posterior talofibular ligaments. Complete removal of the fibular fragment can be effected by cutting the remaining soft tissues, including the calcaneofibular ligament at the distal end; or else the fibula may be rotated downward and permitted to protrude from the wound until it is finally replaced as a bone graft to bridge the ankle joint.

D An incision is made in the periosteum over the lateral aspect of the tibia, just posterior to the attachment of the interosseous membrane. The distal portion of the tibia is exposed subperiosteally. At the same time, the proximal attachment of the ankle joint capsule is separated from the tibia and reflected with the mesial flap of soft tissues.

Next, the attachment of the capsule to the talus is severed and the adjacent portion of the body and neck is exposed subperiosteally. The entire anterior surface of the tibia and ankle joint and of the anterior aspect of the body and neck of the talus is now exposed. The posterior aspect of the tibia and talus may similarly be exposed by raising a periosteal and capsular flap.

NOTE: This incision provides an excellent exposure of the ankle joint. The anterior tibial artery and the deep branch of the peroneal nerve are not endangered as long as the anterior dissection is kept subperiosteal and inside the capsule of the ankle joint. The peroneal tendons are retracted posteriorly out of the way.

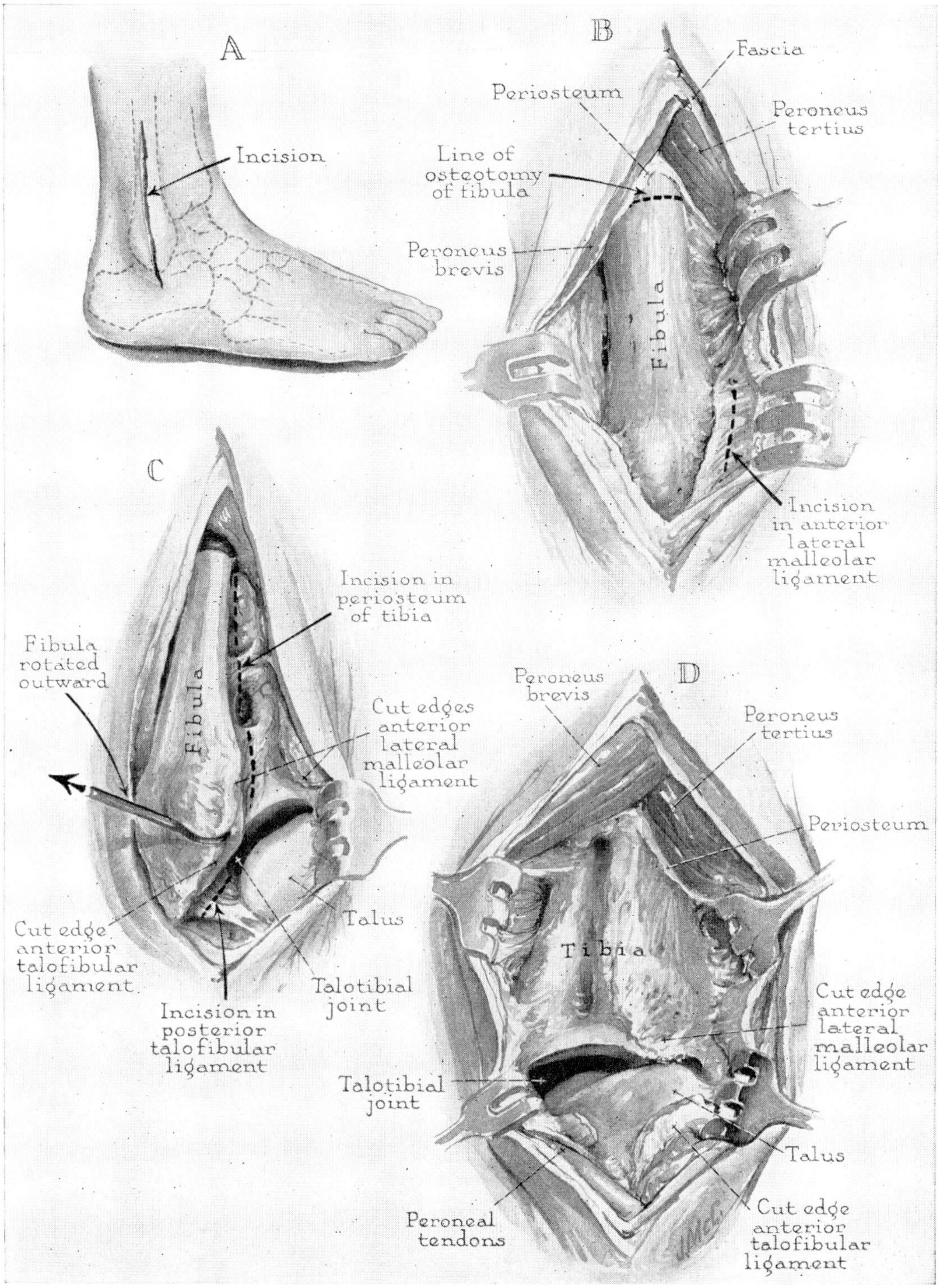

Exposure of the ankle joint through a lateral transfibular incision

EXPOSURE OF THE TALOTIBIAL, TALONAVICULAR, CALCANEO-CUBOID AND TALOCALCANEAL JOINTS THROUGH A LATERAL LEG AND FOOT INCISION, WITH OSTEOTOMY OF THE FIBULA

Indication: 1. Panastragalar Arthrodesis

Plate 166: Description of Procedure

A The incision is made over the distal third of the fibula and, at the lateral malleolus, it curves obliquely onto the dorsum of the foot, to terminate near the second cuneiform bone. The skin margins are widely undercut and retracted.

B The next incision opens the deep fascia in line with the fibula and the fascial flaps are developed and retracted. The lateral end of the transverse crural ligament is also severed. The peroneal tendons are identified posteriorly to the fibula.

C The peroneus tertius muscle, which is located just anterior to the distal end of the fibula, is mobilized and retracted medially. The distal fourth of the bone is exposed subperiosteally. The next incision is made through the cruciate ligament and the fascia over the sinus tarsi and adjacent extensor tendons, as illustrated. (Procedure continued on Plate 167.)

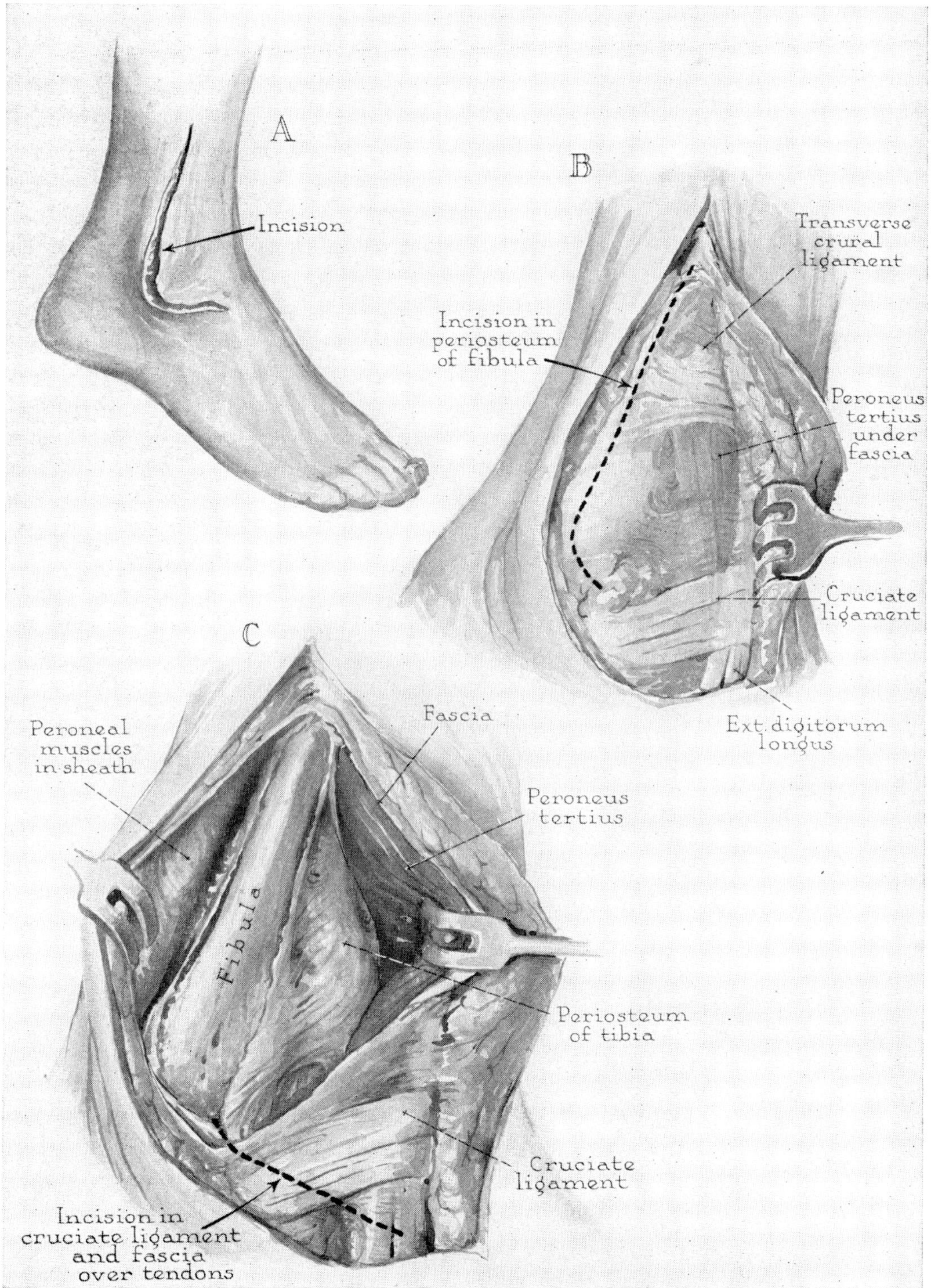

Exposure of the talotibial, talonavicular, calcaneocuboid and talocalcaneal joints through a lateral leg and foot incision with osteotomy of the fibula

EXPOSURE OF THE TALOTIBIAL, TALONAVICULAR, CALCANEO-CUBOID AND TALOCALCANEAL JOINTS THROUGH A LATERAL LEG AND FOOT INCISION, WITH OSTEOTOMY OF THE FIBULA *(Continued)*

Plate 167: Description of Procedure

D An oblique osteotomy of the fibula is made for the purpose of separating the distal fourth of the bone from the proximal three-fourths. The lower fourth is rotated externally out of the wound and removed after being separated from the soft tissues and ligaments.

E The sinus tarsi is now identified and its fatty tissue is removed. An incision is made along the lateral surface of the tibia, just posterior to the attachment of the interosseous membrane. The anterior and lateral surfaces, together with the supra-articular region, of the tibia are next exposed subperiosteally. The proximal attachment of the ankle joint capsule is then separated from the tibia and from its distal attachment to the body of the talus, and the soft tissues are retracted medially to obtain maximum exposure.

F An incision is now made transversely across the calcaneus, just proximal to the calcaneocuboid joint, in order to separate the origin of the extensor digitorum brevis muscle and the capsule of the calcaneocuboid joint. They are next reflected downward to obtain adequate exposure of the joint.

The talonavicular joint is exposed by a lateral incision which traverses the periosteum over the lateral aspect of the neck of the talus, and extends through the capsule of the talonavicular joint to end at about the midportion of the navicular bone. This flap is then raised to expose the talonavicular joint. The talocalcaneal joint has been exposed in the floor of the sinus tarsi.

NOTE: This incision offers a wide exposure of all the joints which border on the talus. Important arteries and nerves are avoided if the dissection is kept subperiosteal. The distal fourth of the fibula is replaced during the closure of the wound as a lateral bone graft to bridge the ankle joint.

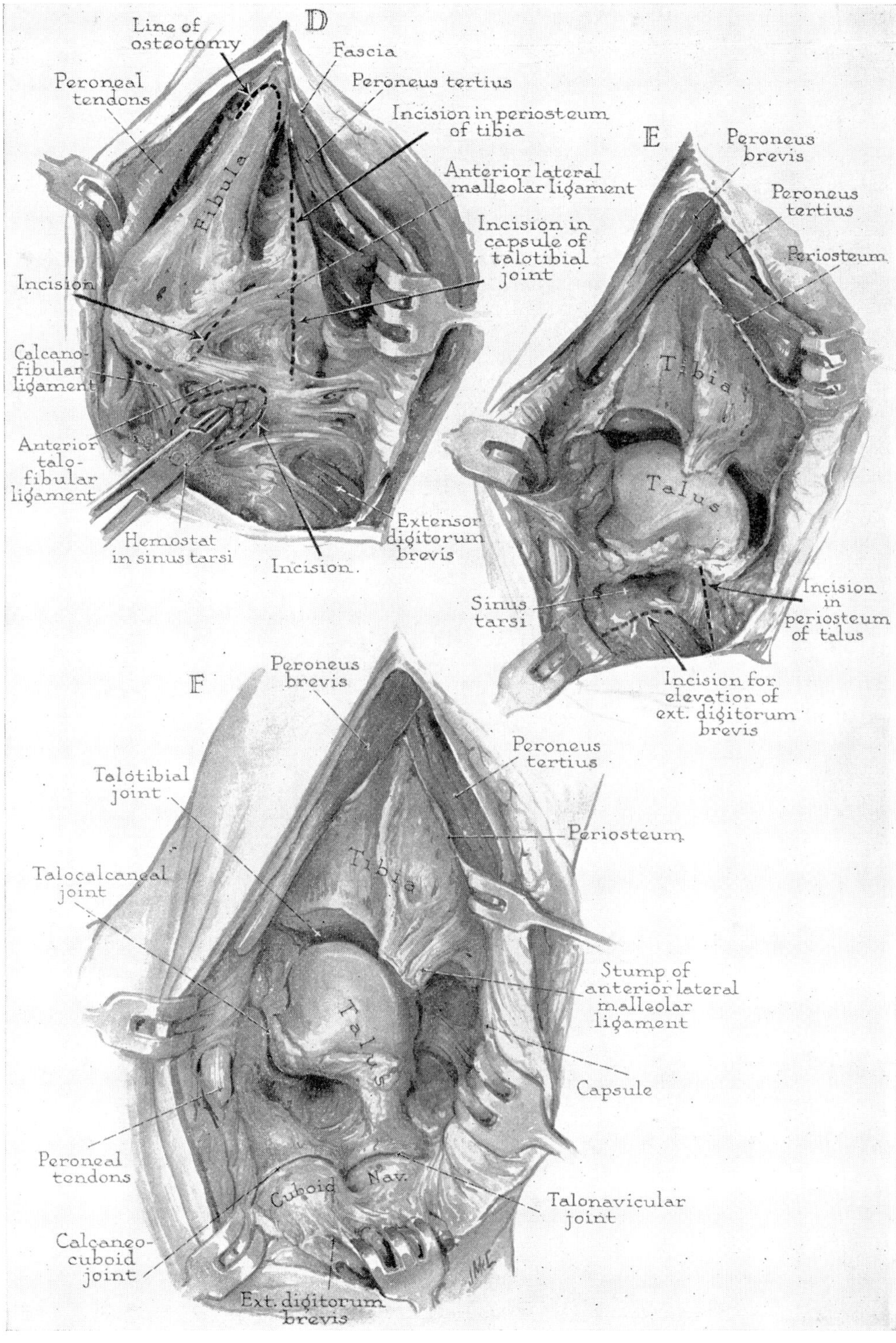

Exposure of the talotibial, talonavicular, calcaneocuboid and talocalcaneal joints through a **lateral** leg and foot incision, with osteotomy of the fibula

EXPOSURE OF THE MEDIAL ASPECT OF THE ANKLE JOINT AND THE ADJACENT PORTION OF THE BODY OF THE TALUS THROUGH A MEDIAL INCISION, WITH OSTEOTOMY OF THE MEDIAL MALLEOLUS

Indication: 1. Treatment of Osteochondritis Dissecans and Other Benign Lesions of the Medial Aspect of the Talus Which Cannot Be Approached through an Anterior Incision

Plate 168: Description of Procedure

A A skin incision, approximately 4 inches long, is made over the medial aspect of the ankle, the midpoint of the incision being centered over the malleolus.

B The deep fascia is opened, the wound margins are retracted to either side, and the malleolus is exposed subperiosteally.

C The capsule of the ankle joint is detached from the anterior margin of the malleolus to give access to the interior of the joint. The medial collateral ligament of the ankle is identified in the lower portion of the incision. The posterior tibial tendon is located posteriorly to the medial malleolus and ligament; it must be protected from injury.

D The medial malleolus is osteotomized at the level of its junction with the shaft of the tibia and rotated downward through 90 degrees to bring into view the ankle joint and the adjacent portion of the talus. By forcibly abducting the foot, the entire superior surface of the talus and of the articular surface of the tibia can be exposed.

NOTE: In closure of the wound, the medial malleolus is accurately reduced and maintained in its normal relationship to the shaft of the tibia by means of a single metal screw. No important arteries or nerves are encountered in this exposure.

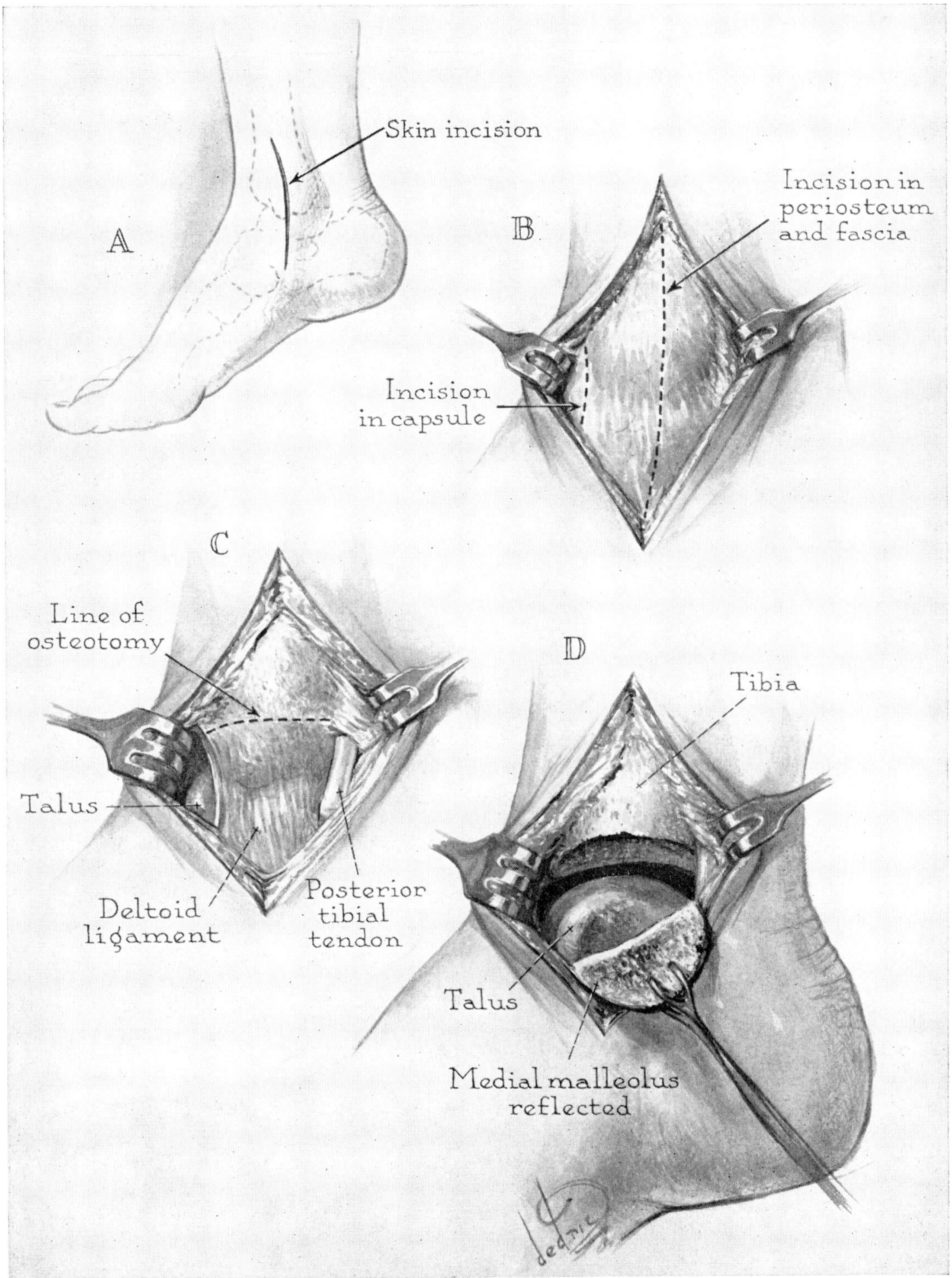

Exposure of the medial aspect of the ankle joint and the adjacent portion of the body of the talus through a medial incision, with osteotomy of the medial malleolus

EXPOSURE OF THE DISTAL PORTION OF THE ANTERIOR SURFACE OF THE TIBIA, THE ANKLE JOINT AND THE MEDIAL MALLEOLUS, THROUGH AN ANTERIOR TIBIAL, MEDIAL MALLEOLUS INCISION

Indications: 1. Open Reduction of Comminuted Fractures, Involving the Distal Shaft, the Articular Surface and the Medial Malleolus of the Tibia

2. The Incision Can Be Used in Whole or in Part for the Surgical Management of Other Lesions Occurring in This Region of the Tibia

Plate 169: Description of Procedure

A The skin incision, approximately 4 1/2 inches long, begins 1 inch distal to the medial malleolus; it first is directed upward and across the center of this bone and then curves onto the medial surface of the tibia to end at the desired distance proximal to the ankle joint.

B The major saphenous vein, which crosses the midportion of the field in an oblique, medial and upward direction, may be sacrificed if necessary, or mobilized and retracted to one or the other side of the wound.

C The periosteum is incised in line with the skin incision, and carefully raised medially and laterally to obtain adequate exposure of the tibia.

D The ankle joint is opened by cutting the proximal attachment of the capsule from the distal anterior margin of the tibia and malleolus. The tip of the medial malleolus can be exposed by separating the overlying deltoid ligament in line with its fibers, so that a metal screw can be introduced through the malleolus and into the adjacent tibia.

NOTE: In reflecting the skin flap laterally in the upper portion of the wound, it is necessary to look for and protect the superficial (sensory) branches of the peroneal nerve. The anterior tibial artery and the deep branch of the peroneal nerve are located superficially to the periosteum between the tendons of the anterior tibial and extensor hallucis longus muscles. The entire anterior surface of the supra-articular portion of the tibia, including the medial malleolus and the ankle joint, can be exposed by this incision.

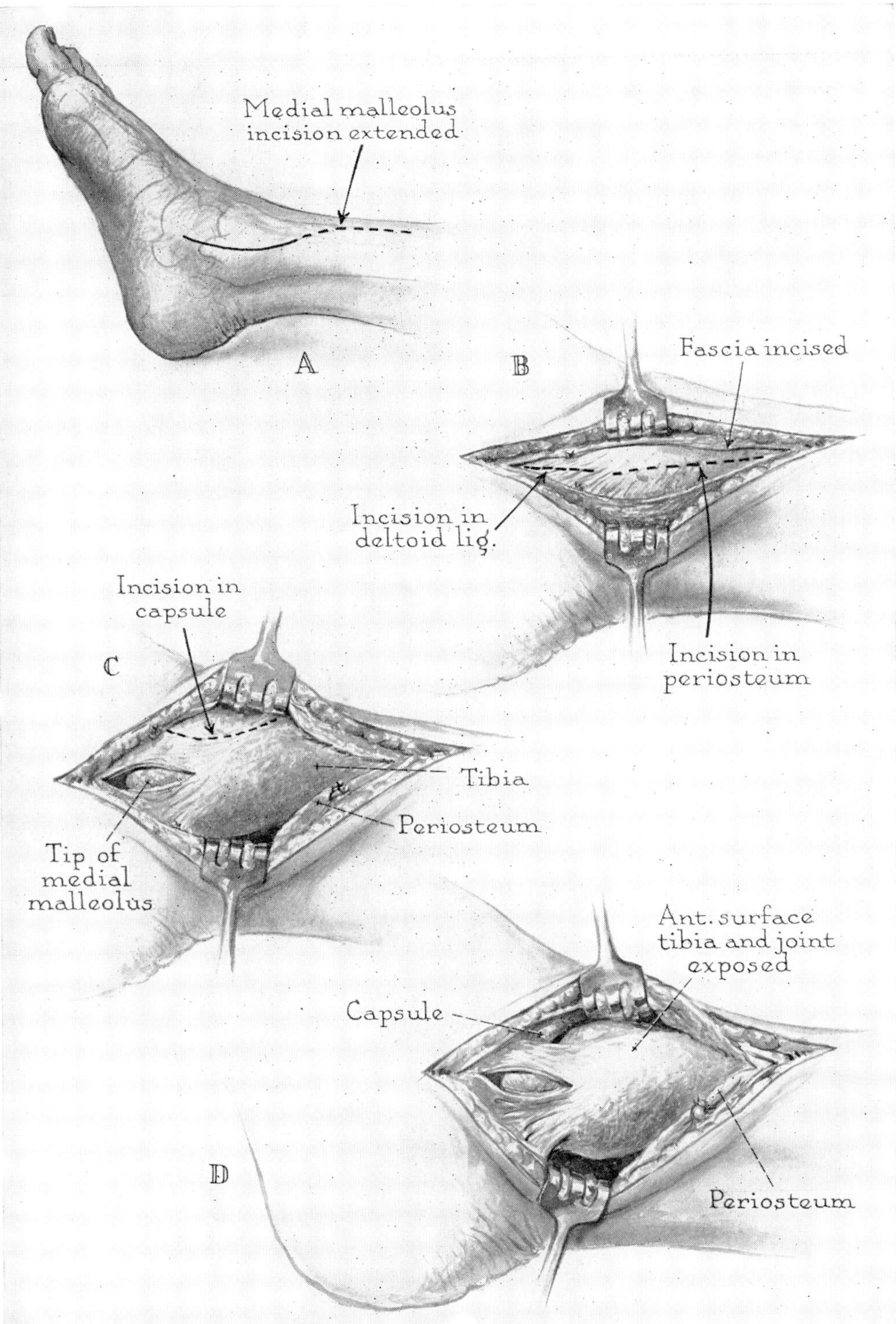

Exposure of the distal portion of the anterior surface of the tibia, the ankle joint and the medial malleolus through an anterior tibial, medial malleolus incision

EXPOSURE OF THE MEDIAL MALLEOLUS OF THE TIBIA AND THE ANKLE JOINT THROUGH A MEDIAL INCISION

Indications: 1. Open Reduction of Recent Fractures of the Medial Malleolus

2. Treatment of Un-united Fractures of the Medial Malleolus

Plate 170: Description of Procedure

A The skin incision, about 3 inches long, begins 1 inch distal to the medial malleolus and extends upward centrally over this bone for the required distance.

B The skin margins are undermined and retracted. The periosteum is incised and elevated to expose the medial malleolus and the adjacent portion of the tibia.

C The deep fascia is opened in the distal fourth of the wound to expose the deltoid ligament of the ankle joint. The small artery which crosses the field must be ligated.

D The lower portion of the malleolus is hidden beneath the deltoid ligament. By incising this ligament centrally in line with its fibers and then separating the margins, adequate exposure can be obtained for the introduction of a screw into the tip of the medial malleolus. The medial aspect of the ankle joint can be explored and the articular surface of the malleolus can be made visible by opening the capsule directly anterior to the deltoid ligament and the medial malleolus.

NOTE: The posterior tibial tendon passes along the posterior and inferior aspects of the medial malleolus, and both it and its tendon sheath must be protected from injury.

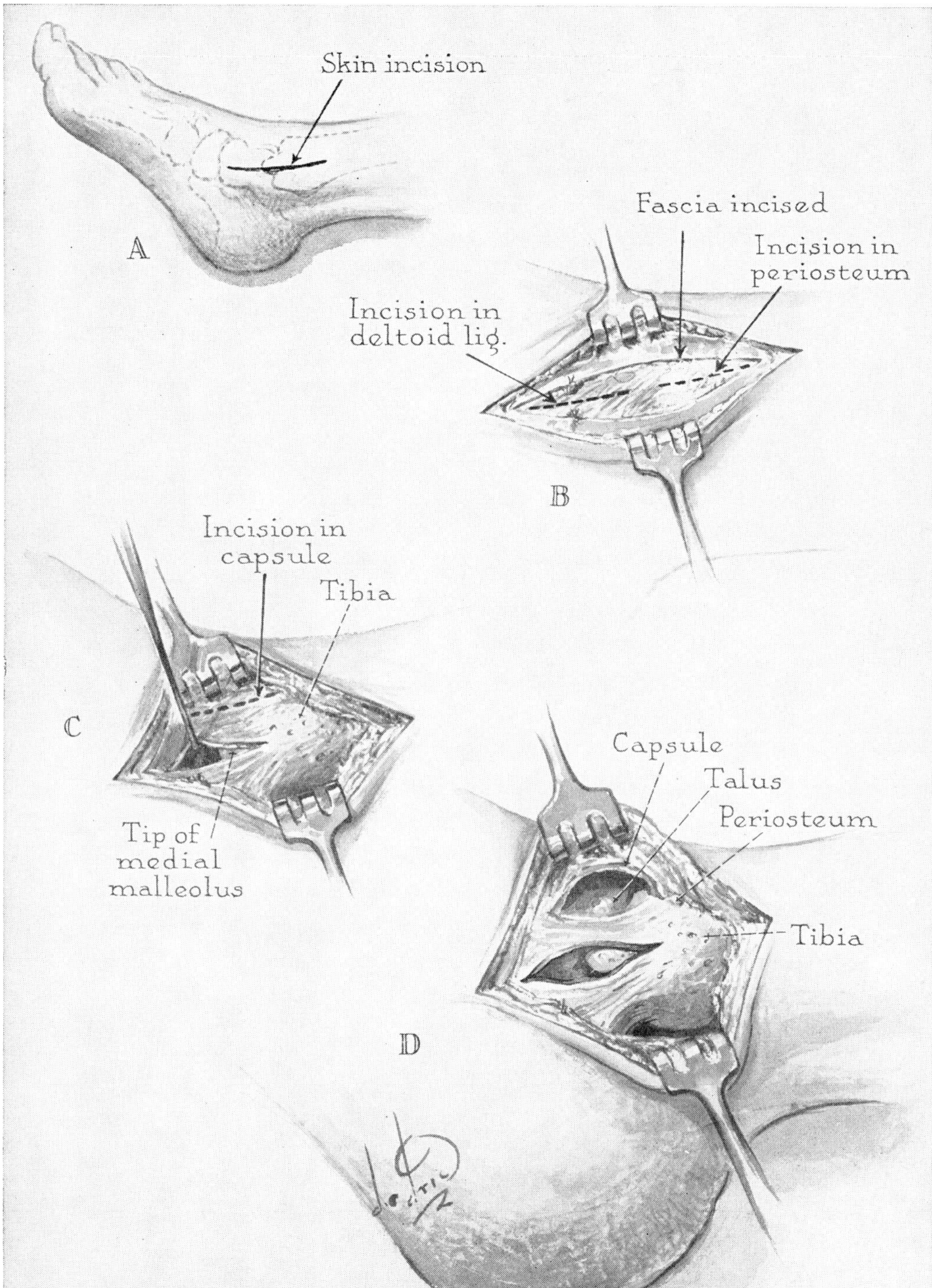

Exposure of the medial malleolus of the tibia and the ankle joint through a medial incision

EXPOSURE OF THE TALONAVICULAR, CALCANEOCUBOID AND TALO-CALCANEAL JOINTS THROUGH AN OBLIQUE TARSAL INCISION

Indication: 1. Triple Arthrodesis of the Foot

Plate 171: Description of Procedure

A An oblique incision begins near the second cuneiform bone and extends backward to end just distal and posterior to the lateral malleolus.

B The deep fascia is opened and the tendons of the peroneal muscles are identified and protected at the posterior extremity of the wound. The cruciate ligament is incised as the fascia is cut. The tendon of the peroneus tertius muscle forms the medial margin of the incision.

C The fat in the sinus tarsi is incised and developed into two flaps, which are retracted proximally and distally, as illustrated. The exposed bones which form the sinus tarsi are denuded of their periosteum. The talocalcaneal joint now lies exposed deep in the wound.

D Exposure of the calcaneocuboid joint is obtained by reflecting the extensor digitorum brevis muscle downward and forward from its origin on the anterolateral portion of the os calcis. The capsule of the calcaneocuboid joint is opened and raised from the adjacent bone. The periosteum is now elevated from the lateral and superior aspects of the neck of the talus. The capsule of the talonavicular joint is then opened by a linear incision and the articular surfaces are exposed by mobilizing the capsule and adjacent periosteum from the joint margins.

NOTE: No important nerves or vessels are encountered in this exposure, although some minor sensory branches of the peroneal nerve may be severed by the incision.

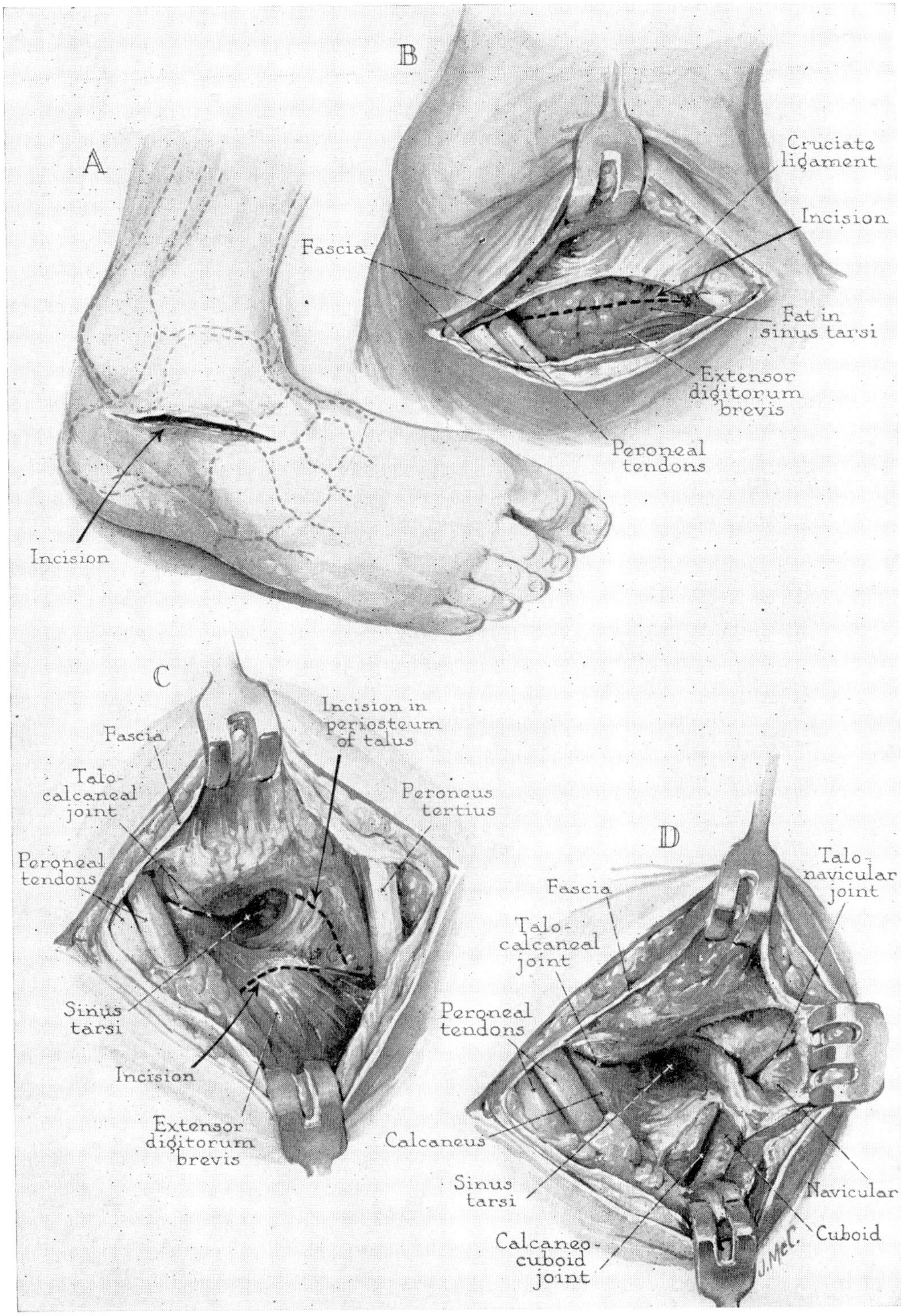

Exposure of the talonavicular, calcaneocuboid and talocalcaneal joints through an oblique tarsal incision

EXPOSURE OF THE TALOCALCANEAL JOINT THROUGH A POSTERIOR LATERAL INCISION, WITH FORWARD REFLECTION OF THE PERONEAL TENDONS

Indication: 1. Open Reduction of Depressed Fractures of the Articular Surface of the Os Calcis at the Talocalcaneal Joint

Plate 172: Description of Procedure

A The skin incision begins 1 1/2 inches below and posterior to the lateral malleolus, and gently curves upward so as to parallel the peroneal tendons.

B The deep fascia is incised, the peroneal tendons are identified and their tendon sheath is opened. The superior peroneal retinaculum, which normally prevents displacement of the tendons from behind the lateral malleolus, is sectioned.

C At the lower portion of the wound the inferior peroneal retinaculum, which holds the peroneus brevis tendon against the lateral aspect of the os calcis, is cut. In a similar manner, the inferior peroneal retinaculum over the peroneus longus tendon is opened. The peroneal tendons are freed from their tendon sheaths and then are reflected anteriorly to the front of the lower end of the fibula, as shown in Illustration D. (Procedure continued on Plate 173.)

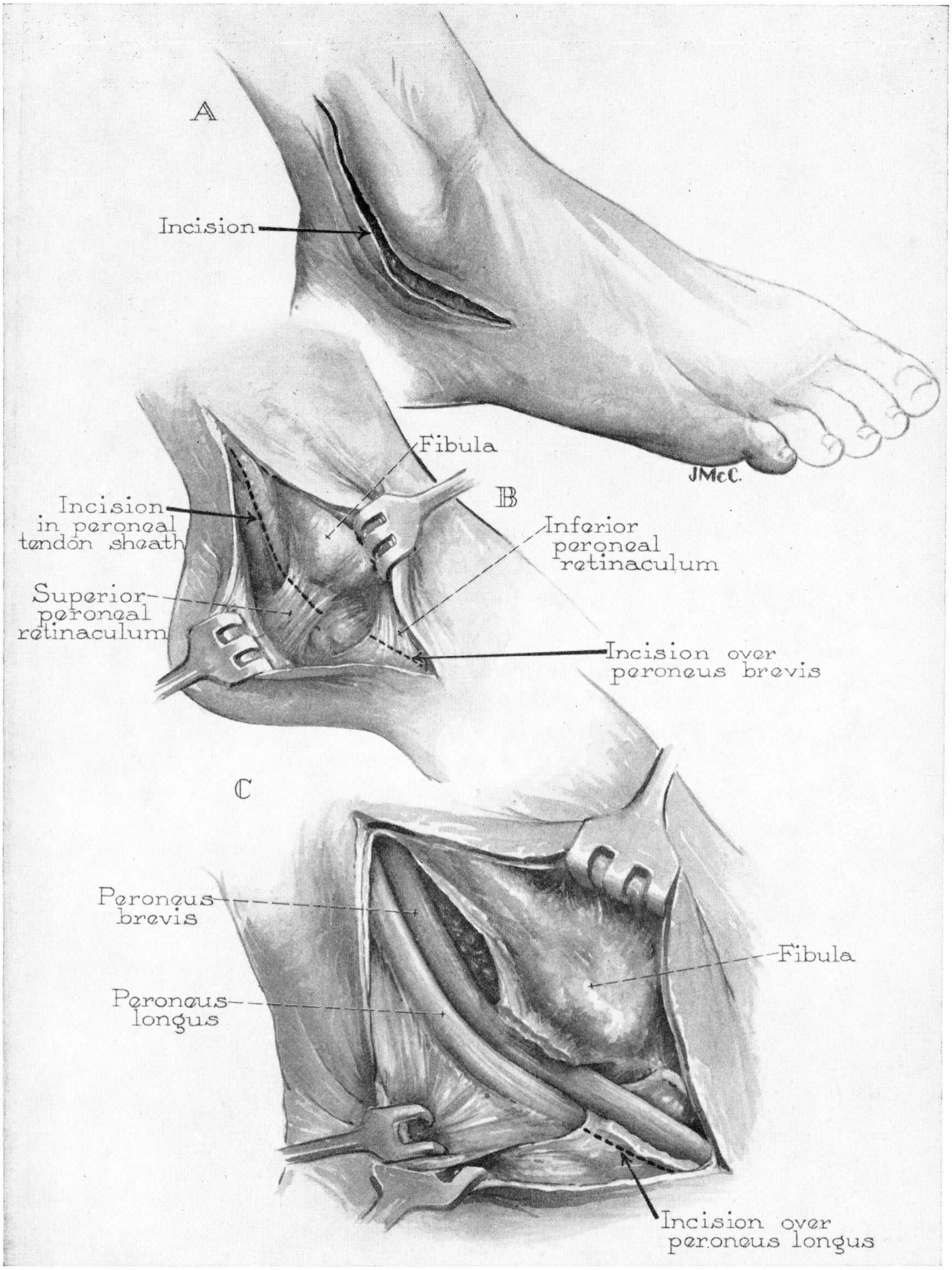

Exposure of the talocalcaneal, joint through a posterior lateral incision with forward reflection of the peroneal tendons

EXPOSURE OF THE TALOCALCANEAL JOINT THROUGH A POSTERIOR LATERAL INCISION, WITH FORWARD REFLECTION OF THE PERONEAL TENDONS *(Continued)*

Plate 173: Description of Procedure

D The calcaneofibular ligament is next exposed. It runs from the lateral malleolus downward and backward to gain its attachment onto the os calcis. The ligament is continuous with the capsule of the talocalcaneal joint, so that a linear incision will cut both.

E The severed ligament and capsule are retracted to expose the joint; the adjacent lateral surface of the os calcis is exposed subperiosteally in order to obtain more room.

NOTE: Comminuted fractures of the os calcis usually involve some fragmentation of the trochlear process and of the surrounding bone. The interior of the os calcis can be exposed by retracting the fractured fragment of lateral cortex out of the way. The wound is closed anatomically in the reverse order to that in which it was opened. It is important to replace the peroneal tendons accurately, and to restore the continuity of the calcaneofibular ligament and of the superior and inferior peroneal retinacula.

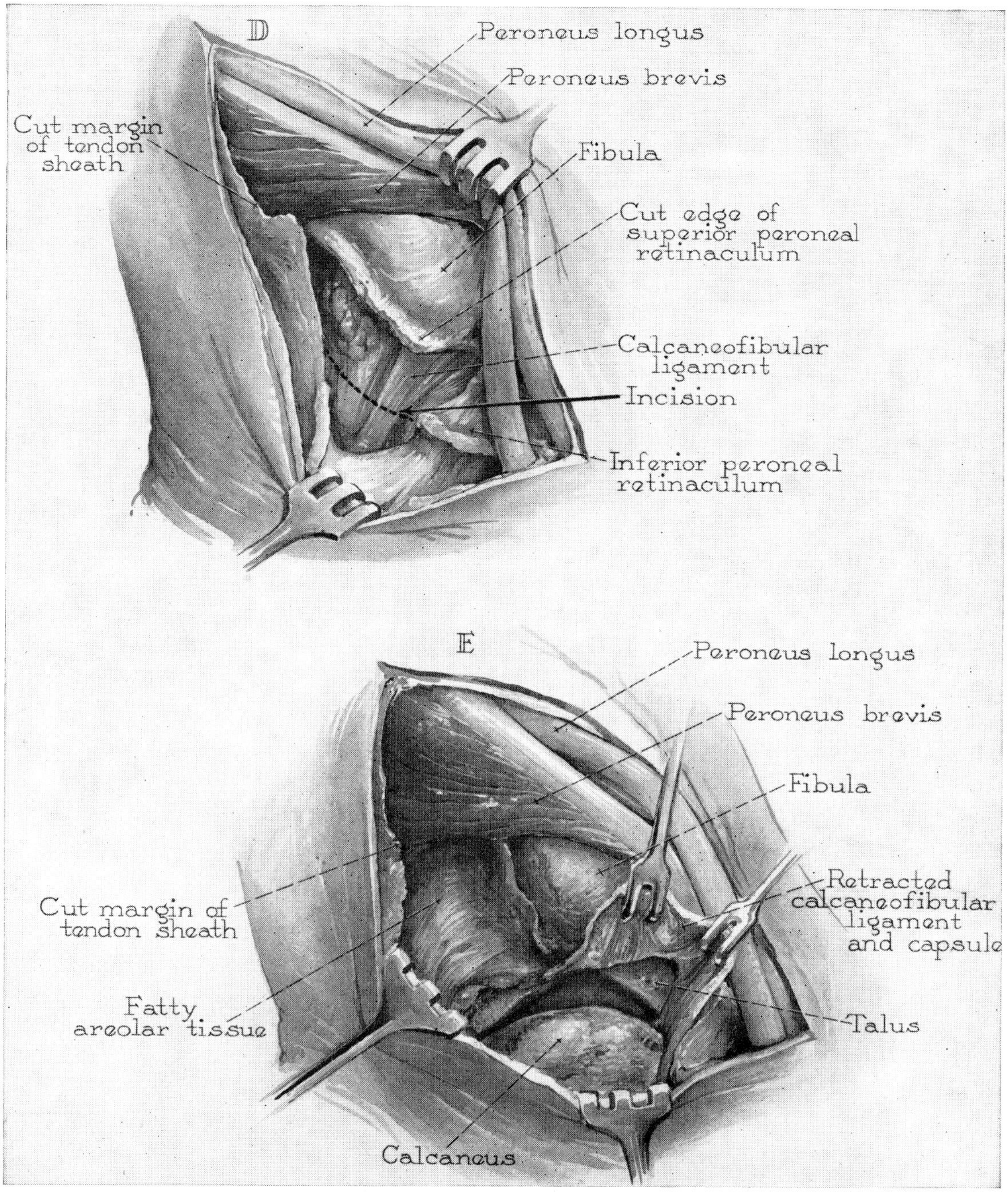

Exposure of the talocalcaneal joint through a posterior lateral incision, with forward reflection of the peroneal tendons

EXPOSURE OF THE TALOCALCANEAL JOINT THROUGH A LATERAL, OBLIQUE, TARSAL INCISION

Indication: 1. Arthrodesis of the Talocalcaneal Joint

Plate 174: Description of Procedure

A The foot is placed on a sandbag with the extremity in marked internal rotation. The incision begins 1 inch distal to the tip of the laterel malleolus and extends obliquely downward and forward across the sinus tarsi to end in the region of the second cuneiform bone. The skin margins must not be undercut, for it might interfere with the local circulation. Adequate retraction can be obtained, however, because of the loose attachment of the skin to the underlying tissues.

B The deep fascia is incised parallel with the skin incision. The cruciate ligament will be cut in the anterior portion of the wound, where it can easily be identified as a band of thickened fibers of the deep fascia. The peroneal tendons in the posterior extremity of the wound are next exposed; they must be preserved by being retracted posteriorly out of the way. An oblique incision is made through the fat in the sinus tarsi, as marked in the illustration, which is undercut proximally and distally to develop two flaps, which then are retracted.

C The dissection proceeds subperiosteally, to expose the adjacent portion of the talus and the calcaneus bones; the remaining fatty tissue is at the same time removed from the sinus tarsi. The talocalcaneal joint is easily seen by inverting the heel. Additional exposure can be obtained by stripping the capsule from the lateral margins of the joint and by firmly retracting the peroneal tendons posteriorly.

NOTE: It is also possible to start this exposure with a longitudinal incision, which is centered over the sinus tarsi; however, the oblique incision here described permits a wider exposure of the wound, although there is a slightly greater tendency for necrosis of the skin margins, especially if they have previously been traumatized or are not accurately approximated during closure.

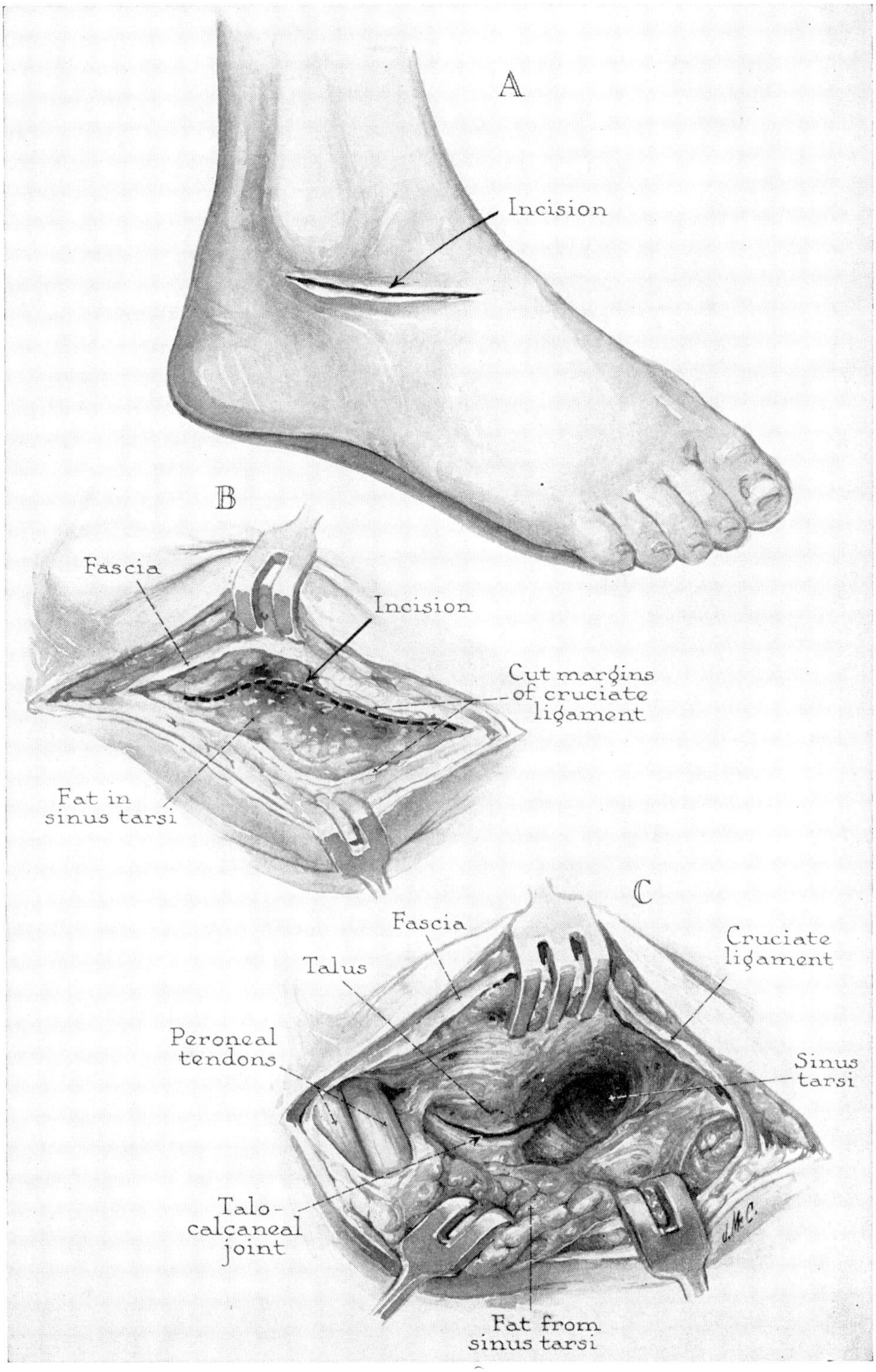

Exposure of the talocalcaneal joint through a lateral, oblique, tarsal incision

EXPOSURE OF THE CALCANEOCUBOID JOINT THROUGH A LATERAL INCISION

Indication: 1. Arthrodesis of the Calcaneocuboid Joint

Plate 175: Description of Procedure

A The calcaneocuboid joint is located at the lateral side of the foot. It lies just distally and slightly posteriorly to the sinus tarsi and the anterior process of the os calcis, which can easily be palpated; this process serves as the landmark for the exposure. The skin incision centers over the articulation, and is about 1 1/2 inches in length.

B The deep fascia is mobilized to expose the peroneus brevis tendon and the extensor digitorum brevis muscle beneath its fascia.

C The fascia and periosteum are incised at the inferior margin of the extensor digitorum brevis muscle. The end of the anterior process of the calcaneus and the cuboid bone are exposed by retracting upward the soft tissues, including the previously mobilized muscle and capsule, as shown in the illustration. It is not necessary to disturb the peroneus brevis tendon, unless it is necessary to expose the inferior aspect of the joint.

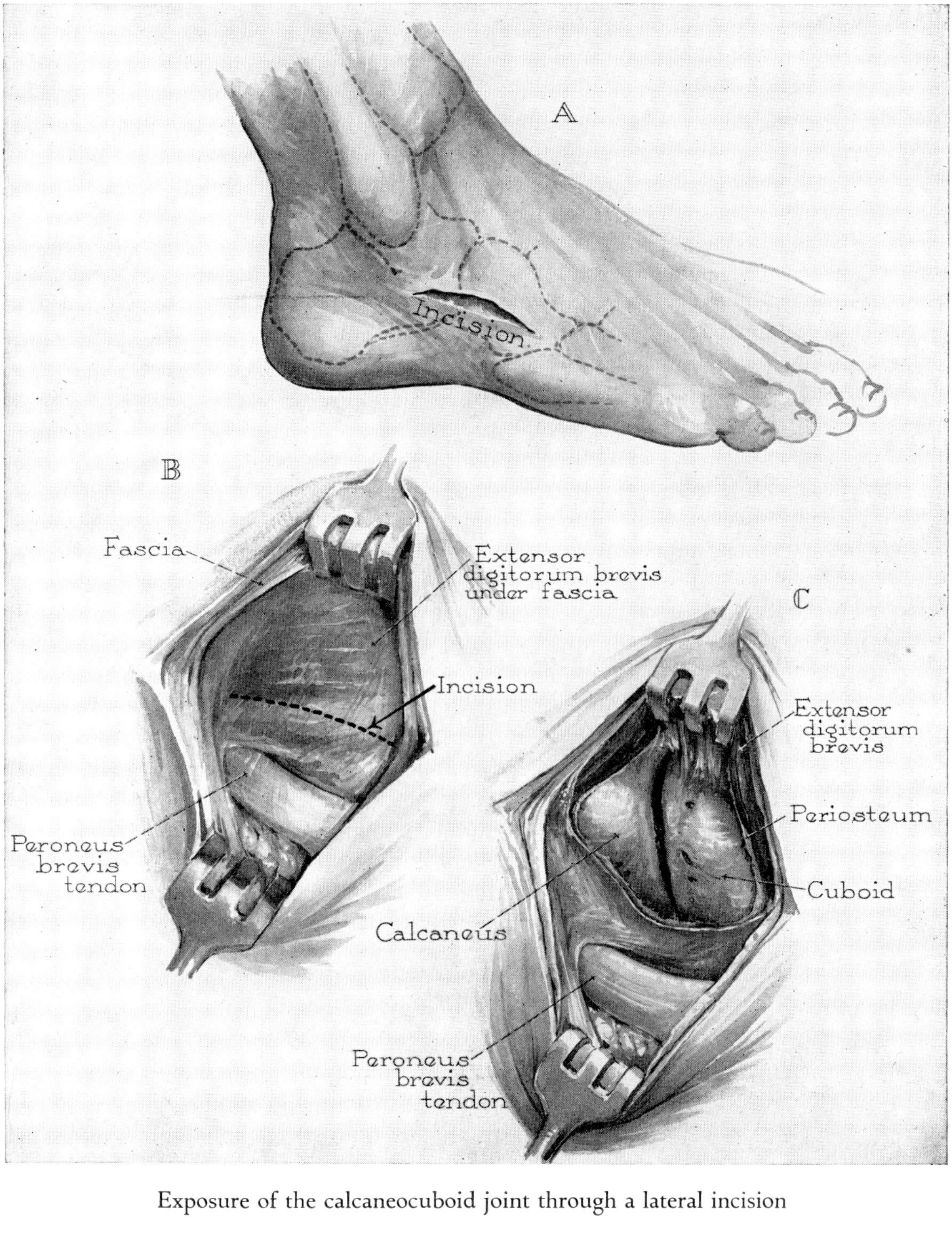

Exposure of the calcaneocuboid joint through a lateral incision

EXPOSURE OF THE TALONAVICULAR JOINT THROUGH A LINEAR DORSAL INCISION

Indication: 1. Arthrodesis of the Talonavicular Joint

Plate 176: Description of Procedure

A The skin incision, about 3 inches long and centering over the talonavicular joint (identified by palpation), is made in a direction parallel with the lateral margin of the anterior tibial tendon. The skin is retracted, and the transverse crural ligament above, and the cruciate ligament below, are identified.

B The next incision is made through the deep fascia and the transverse crural and cruciate ligaments. The anterior tibial tendon is present along the inner aspect of the wound, and the extensor hallucis longus tendon can be seen laterally. A layer of fatty tissue lies below the deep fascia and ligaments.

C This layer of fatty tissue is incised parallel with the skin incision, and the margins are retracted so that the capsule of the talonavicular joint can be identified. Next, a linear incision is made through the capsule, and the edges are retracted to expose the joint surfaces. A wider access to the joint can be obtained by raising the capsule and adjacent periosteum for the necessary distance. It should be noted that the navicular bone is relatively short, and that consequently the navicular-first cuneiform joint may be opened if the periosteum is stripped too far distally. The dissection can be extended proximally to denude the head and neck of the talus, but care must be exercised not to open the capsule of the ankle joint.

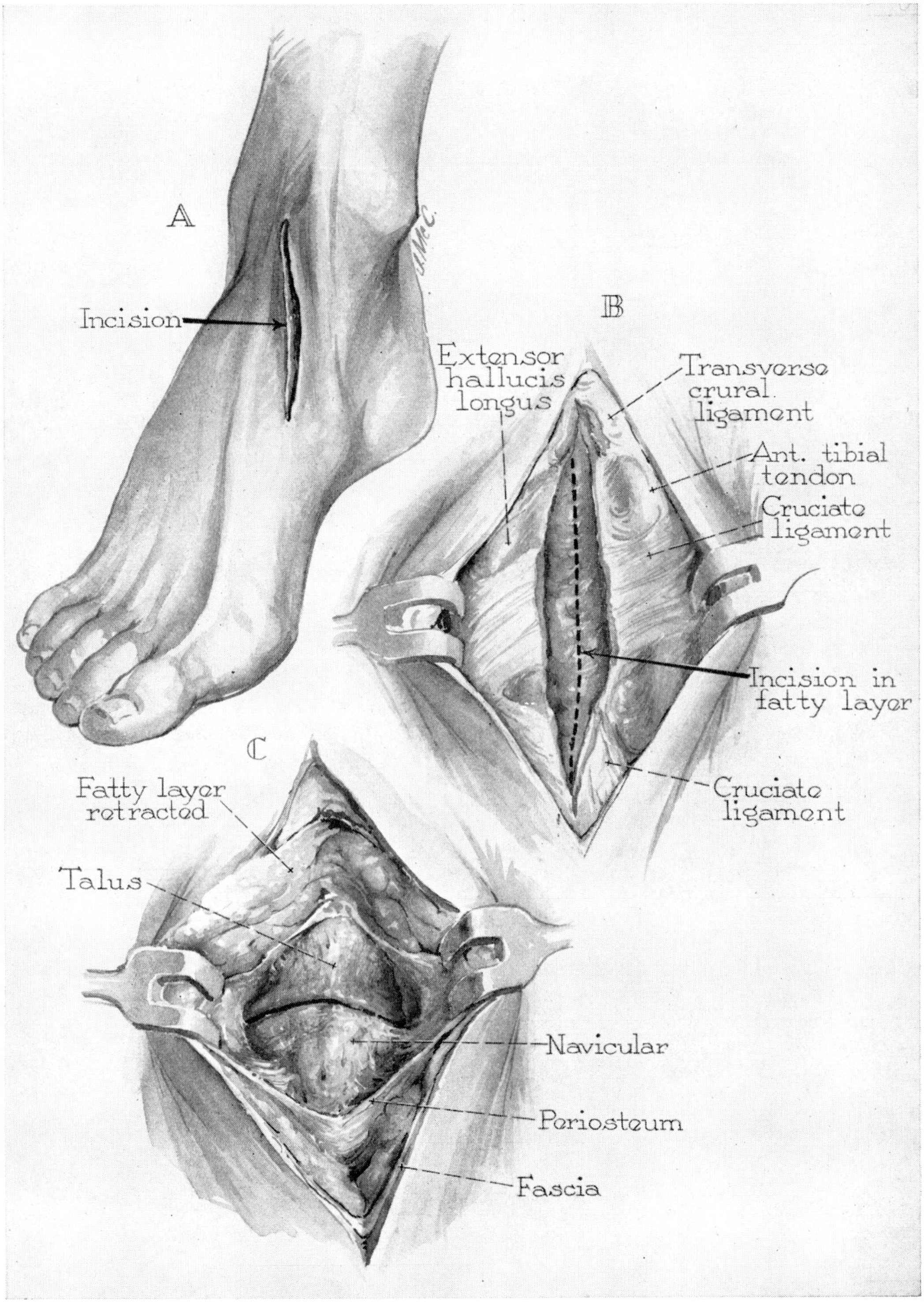

Exposure of the talonavicular joint through a linear dorsal incision

EXPOSURE OF THE LATERAL SURFACE OF THE OS CALCIS THROUGH A CURVED LATERAL INCISION

Indications: 1. Removal of Benign Tumors

2. Partial Ostectomy for Chronic Osteomyelitis

Plate 177: Description of Procedure

A The skin incision, approximately 3 inches long, is centered over the lateral aspect of the tuber portion of the os calcis at the site of the lesion. The incision is slightly arched and is posterior to the peroneal tendons.

B The skin margins are widely undercut, especially on the posterior side, and the flaps are firmly retracted to give optimum exposure.

C The fascia and periosteum are cut and the calcaneus is exposed subperiosteally.

NOTE: The authors prefer this approach to the os calcis, as against the heel-splitting incision, for the treatment of chronic osteomyelitis.

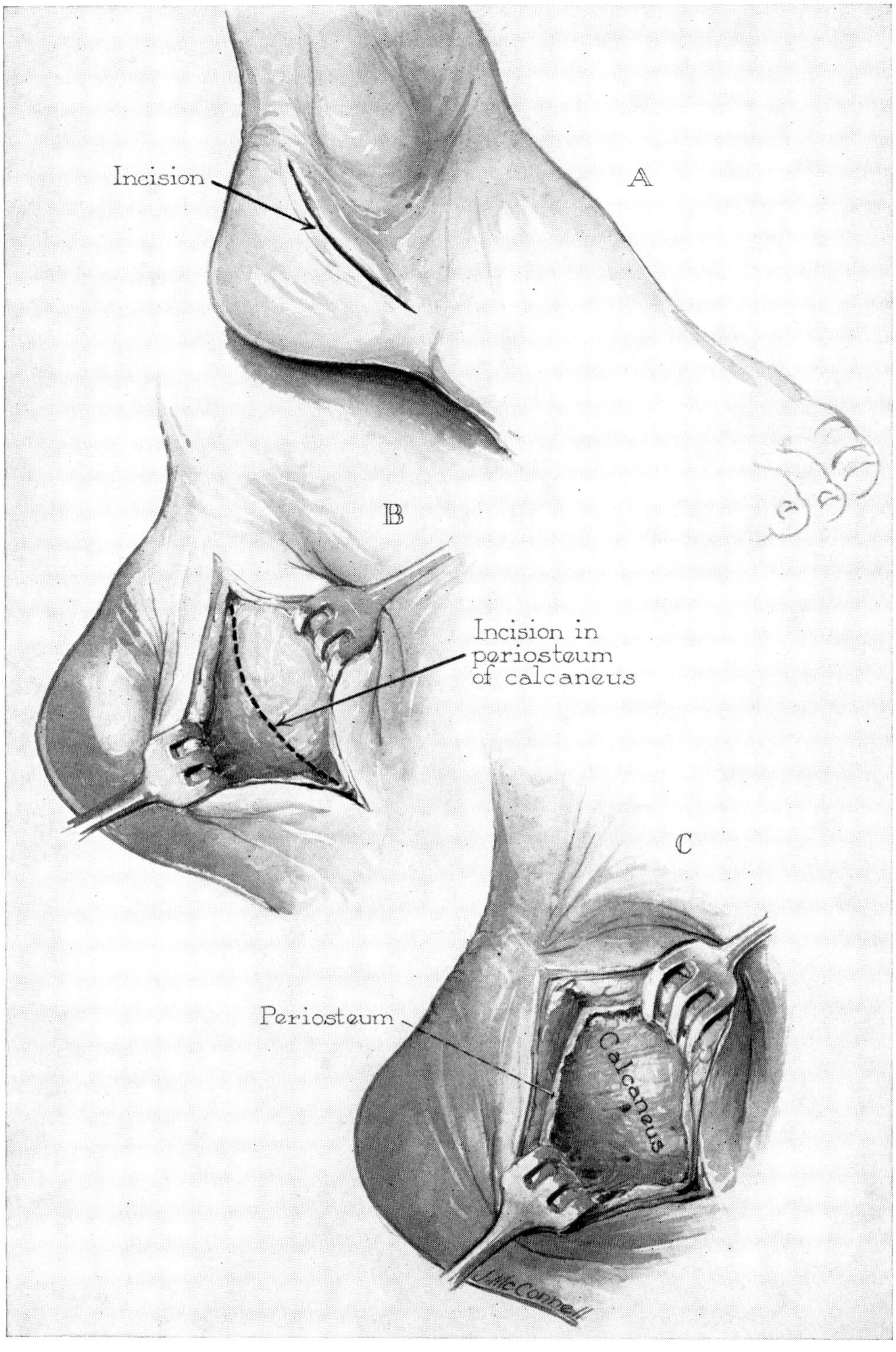

Exposure of the lateral surface of the os calcis through a curved lateral incision

EXPOSURE OF THE INFERIOR SURFACE OF THE TUBER PORTION OF THE OS CALCIS THROUGH A MEDIAL PLANTAR INCISION

Indications: 1. Fasciotomy of the Plantar Aponeurosis

2. Partial Ostectomy of the Os Calcis

3. Resection of Benign Tumors

Plate 178: Description of Procedure

A The incision, approximately 2 1/4 inches long, begins just short of the back of the heel, and extends forward along the line of junction of the plantar skin of the foot and that of the side of the heel. The skin margins are undermined and retracted to expose the deep fascia. The latter then is incised and the inferior margin of the abductor hallucis is identified.

B The abductor hallucis muscle is mobilized and retracted upward. The dissection is carried through the fatty tissue in the direction of the os calcis, which can be easily palpated. The plantar aponeurosis is cleared of the overlying fat, and its attachment to the inferior portion of the os calcis is developed.

C The plantar aponeurosis and its attached muscles are separated from the os calcis and both are retracted downward in the direction of the toes. The abductor hallucis is firmly retracted upward, and the inferior surface of the calcaneus is exposed, to the degree desired, by reflecting the periosteum with the attached soft tissues from the surface of the bone.

NOTE: The length of the incision depends entirely on the surgical objective in view. A fasciotomy of the plantar aponeurosis, for example, does not require quite as long an incision as has here been described. It may also be noted that the abductor hallucis muscle may not be encountered if the incision is placed near the plantar surface of the heel and the deep dissection is kept in that plane.

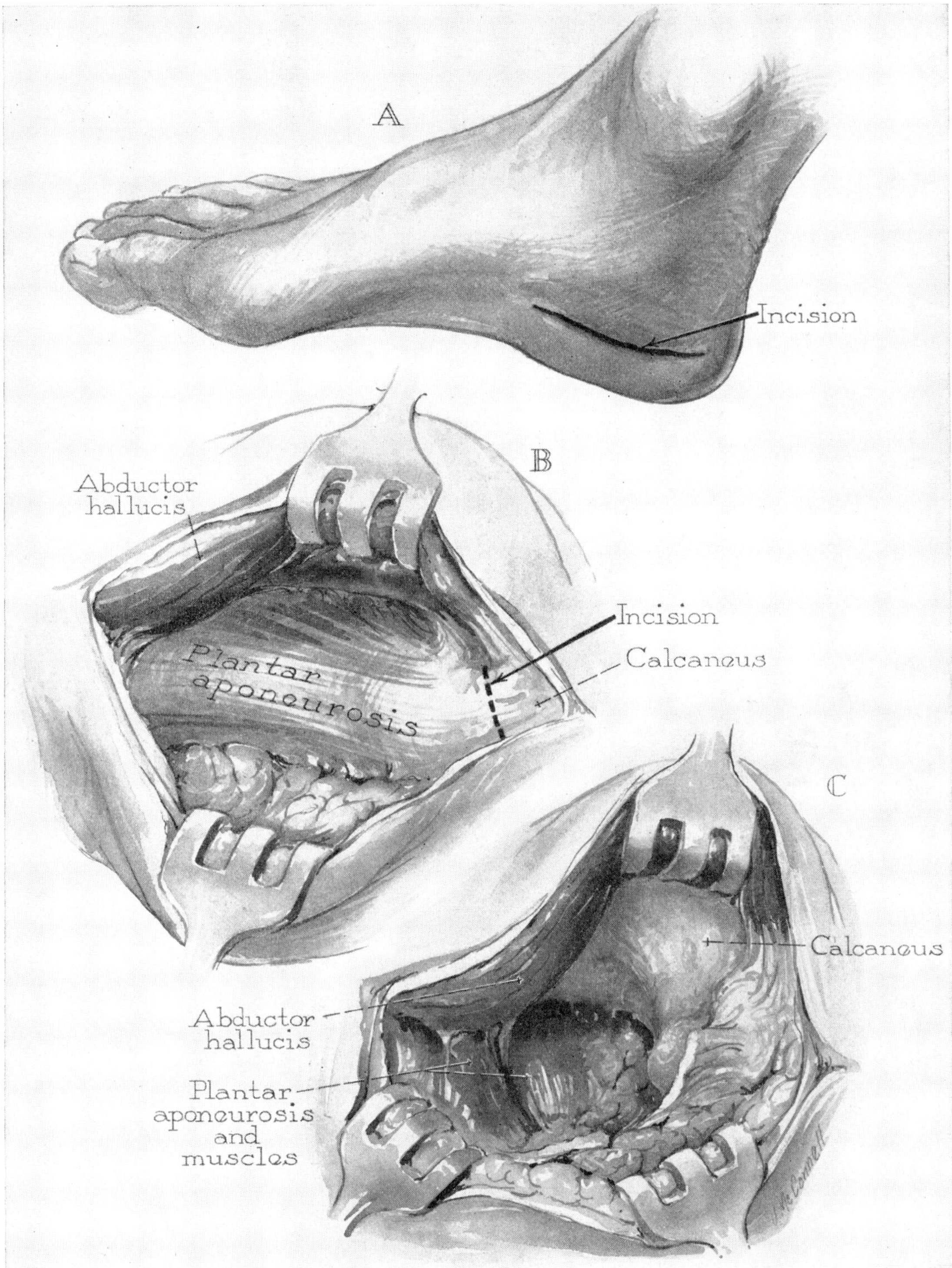

Exposure of the inferior surface of the tuber portion of the os calcis through a medial plantar incision.

EXPOSURE OF THE OS CALCIS THROUGH A CIRCUMFERENTIAL HEEL INCISION

Indications: 1. Removal of Benign Tumors

2. Open Reduction of Avulsion Fractures

3. Partial Ostectomy for Some Cases of Osteomyelitis

Plate 179: Description of Procedure

A The patient is placed on the operating table in the prone position to facilitate the surgical procedure. The skin incision is made around the back portion of the heel, along one of the skin creases.

B The skin flaps are undercut to permit wide separation of the wound.

C The periosteum is cut directly distal to the attachment of the Achilles tendon, and then is reflected from the posterior surface of the calcaneus.

D The dissection is continued distally either by cutting the plantar aponeurosis and the muscles to the os calcis or by stripping these structures from the bone with an osteotome. The body of the bone can be exposed on its inferior surface by freeing it subperiosteally.

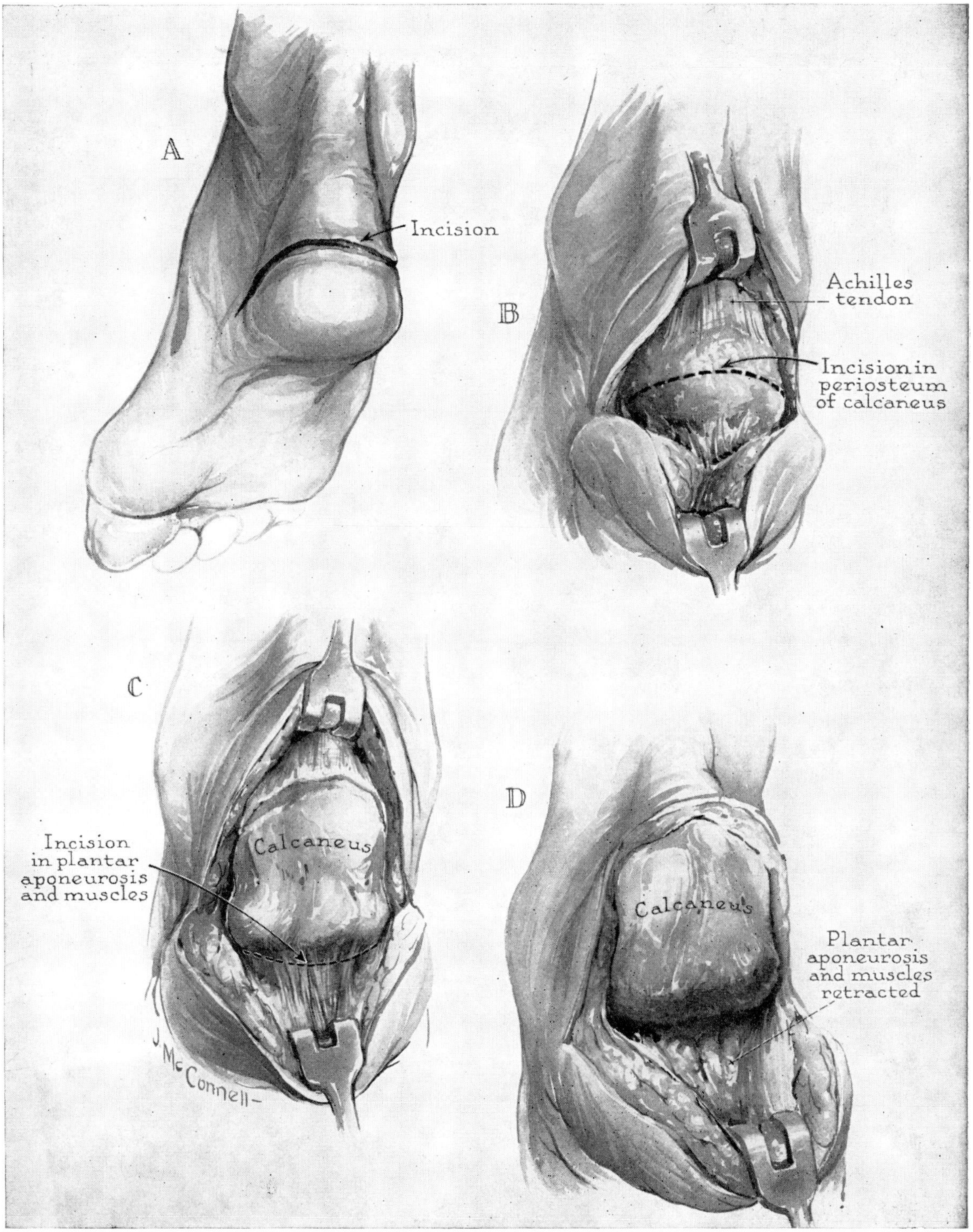

Exposure of the os calcis through a circumferential heel incision

Index

I

O

T